Endorsements for *The Practical Handbook* (

It's a pleasure to see such an eclectic mix of contributors in this practical handbook on living with dementia. The variety and expertise, both from people with lived experience themselves and from professionals in the field, give the reader a rich recipe of ideas and thoughts on how to enable others to live with dementia. As we all know, or should know, one size doesn't fit all, and the book offers a variety of approaches that can be adapted to fit the person's practical and emotional needs. I always say, when I got a diagnosis of dementia, so did my daughters, and both sides are equally important in their need for support and education. Thankfully, this book offers the holistic support for which many would be grateful.

Wendy Mitchell, author of *Somebody I Used to Know* **and** *What I Wish People Knew About Dementia*

Filled with personal accounts and the most up-to-date research in the field, this book is a brilliant example of the possible – of what can be achieved when those living with dementia, their carers and specialists collaborate, deconstructing the patient–doctor relationship, with agency shifted from the disease to the person. This is a wonderful collaboration and an important contribution to the literature of dementia and person-centred care.

Rod Kersh, consultant community physician and Divisional Director, Therapies, Dietetics and Community Care, Rotherham NHS Foundation Trust

The breadth of this practical handbook means that it offers something of value not only for people living with dementia, family carers, health or social care professionals, creative practitioners and volunteers, but also for many other individuals interested in the challenges of dementia and how to live with a chronic, life limiting illness whose prevalence is forecast to increase steeply across all ageing populations. All readers should read Part One, which hits the right note from the beginning as people with lived experience and family carers recount and reflect on their dementia journeys and candidly share what they have learned – small but perfectly formed pieces of advice that have made a real difference to their lives. The chapters that follow offer a constellation of different resources for organising and providing care and support for people with dementia, including creative approaches that contribute to the health and wellbeing of individuals and carers.

Maria S Pasiecznik Parsons, Chief Executive, Creative Dementia Arts Network, Bristol

Compared with the vast literature on how to diagnose dementia, there is a yawning gap when it comes to information about what to do after a diagnosis. Yet, there may be many years of life to live after a diagnosis has been made. Far too often, people living with dementia and their carers are left lonely and empty, with nothing to tell them how to move forward. This unique, invaluable book succeeds in filling the void. Beginning, appropriately, with the voices of people living with dementia and their carers describing how they live their lives, it goes on to consider different aspects of caring right through life up to the time when palliative care becomes necessary. The third section considers how to support people living with dementia, with a welcome emphasis on how to maintain communication. The valuable last section on creative approaches describes numerous ways – from dance to poetry, from yoga to mindfulness – in which people with dementia can find fulfilment. Well written and easy to read and providing excellent references, this book is an essential read for anyone concerned with care after a diagnosis of dementia.

Nori Graham, emeritus consultant in the psychiatry of old age, specialist advisor in mental health and dementia for Care UK and Vice President of the Alzheimer's Society.

Much of what makes dementia scary or uniquely distressing is not the illness itself but the way we view it as a society and treat people living with it. Running through this intelligent, dynamic, optimistic book is the insistence on the selfhood and uniqueness of every person living with dementia. In every chapter, it offers a helping hand – practically, psychologically, emotionally; on the value of creativity, mindfulness, advanced planning, hospital admissions, end-of-life care and so much more – to those affected by dementia and to their carers, and in so doing shines a light on what it is to be human.

Nicci Gerrard, campaigner, novelist, author of *What Dementia Teaches Us About Love* and co-founder of John's Campaign

The Practical Handbook of Living with Dementia

Edited by
Isla Parker, Richard Coaten
and Mark Hopfenbeck

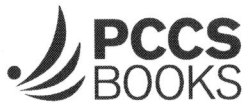

PCCS BOOKS

First published 2022

PCCS Books Ltd
Wyastone Business Park
Wyastone Leys
Monmouth
NP25 3SR
contact@pccs-books.co.uk
www.pccs-books.co.uk

The Practical Handbook of Living with Dementia

British Library Cataloguing in Publication data: a catalogue record for this book is available from the British Library.

ISBN Paperback 978 1 915220 16 5
ePub 978 1 915220 17 2

Cover design by Jason Anscomb

Typeset in-house by PCCS Books using Minion Pro and Myriad Pro
Printed in the UK by 4Edge, Hockley

Contents

PART THREE – SUPPORTING PEOPLE LIVING WITH DEMENTIA

PART FOUR – CREATIVE APPROACHES TO DEMENTIA

Acknowledgements

The editors would like to acknowledge and thank all the contributors for their work in making this a new and vibrant addition to the literature and to the field. This book was created in the midst of the global pandemic, and a great deal has happened during these Covid years for people living with dementia and their professional and family carers. Despite the added burden the pandemic put on the chapter authors, they have graciously contributed their time to create this handbook, which we hope will be a source of practical help and innovative ideas for years to come.

We would also like to express our gratitude to the many unnamed yet vital individuals who, over the years, both nationally in the UK and internationally, have worked with all the authors, informing their practice, knowledge and experience, which now features in these pages. Richard in particular would like to thank the many colleagues and people he has had the honour and privilege to work with in West Yorkshire while serving in the NHS and beyond, both nationally and internationally. They have all taught him so much over the years about what best practice in the care of people living with dementia really means and given him the confidence to be able to contribute to this publication.

Foreword

Steven Sabat

'What's more important, love or money?'
'Love, definitely.'

This question and the immediate answer given by a resident in a care home for people living with dementia reveal something fundamentally important about the man who answered and the person who asked the question. The exchange comes from a film about the Ella and Ridley Jacobs House residential care home in north London, run by Jewish Care – a film that was made with the residents by Frames of Mind, the innovative digital arts project described in Chapter 31.[1] The question is not part of a standard neuropsychological test. Such tests are often given to people living with dementia and include questions for which there is one, and only one, correct answer, sans explanation. This question, however, drew instead on the man's decades of accumulated wisdom, allowing him to share his thoughts about something he found especially meaningful, without the anxiety that often accompanies being tested in a clinic.

There is a world of difference between asking someone to name objects, recount the date and day of the week, repeat odd sentences and perform mathematical calculations out of context, as people with suspected dementia are often asked to do in clinical tests, and engaging them in conversation about what truly matters to them in life. How people with dementia engage with others certainly can reveal evidence supportive of their diagnosis. The form of engagement can also reveal ample evidence of the humanity, wisdom and creativity they share with people otherwise deemed healthy. The differences in the forms of engagement are reflected in Martin Buber's distinction between 'I-It' and 'I-Thou' relationships (Buber, 1937).

---

1. The film, *Daringly Able*, can be found at http://salmagundifilms.co.uk/Working-with-Dementia

I-It relationships are characterised by their detachment, cool affect, abstract understanding and keeping a safe distance from the other person. Such relationships are objective, task-oriented and about fulfilling duties; they involve either not hearing the 'other' person's voice and feelings or minimising them. This characterises what is sometimes called professional comportment, wherein the professional tells the 'patient' what to do and ticks off appropriate boxes on a form, asking the scripted questions in the scripted manner.

In I-Thou relationships, you move toward the other person; you are open and vulnerable, spontaneous and personal, person-oriented; you listen closely to what the other person says and respond openly. These relationships are not about naming things and quantitative; they are qualitatively oriented. They're about engaging with the other, hearing their voice, and being with another person in order to understand their point of view, fears, anxieties, hopes and sense of humour. Indeed, these relationships are crucial to person-centred care.

This book contains a plethora of examples of insightful person-centred care. It illuminates the multiple strengths possessed by people living with dementia – strengths that, when engaged, can help to create good moments and even good days. It is a clear statement that people living with dementia share numerous valued qualities and creative abilities with the human family to which they belong. As such, it is presented as an alternative to what Oliver Sacks called, 'treating the disease the person has' (Sacks, 1985). It invites the reader to engage in 'I-Thou' relationships with 'the person the disease has', in Sacks' words, and thereby speaks to, and helps reveal, the best in all.

References

Buber, M. (1937). *I and thou.* (R. Gregor Smith, Trans.). T. & T. Clark.

Sacks, O. (1985). *The man who mistook his wife for a hat and other clinical tales.* Summit Books.

Introduction

The Courtyard in September
We're sitting in the courtyard on a lovely afternoon.
The sky is blue and there's one white cloud.
The four walls round us are sentinel still,
Half in shadow and half in sun.
A plane flies over, disturbing the peace,
But the courtyard is still, silent and sleepy.

Birds sang in the tree. Then the courtyard was 'sentinel still', as Vera, my granny, said. These were her words, not mine. I just wrote them down. The words drew us closer. Vera had only eaten two mouthfuls of the éclair in front of her. She had very little appetite. I watched as she took another sip of her tea through a straw. I remember each of these moments – it was the last time that we would write a poem together.

§

As Steven Sabat explains in his Foreword to this handbook, 'I-Thou' relationships help tremendously when we are supporting people living with dementia. Six years later, this afternoon with my granny remains vivid in my mind, and I am grateful to the workshop that I attended two years previously in Oxford Town Hall, when John Killick shared with me his method for creating poems with people living with dementia. Killick has worked extensively on communication in this field. He has published seven books on the subject, often with the emphasis on creativity. I drew on Killick's method for writing poetry with my granny (see his Chapter 34 in this book, and my own Chapter 3) when I co-facilitated 20 poems with Vera in the period shortly before she died. This arts-based therapy approach fostered compassion, creativity and growth for Vera as she lived with dementia.

I did not have a traditional granddaughter–grandmother relationship with Vera, as I was brought up by my grandparents and had no contact with my biological father in my childhood. And yet I was not her carer in a traditional sense. Vera did not expect this; she wanted me to get on with my life. I was in my early 30s at the time, a graduate student, and I lived more than two hours away by train. I only visited Vera once or twice a month. Vera also received regular visits from her two daughters, who lived close to her care home. I did try my best, though, to develop different arts-based therapies that Vera enjoyed, so as to make a connection, and I turned to puppetry and music to do this.

It was during the long train ride back to Oxford after the above poem was written that it occurred to me to edit a 'practical handbook of dementia'. I wanted to improve the field by showcasing some of the latest and best-practice approaches and examples in many different and complementary areas, written by and for professionals and carers.

Dementia is one of the biggest challenges of our time. As Age UK says on its website:[1] 'Dementia is a term used to describe a collection of symptoms that occur when certain diseases or conditions affect the brain.' A person with dementia may have problems remembering things that have happened recently, or the names of people or objects. They may forget where things are kept, such as the tea and milk that they need to make a cuppa. They may feel that their thinking is muddled and struggle to follow conversations. When they visit a familiar place, they may get confused and lost. They may also get irritated or short tempered and lose interest in their hobbies. These are just some of the signs that a person is living with dementia. No person living with dementia is the same as another. Dementia affects individuals very differently.

The number of people living with dementia worldwide is currently estimated at 47 million and is expected to increase to 75 million by 2030 (World Health Organization, n.d.), as growth in population and increased longevity means more people live into older age. In the UK alone, there are currently 850,000 people living with dementia, which is more than ever before.

In *The Practical Handbook of Living with Dementia*, people living with dementia, carers, health professionals and therapists have come together to offer families caring for people with dementia more choice by providing practical suggestions as to what may help them to live with dignity in the community and in care settings.

We (me and my co-editors, Richard Coaten and Mark Hopfenbeck) really appreciate the time and effort our authors have put into writing helpful, practical chapters.

We suggest you dip into the chapters that interest you, so that you can find out more about different support and helpful approaches that are available. We recommend a holistic approach: that is, we advise you to think about the

---

1. www.ageuk.org.uk/information-advice/health-wellbeing/conditions-illnesses/dementia/understanding-dementia/

physical, psychological, emotional, environmental and social factors in dementia. Everything is connected. We believe that a holistic approach that integrates the body, emotions, mind and spirit of the person living with dementia produces a better quality of life, where they can flourish.

The Practical Handbook of Living with Dementia begins with chapters by Keith Oliver and Gail Gregory, who both write movingly about practical strategies that they use to live well with dementia. Part 1, 'The voices of people with dementia and their carers', also includes chapters written by carers, including a daughter, a son and a husband, who write about practical ways in which they have compassionately supported loved ones with moderate to advanced dementia.

Part 2, 'Caring for people with dementia', outlines what help is available to people with dementia and their families from varied sources. Readers are also introduced to why values-based practice is relevant and important in dementia care, and how it can be applied. Further chapters describe why advance care planning is helpful in discussing and recording a person's priorities and wishes for future care and treatment. Even in the advanced stages, genuine attention, nearness and human contact may foster comfort and contentment in people with dementia.

In Part 3, 'Supporting people living with dementia', different health professionals give advice as to what help and support can be offered to people living with dementia. Advice is offered on diet, overcoming speech and swallowing difficulties, improving sleep, and how to relate well to a person with dementia when they spend time in hospital. Advice is also given as to how they can be supported in employment and what technology and interior design in a home or care setting can help people with dementia to remain independent. They are also encouraged to try gardening, and to visit a 'memory café' for people with dementia, where they can socialise with others. Another chapter looks at some of the practical issues to consider when working with carers and people living with dementia from black and minority ethnic backgrounds.

Finally, in Part 4, on 'Creative approaches to dementia', artists, a dancer, a poet, a musician, film-makers, care staff and therapists write chapters about arts-based approaches to foster compassion, creativity and growth. How does the ability to play with language, poetry, movement, music, dance, song and reminiscence and interaction with a clown help the person with dementia? There are also chapters on yoga and mindfulness, and visiting museums, where the person can interact with objects that help them to connect with earlier memories and with others.

We hope that you will find the chapters useful, informative and interesting.

Isla Parker

Reference

World Health Organization. (n.d.). *Dementia*. Fact sheet. [Online]. www.who.int/news-room/fact-sheets

Part one

The voices of people with dementia and their carers

1 The me in dementia

Keith Oliver

As a society, we tend to feel comfortable pigeon-holing people by labels. For example, in my case, the labels are teacher, headteacher, parent, grandparent and, more latterly, person with dementia. Formerly, many would say, 'I knew you were a teacher before you told me.' Nowadays I am often labelled as a person with dementia, service user or by the much worse label, dementia sufferer, all of which can at times generate looks or comments of disbelief from those issuing them as I do not conform to the stereotypical image of a person with dementia.

I often think about a quote from W.C. Fields, who is said to have said, 'It ain't what they call you. It's what you answer to.'

Taking this quote and thinking about how I see myself by way of labels relating to living with dementia, while all have some accuracy and use for professionals, labels that I've carried for much longer, such as married, parent, teacher, headteacher, and indeed person with a name, are, I feel, better ways of identifying me. I still get a sense from time to time that some professionals and members of the public see people like me as a person with dementia rather than a person. Thankfully these views are being challenged and through awareness raising, education, training, and conferences, the tide is turning. Kitwood summarises this brilliantly in outlining the 'uniqueness of persons' (Kitwood & Brooker, 2019).

If you consider to be true the expression 'If you've met one person with dementia, you've met one person with dementia', alongside stating that everyone either with or without dementia is a unique individual, this provides us with cause to celebrate, and yet, when seeking to provide care, one can feel challenged. The stereotypical portrayal of dementia is accurate for some people, especially in the later stages, but certainly not for all.

With the support of my wife, Rosemary, and undergraduate supporters Lucy, Lydia and Jess, I intend to outline how, with the love as outlined in the Kitwood flower and the support of family and friends, there is more chance of the 'me' inside dementia – the 'me in dementia' – remaining the dominant force as the condition develops.

Figure 1.1: The Kitwood flower (Kitwood & Brooker, 2019, p.98)

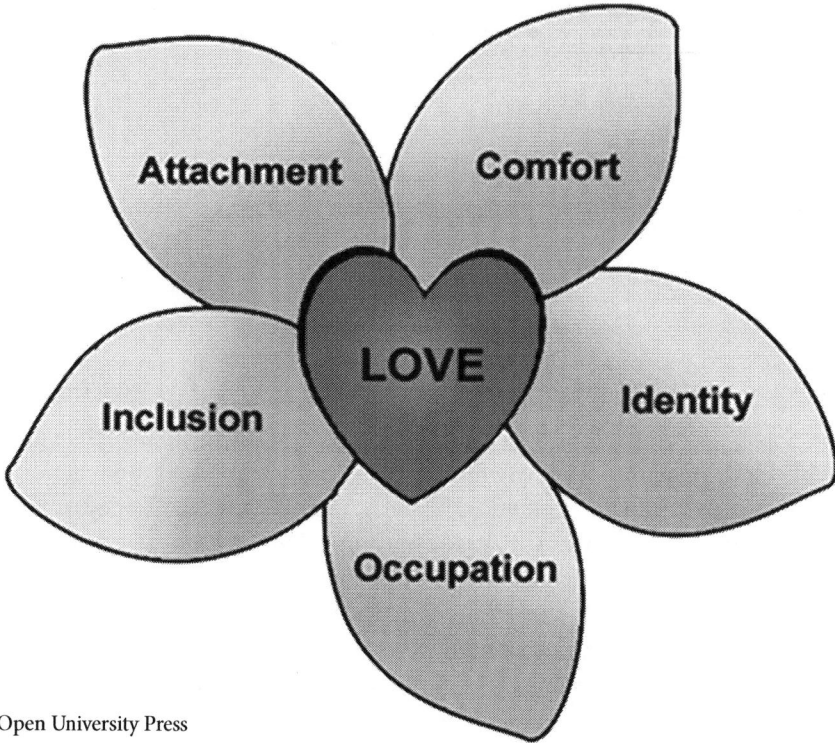

© Open University Press

Learning point 1

Before you read any further you may like to consider the following:

- Have you ever been described with a label?
- Have you ever thought of someone else as a label?
- How did you feel about this?
- How do you feel about the Kitwood flower (Figure 1.1) in terms of dementia care today?

I was born in Nottingham in 1955 and moved south to Kent as a young teacher in 1981. Since then, I have settled in the Canterbury area with my wife and family. I taught in a range of primary schools and became the head of a school in Dover in 1995, moving to a larger school in Canterbury in 2000. I loved the job and engaged readily and happily with the full school community of children, parents and governors. In 2008, I felt I needed a new challenge as I always sought 'new mountains to climb', so I took on the role of advising the 23 primary schools in the Canterbury area for a two-year secondment (Oliver, 2016). My health up until this point had generally been good, especially my mental health. Any stress that came with my career or life generally, I readily diverted into a positive. I was never depressed and never needed to speak to anyone about anxiety or stress in my life. I was often regarded as a rock for other people to lean upon – a role I was comfortable with. However, between 2006 and 2010, I did experience a number of physical health challenges around sinus infections, thyroid problems and urinary tract infections, and in retrospect I can see that some did have a relatively small but noticeable impact on my cognitive functioning at the time. But none of them prepared me for what was to confront me in 2010.

Early in 2010, I experienced a number of unexplained falls and felt at times that I was walking on a ship in rough seas. With encouragement from my wife, I went to see the GP, expecting to be told that I had an ear infection. Her examination suggested this was not the case, but she gave me antibiotics and told me to return in a week if I felt no better. I was back there one week later as there had been another fall and I was now experiencing greater difficulty concentrating at work and at home. The GP carried out further tests on my balance and cognitive functioning and referred me for an fMRI scan, which took place two weeks later. I had no indication why she sent me for the scan. In retrospect, I'm surprised that I failed to ask her. I have written at length about this in the book *Welcome to Our World* (Saints et al., 2014).[1] The scan was followed by an appointment with a neurologist, who gave my wife and me two shocking pieces of information. First of all, he explained the good news – that the GP's suspicions of a brain tumour were unfounded; the bad news was that the scans and the questions that the neurologist and GP had asked suggested that I was developing Alzheimer's. I was 54 years of age and I had never met anyone younger than 75 who had received a diagnosis of any form of dementia.

I have a long-term relationship with dementia, first through my mother, whose 'journey into the fog' began in the 1970s, when she was in her early 40s and was diagnosed with bi-polar disorder, or manic depression, as it was cruelly labelled. This, coupled with Alzheimer's disease in her mid-70s, made life difficult for her and, at times, to be honest, for me too. Despite the latter, the key was to maintain her needs at the centre. With this experience in mind, while I was not scared at the time of my diagnosis, I was confused, as I had no understanding of young onset dementia or the impact it was going to have on me.

This suggested diagnosis was followed by blood tests, a PET scan and five lengthy assessment appointments at the local memory clinic (Warner & Graham, 2018, p.62). The results of all of these were consistent with a confirmed diagnosis of Alzheimer's disease, delivered on New Year's Eve 2010. There were no celebrations for us that night to see in the New Year.

---

1. I was delighted to see mention of this book in the work of Mary Jordan and Dr Noel Collins, who used the words of those with dementia to endorse their book *The D Word: Rethinking dementia* (Jordan & Collins, 2017, pp.48–50). This book, written by a psychiatrist and a third-sector worker, attempts to challenge the medical model of treating people with dementia.

Learning point 2

- What would your feelings be if this happened to you?
- Consider the impact that such a diagnosis might have on someone aged 54 and their family.
- How could you be best supported at this time?

To be told you have dementia challenges so much about one's views of oneself. The weeks and months immediately after the diagnosis were probably the hardest time. Surprisingly, I was not depressed, because depression had never been part of my make-up. I was certainly worried and frustrated that a career I was enjoying was almost certainly going to come to an end. I was also bored, because I was used to being busy, and confused because I thought I was the only person anywhere to be diagnosed in their mid-50s and oblivious to the impact dementia was going to have on me. My coping strategy was to think 'Information is power', so I began to read both personal stories and medical texts about dementia, especially young onset dementia – i.e. dementia affecting those before the age of 65. Among the most notable were *Dancing with Dementia* (Bryden, 2005) and the ground-breaking novel *Still Alice*, which was later made into an Oscar-winning movie (Genova, 2007).

After three or four months in this wilderness, where my feelings about the 'me' in dementia had few positive connotations, I was fortunate to attend with my wife a Living Well group for two afternoons. Here we met other people with young onset dementia and their partners, and we realised we were not alone. My exit from my career was now complete and a pension secured, which took a lot of pressure off me, and I met Reinhard Guss, a clinical psychologist. Over time, he became a friend, ally and collaborator on many projects that have given me a new sense of purpose in life and an understanding that the 'me' in dementia is not totally negative.

> My appearance is largely the same, and when I am remembering to do my balance exercise my walk seems the same. Whilst words sometimes confound me, my voice remains unchanged; despite all of this I feel fundamentally different, and central to this is that my thinking is now almost always emotionally dominated. (Oliver, 2019, p.25)

Since living with dementia, I sense the 'me' is changing. Formerly, as a headteacher, parent, husband etcetera, the cognitive element of my thinking was always strongest and the emotional was secondary. If one viewed this as a balance scale, for some time now the scales have tipped heavily towards the emotional. Always close to the surface are feelings of happiness, sadness, being scared, anxious, relieved and, essentially, frustrated. For many, frustration understandably boils over and is displayed in their behaviour, which many would term to be 'challenging'. Unfortunately, one consequence of this is that the person is viewed as 'challenging'. For me, the person most challenged by my behaviour is me, next is my wife, before this cascades out towards others.

I hope that any behaviour I display that is seen as challenging can be traced back to a cause, which can then be addressed to enable me to express myself and my needs appropriately.

One emotion that I never feel is anger, which surprises some people. Having seen the results of angry outbursts from both children and adults, and at times having had to manage these situations, an old expression comes to mind: 'Anger is like drinking poison and expecting the other person to die.' Having said that, there are times when my dementia makes me feel guilty – both for what I have done or failed to do and said or failed to say. All of which is very different from the me you would have met nine years ago, and the only possible explanation in my mind for this is the dementia.

In order to address the negative emotions and enhance the positives, I look for support. The biggest difference for me now is that I don't just see support with my eyes or hear it with my ears. When support is most effective now, I feel it with my heart. For me now, it is no longer sufficient for people to merely care; I need to see and feel they care in order to feel safe, secure and supported emotionally, physically and psychologically. I know how lucky I am to live as well as I do, and the more support I have, the luckier I am. My current care plan (Table 1.1) clearly shows how my desire to live well is based upon support. It is a proactive document, in the sense that it works best on the days when I am functioning quite well, and it has been useful in avoiding the need to seek crisis support, which is often what care plans are designed for. The plan was devised by me and my consultant, and I often say of it, 'It took me four years to get and 10 minutes to write.' This is because its predecessor appeared to focus solely on my medication.

The care that is shown through the plan is person centred and passionately delivered, and I wish this to be continued throughout my dementia journey by professionals, friends and family, and for them to be both truthful and honest with me without being blunt and demeaning. I am reminded of Maya Angelou, who said that, if you're brutally honest with people, they forget the honesty but are left with the brutality.

Life for me is about the journey, not the destination. Ever since being diagnosed, I have advocated and tried to live the maxim of living in and for the day. So often textbooks, the media and some professionals focus on the progressive element of dementia and the decline of the individual. When first diagnosed, that was the bulk of the literature that I was exposed to. While awareness of living with dementia is increasing – indeed, awareness of living well with dementia, rather than dying with dementia – there is still a considerable way to go. I recently encountered this when I saw a former headteacher colleague at Canterbury railway station. He hadn't seen me since my retirement eight years previously, and his opening statement was, 'Hello Keith, I thought you were dead!' The brief conversation that followed clearly

Table 1.1: My care plan

Patient/Service User: Keith Oliver   Care coordinator / Consultant: [Named individual]   GP: [Named individual]   Review Date: 07 March 2022

Activity	Delivery (How)	Location (Where)	Purpose (Why)	Professional (Who)	Interval (When)	Impact (Outcome)	Timeframe and review (start and finish date)
Time with those closest to me	Creating balance and quality time together	Kent	Maintain a good life balance and positive relationship	Rosemary	One weekday and weekends (minimum)	Better wellbeing for both	Indefinite
Outpatient review	One-to-one with Rosemary for part of the appointment	Lifesize video call or face to face as needed	Monitoring	[Named individual]	Every 4 months	Being cared for, monitored, check of my health, source of person-centred clinical specialist advice	Indefinite
Forget-Me-Nots/Envoy/Ambassador	Meetings, conferences, reading, advising, consulting with support of Rosemary and students	Video call (Zoom, Lifesize, Microsoft Teams) Canterbury London	Maintain self-esteem, self-worth and sense of value through contribution	[Named individual], students and volunteers supervised by Clare Streeter	Monthly and as required	On me On the work Connectedness Support to manage demands and debriefing and processing.	6-monthly review with [named individual]
Medication	Galantamine MR 24mg and Memantine 10mg once daily		Reduce symptoms of Alzheimer's disease	Supplied by [named individual]	Collect every two months	Maintain function without adverse side effects	Indefinite
Primary care dementia review	One to one	Remote consultation or GP surgery	Check BP and needs	[Named individual]	Annually	Maintain physical health and stable blood pressure	Indefinite

Body Well	One to one	Blean	Spinal treatment and muscular and joint massage	[Named individual]	Weekly spinal adjustment; additional as necessary	Holistic lifestyle; sharing experience with Rosemary	Review in 6 months
Support from key friends	One to one		Emotional support to and from key friends	Limited due to Covid pandemic		Manage difficult emotions	Indefinite
Social walking	One to one with PPE/distancing	Familiar local routes	Physical and mental exercise	Volunteers (students)	Three weekly		Review
Talking therapy	60 mins per session – person-centred therapy	Face to face at Lombard House	Regular forum to share concerns and develop strategies	[Named individual]	Every 3 weeks	Coping strategies to deal with anxiety and dementia and maintain selfhood	Ongoing with review as needed
Inter-generational support from psychology students, volunteers	Formal and informal meetings	Canterbury and events as needed	Support with project work and travel, positive conversations, connecting with former roles	Pool of students/ volunteers with supervisors	Once or twice per month	**On me** –helping young people, enrich their placement, offer guidance, experience, friendship **On them** – being a recipient of the above, encouragement, interest	Annual review

Crisis / urgent response plan

If you need to reach out and ask for help between appointments, you may want to take up the following options:

1) **Between 8.30am and 5pm Monday – Friday** – contact [named individual] – if no one is available to answer the phone straight away then please leave a message and this will be picked up within a short period of time and responded to. This may lead to you being transferred for a discussion with the duty clinician (a nurse or occupational therapist). If needed, they can see you that day or may suggest an alternative response. This could include a telephone call from [named individual] at a given time, and/ or by an earlier appointment or home visit. Alternatively, a call can be requested from [named individual].

2) **Out of hours** call KMPT Single Point of Access number on [...] – calls are handled by clinical staff, and they can listen and discuss issues and arrange next working day response from Canterbury CMHTOP/Gregory House team.

showed that he thought no one with Alzheimer's could possibly survive eight years after diagnosis, and certainly not still be living as well as I was attempting to do.

I recognise the importance for me and others with dementia in remaining independent. Having said that, it is crucial that we take this further and seek to support people to remain interdependent, as one consequence of having dementia is difficulty establishing, maintaining and expanding one's social network. For me, the best thing about the past nine years has been forming associations and friendships with people who have dementia and those who seek to care for and about us as volunteers and professionals. Support for this has been through the Dementia Engagement and Empowerment Project (DEEP), which Forget Me Nots – the group in Kent that I helped establish in November 2012 – is aligned with. When I think back to 2011 and being steered towards retirement, I could never have possibly imagined the opportunities to explore the positive aspects of the me in dementia that being part of this network has provided. Meeting and sharing hopes, aspirations and concerns with others living with dementia, alongside some stimulating projects that we have undertaken, has been so rewarding and helped stave off challenges to my self-esteem. Among them is my dear friend Wendy Mitchell, who, in her bestselling book *Somebody I Used to Know*, kindly wrote about the positive impact of watching the film about me on YouTube entitled *Keith Oliver's Story* (Mitchell, 2018, pp.45–46).

I have tried to maintain a sense of pride in my appearance but the me in dementia may now dress a bit differently from the former me. I now rarely wear a suit and tie, and grey, brown and dark blues are replaced by reds, greens and bright colours. Soon after diagnosis, I realised I struggled to remember if I had cleaned my teeth, shaved or combed my hair. Consequently, I devised a system whereby I get all I need out of my cupboard and, as the things are used, they are put back into a box and then returned to the cupboard, so it is clear to me when I have completed these tasks.

Learning point 3

If you had a diagnosis of dementia:

- How would you aim to stay connected with others and participate in society?
- Accepting and seeking help – who/how would you ask for help?
- What do you see are the issues of seeking to be independent/interdependent and what are the benefits and challenges of that?

If you were caring for someone with dementia:

- How would you seek to separate behaviours that are challenging from the person?
- How could you help someone with dementia overcome their frustration before it manifests into becoming challenging behaviour?

I began this chapter by expressing my thoughts on people being labelled by others – and at times, I suspect, by oneself. Over the past nine years not just labels but roles have been attached to and associated with me, and these give me a great sense of pride and surprise in reflecting on some of the achievements the me in dementia has been identified with. First of all, in 2012, I took up the role of Kent and Medway Dementia Envoy, which, with the help and encouragement of clinical psychologist Reinhard Guss and a succession of placement students, I devised, developed and have been party to extending to three other enthusiastic people with dementia. I look at the eminent list of Alzheimer's Society Ambassadors and since 2015 I am honoured and humbled to share the role with them. The epithet of author is something I only dreamt of as a teenager who had aspirations to write and publish and had to wait 45 years to realise.

I have always viewed with interest the work of the United Nations but would never have imagined having the opportunity of being one of the first people in the world with dementia to address the UN Convention on the Rights of People with Disabilities, in Geneva in 2018. So often people are written off when their 'me' becomes part of dementia and when dementia becomes a part of them. I am the proof, and there are many others too who dispel and challenge this. When I was diagnosed, the old me was successfully studying for a master's degree at my local university. At the time I thought my future was bleak and the words of my supervising professor have stayed with me. He simply said, on hearing of my diagnosis, 'Well, we'd better call it a day.' And I did. I accepted this totally as, like him, I thought there was no alternative. Time and events have shown that he and I were wrong.

To close, I have tried to bring you, the reader, into my world so that you can gain a sense of the 'me in dementia'. To allow me to live as well as possible, an important part of my life is intergenerational friendships and working – which, I suspect, is based on my former life in education. Sharing my inner thoughts like this is never easy, and I am indebted to Lydia, Jess and Lucy, who along with Rosemary have been a great source of support with writing this. By doing this together, we have explored some of the strategies and challenges that face me from day to day, and how, with person-centred support, it has been possible for me to live reasonably well. I am both surprised and proud of what I have achieved, with support, over the past nine years, but I know that there is still a lot to do to enable the 'me in dementia' to call it a day and hand over the baton.

This chapter was written by me with the outstanding support of Lydia Smith, Jess Shaw and Lucy Jobbins, all undergraduate students at the University of Kent, alongside Rosemary, my wife and diligent first reader.

References

Bryden, C. (2005). *Dancing with dementia*. Jessica Kingsley Publishers.

Genova, L. (2007). *Still Alice*. Simon & Schuster.

Jordan, M. & Collins, N. (2017). *The D word: Rethinking dementia*. Hammersmith Health Books.

Kitwood, T. & Brooker, D. (Ed.) (2019). *Dementia reconsidered revisited. The person still comes first* (2nd ed.). Open University Press.

Mitchell, W. (2018). *Somebody I used to know*. London: Bloomsbury.

Oliver, K. (2016). *Walk the walk, talk the talk*. Forget-Me-Nots.

Oliver, K. (2019). *Dear Alzheimer's: A diary of living with dementia*. Jessica Kingsley Publishers.

Saints, M.J., De Frene, B. & Jennings, L. (Eds.). (2014). *Welcome to our world: A collection of life writing by people with dementia*. Forget-Me-Nots.

Warner, J. & Graham, N. (2018). *Understanding Alzheimer's disease and other dementias* (2nd ed.). Jessica Kingsley Publishers.

2   Poetry and crafting for people living with dementia

Gail Gregory

When you get a diagnosis of dementia, many people tell you, 'You won't be able to do the things that you used to, you know.' That may be so. I live with dementia, and I have found that living with dementia has opened up my world to a whole load of new things I never did before or haven't done for a long time.

Writing poetry as a therapeutic activity

Lockdown for me was quite useful in a way, in that it made me want to write poems. Poems are a way of expressing my feelings; instead of keeping them locked inside, I can release them and sometimes share them with the outside world. I think I wrote my first poem just after my diagnosis of dementia, when I was in my early 50s. I shared the poem with my family, who said that it was really good. I just thought that they were being kind. Then I started to share my poems on Facebook. That was when people commented on how brilliant my poems were. People could relate to my poetry. Some people said: 'Your poems are so full of feeling.'

My poems were helping me to get my feelings out. They were also touching others. I once read one of my poems at a meeting where there were healthcare professionals present. You could have heard a pin drop… it was like the room was empty. I think that was when I knew that my poems had quite an impact – I could actually get my feelings across more effectively than when I had a conversation, because people actually listened to my poems. In the 'dementia world', you do find that people stop listening to you, so in a way my poems offered a way of being heard again. My poems touched people. They could feel what I was feeling. For a few minutes, people were on my dementia journey *with me*.

To think that my English teacher said that I was 'useless at writing poetry'. Dementia has encouraged me to write poetry. Writing poetry has made me feel more confident, so I write more poems. I get a tremendous feeling of achievement.

Writing poems has become a way of releasing my anger and frustration at the hurdles that I have faced throughout my dementia journey. Each time I have a bad experience about how I am feeling on a particular day, I write a poem. I wrote quite a few poems after my diagnosis of dementia, as I had no one to talk to who understood. A feeling of loneliness seemed to take over.

So, when lockdown was introduced, I suppose it was like having a repeated diagnosis of dementia. The isolation and loneliness cloud loomed over me again. I had overcome this once, so I could overcome it again. Here is a poem that I wrote about my experience of lockdown.

We're in lockdown

We're in lockdown
It feels kinda funny
We can't go out spending paper money
We have to use the square plastic card
Remembering the number can be really quite hard

We're in lockdown
So, no family gatherings
I love sitting round all jibber-jabbering
I miss them all which is really quite sad
But it's not forever so it's not too bad

We're in lockdown
Shop shelves looking empty
We were all told that there would be plenty
Plenty of prunes – the things I don't like
There's no toilet rolls, can't go for a shite

We're in lockdown
The streets are so empty
No backed-up traffic and there used to be plenty
No flashy cars racing down the roads
Or the rumbling of wagons with big heavy loads

We're in lockdown
Time to learn something new
I wish you were here, so I could show you
The things I have made, the things I have done
At this moment in time our life just goes on
We're in lockdown

Just smile your way through it
Don't let this virus beat you to it
Just keep on going right to the end
So we can be with our family and friends

Lockdown, what a strange time! It took me time to adapt to a new routine and change. No longer could my husband and I go for our coffee breaks in our local café… have our Sunday morning brunch treat… attend our local Tuesday dementia group. Everything changed overnight, and it was a massive change. When you have dementia, change is a major disruption to your normal routine, and it upsets your body clock and your equilibrium.

Learning point 1

- Have you tried writing poems? What subjects have you written about?
- Have you shared your poems with your family or friends?
- Does writing poems help you to express your feelings?

The one thing in my daily routine that didn't change was walking my dogs, Toby and Charlie. Every day I walk Toby, my Scottish Terrier, who is very energetic and needs to burn off energy. I don't need to walk Charlie, my very lazy King Charles Spaniel, quite as often. Walking helps me to get my routine going at the start of my day. It gets me out of the house. It is also exercise.

Standing on the beach listening to the sea is my favourite activity. It is such a calming place. I love listening to the waves as they lap gently against the shore. I even enjoy watching the sea on the days when it is not calm and seeing the white foamed curling waves crash onto the shore or against the sea wall, with the waves lifting to great heights. I like feeling the sea spray and tasting the salty sea air. It is fascinating. It just captivates me and draws me into the rhythms of the sea, which are invigorating and yet calming. It makes me feel good. Below is a poem that I wrote about my visits to the beach.

Calming place

Where it's calm, I'm meant to be
I love to walk beside the sea
The lapping waves upon the shore
Leaves me wanting to walk some more
The more I walk the more I see this is where I want to be

My daily life is like the sea
Some days it's calm as calm can be
Then the tide changes and it gets rough
Then my day is very tough

Tangled wires inside my head
I think I should have stayed in bed

My cupboard doors all look the same
What's inside? It's not a game

Hide 'n seek is very frustrating
And now I'm stressed my pulse is racing

I think I know where I should be
The calming place beside the sea

Learning new crafts

Crafting and Zoom (online meetings) were also my saviours during lockdown. Crafting took off big time during lockdown, as it was a way of keeping myself busy and filling the long, empty days of nothingness.

I started creating Fairy Houses out of tree logs, and then I moved on to making pebble Fairy Houses. My imagination went into overdrive. In a way, I returned to my childhood of believing in fairies. Before I knew it, I had created a fairy village, with a fairy pond and a fountain. Then I decided to share what I was doing and I made short videos.

The videos were not as easy to master… my iPad kept falling over. I was also mumbling my words and forgetting what I was supposed to be doing next. At first it stressed me out. Then I developed the following strategies to help me:

- I bought a stand for my iPad.
- I always had everything to hand and laid out in the order that I would use them.
- I made notes and put them out of view of the camera.
- I told myself to relax – 'You have dementia, so nothing is going to be perfect.'

The videoing went so much smoother from that point onwards. I am not saying that the videos are perfect, but that doesn't matter. The videos are created by me, and my sidekick (I call Alzheimer's my 'sidekick').

YouTube was a whole different ball game. I also struggled to upload videos at times. But I do find that, if anything stresses me out, I just need to walk away and return later on.

The Fairy House construction was okay when we had the fine sunny days. But when it started raining, I had to look for another craft. That was when I thought about the cards that I used to make years ago. I told myself that, if I could make a Fairy House, I could surely make a card. So that was when I started the card making.

It has been quite testing at times to make cards, but notes, videos and photos help greatly. These are my memory aids now. I always say, 'Never give up!'- 'Keep trying' – 'If you can't do something today, try again tomorrow… tomorrow is a new day!'

So, my card-making really took off. I could spend hours creating just one card. I felt relaxed… I just focused on the card. I got completely lost in the moment, and before I knew it a couple of hours had passed quite quickly. The sense of achievement when I was creating a card was so fulfilling, and yet I was also very relaxed. I watched tutorials over and over again, so as to pick up tips about how I could make the different card folds. This has not been easy, and at times I have had to walk away. I thought that I would never get the hang of some of the card folds, but perseverance, and making lots of mistakes, has paid off. With plenty of practice, and after using lots of paper and card, I have created a card that I am pleased with. Wow, it feels so good when I have the finished product there in front of me. What an achievement! It is quite addictive too, and it leaves me wanting to create more cards!

Learning point 2

Below are links to some of my YouTube videos that I have created to help others to try crafting, and possibly to make cards like mine. Please watch them:

https://youtu.be/OJZJQXQbW3o
https://youtu.be/Nt4sXWsS9IE
https://youtu.be/2oqzQnr_wK4

Don't give up!

For anyone reading my chapter who is living with dementia, please feel encouraged to try new things. Don't give up, as you still have plenty to give. You may misplace things, forget your words and probably lots of other things. The most important thing, though, is to keep trying! Let us do things! Yes, we will make lots of mistakes, but we can also still achieve things.

Write a diary, or even a blog, for you and your family to look back on. It may help them to understand how you actually feel. It is also good to keep your brain active and to keep your words flowing. My spelling is atrocious now, but I don't care; it's me! There is always spell-checker!

Take lots of photos. They are a great reminder of what you have done and where you have been. I use my phone camera as 'a memory tool'. If I'm going on the tram or bus, I always take photos of where I get on and where I get off, and of the surrounding areas. I just take photos of things that I have done and places that I have visited, so that I do not forget them. My photos are a great comfort and reminder of my days.

I'm always finding new strategies to try to assist me, so that I am able to do things for myself, as I have to keep my brain going. Luckily, my hubby supports me, and he does not take over, unless I'm struggling.

If I stop doing things, I will forget how to do things so much quicker. So, my strategy is to carry on. I am hoping that I will retain the information about how to do things for longer.

So, my message is 'Don't give up, and sit back.' Please keep trying.

You can live your life with dementia.

3 Using poetry to support my granny when she had dementia

Isla Parker

My late granny, Vera, was a vibrant, intelligent lady who left school at the age of 15 but spent her life educating herself. She brought up two generations, including me, and many turned to her when they wanted motherly advice. Vera was happily married for more than 50 years and celebrated her Golden Wedding with a party in her and Grandpa's cottage garden. My grandparents enjoyed working together on different projects. My grandpa was a banker, but secretly wished that he had been a farmer. Vera indulged Grandpa's love of the outdoors by helping him to run a flower business, when they dressed window boxes of businesses and flats. When Grandpa died in his early 80s, Vera moved back to a village where we had lived when I was a young child, with her small Westie dog, and there she had a busy life, having her friends over for meals and volunteering as a steward at the local National Trust house – an Elizabethan manor.

Vera regretted having to leave school early, and she enjoyed driving herself to University of the Third Age classes,[1] such as current affairs and astrology courses. She drove a car until the grand old age of 89, when her deteriorating eyesight and her cognitive decline made it unsafe for her to be on the road. At this point, my aunt decided to hide Vera's car keys. She also asked Vera's GP to test her sight, hoping that she would fail. When Vera passed the eye test, my aunt wrote to the Driver and Vehicle Licensing Agency (DVLA) to say that Vera driving a car was a danger to others on the road.[2]

Vera had an older friend called Dorothy, whom she met in her 20s when she worked at an advertising agency as a secretary. Years later, Dorothy (then in her mid-80s) had quite advanced dementia, and I remember her coming over for lunch

---

1. www.u3a.org.uk/

2. For the DVLA rules about driving and dementia, see www.gov.uk/dementia-and-driving

at my granny's with her carer. Dorothy was in tears as she was so disorientated and confused. Vera found the lunch challenging as she tried to keep a conversation going with Dorothy's carer while Dorothy sat there looking bewildered and tearful.

After Dorothy left, my granny said to me, 'Sadly everyone has to go one day, physically or mentally. I hope, when my time comes, I can go physically. It is better that way.' Vera clearly feared Dorothy's predicament would happen to her one day. At this point, I wish that I had spoken to Granny longer about this subject; it might have been possible then to have encouraged members of the family to ask her to put in place a detailed person-centred Advance Directive (please see Chapters 4, 12 and 13 for advice on Advance Directives). Then the family would have known exactly what Vera's wishes were if she were to experience advanced cognitive decline, like Dorothy, who did not even recognise one of her oldest friends. I was in my mid-20s at the time and I did not have any experience of supporting someone with dementia.

In this chapter, I am going to tell you about how I dealt with my own feelings of powerlessness, sadness and fear several years later, as I watched Vera's cognitive decline, by turning to the arts to support her.

Poetry as a therapeutic strategy

Vera and I enjoyed reading poems together when I was a small child. Language clearly poses a significant challenge for people living with dementia. People with dementia who can no longer write can be assisted to do so. The poet John Killick has found that helping people with dementia to write poems can offer them real benefits by enabling them to convey the subjective reality of dementia and restoring their personhood and dignity. Killick has made poetry out of the world of people with dementia for the past 25 years (please see Chapter 34).

After attending one of John Killick's poetry workshops in Oxford several years ago, I began co-facilitating poems with Vera when she developed early-stage vascular dementia. She could still recall early experiences and she enjoyed reminiscing about the past. Co-facilitating the poems also gave my mum and Vera's carers a valuable insight into her experiences, and so helped them to improve Vera's quality of care.

Learning point 1

I used the following process that I learned from John Killick to co-facilitate the poems:

- Vera and I had a cup of tea together. It was important that this was a social occasion, as Vera looked forward to this. I suggested for the poem a theme such as 'the seaside', and we explored this memory together. I wrote down phrases that Vera spoke, to provide memory prompts for us to revisit.

- I suggested to Vera that we started the poem. If she had difficulty

> thinking of a first line, I would ask leading questions: 'What did your grandpa's garden look like? Why did you go there?'
>
> - Sometimes, Vera had difficulty creating new lines of poetry. On these occasions, I used a dog puppet to act out where the poem could go next, which helped to create a flow again. It was important that creating the poem was fun for Vera, and the dog puppet seemed to add to her enjoyment of the process.
>
> - I gave Vera a printed copy of the poem to keep. Vera often put the poem away in her handbag and smiled. It showed that she was pleased with the poem.

Therapeutic benefits

The poems were great for encouraging Vera to speak more. As poetry is often learned by people in their infancy, its rhythms and sounds make it the most memorable language. In this way, poetry is a most helpful medium. Vera could look at the poems when I was not with her and doing this may have reminded her of the memories they described.

I will now present a selection of Vera's poems and discuss each of these in turn to highlight the ways in which these connected Vera to earlier memories and to show why this has therapeutic value.

Grandpa's garden

I ran onto the path and it went sharp.
Bob, the sheepdog was always ready for a walk.
'Come on Bob, shall we go for a walk?'
He perked his ears up and said yes.
We go round the corner of the house,
I can see the Japanese anemones,
They're simple but white flowers and
Backed by the brick wall and the bakery.
I love the smell of freshly baked bread,
It makes me hungry.

Bob jumps up to make sure we're going for a walk.
So we go round the house and straight
Over the busy road until we come to the cemetery.
I like it here; it's quiet and peaceful.
Bob's trotting beside me.

The lonely gravestones make me feel quiet.
I look at the names and sometimes pick up a local family name.
I wonder what they did and how they lived.

Bob never barked in the cemetery,
Because he sensed people were sleeping like logs.
When he wasn't there, he was so lively.
He was a very nice dog.

Vera was a dog lover. My grandparents enjoyed having a sheepdog and then a collie during their married life together. Vera was brought up by her mum, her aunt and her grandparents, as her parents divorced when she was just four years old, which was unusual for that generation. I imagine that her grandpa's dog shared her adventures and brought her a lot of comfort when she was a small child, so it was helpful for the poem to take her back to this early memory. When Vera was living in the care home, a lady brought in a PAT dog (Pets as Therapy[3]) once a week for the residents to stroke and pet. Vera's face would light up during this time, as she had a special bond with the dog. The dog helped her to connect more to her surroundings.

In this poem, Vera and the dog enter a cemetery together. Both are respectful of those who are buried there – the dog doesn't bark, and Vera herself says, 'I like it here.' She is not afraid of death – in her mind 'people are sleeping like logs'. Vera has an interest in what the dead have done in their lives – as she says, 'I wonder what they did and how they lived?' Vera herself at this point had had a very long life, when she enjoyed being a secretary, a gardener, a mother, a granny and a great-granny, so perhaps it was comforting for her to think about these gravestones being records of what people had accomplished during their lives.

In the poem, some of Vera's rich vocabulary remains – she can recall the name of one flower, 'Japanese anemone'. Sadly, in her day-to-day life, Vera had now forgotten many names of flowers, so we both gained pleasure from this moment when she recalled the flower's name.

Learning point 2

- Does your relative or friend with dementia forget names or words? Do they get anxious when this happens? What helps them not to judge themselves harshly for forgetting words or names?

- Does your relative or friend with dementia have an interest (such as gardening, or playing a musical instrument) that helps them to connect to their senses (i.e. touch or smell)? Do these senses help them to feel more present in their surroundings?

A happy time in my childhood was going with my grandparents, brother and cousins to visit my grandparents' holiday cottage in Dorset. One of Vera's poems revisits this earlier time.

---

3. https://petsastherapy.org/

Good morning cows!

Have you lived in a cottage where every morning
The cows come to greet you? No? Well, I have.
Fair weather or foul, they always were there.
They grazed in a field just past our house,
And so rain or shine they had to come down for the milking every morning,
And I would be at my kitchen window,
And every morning they came down
From the grazing to be milked in the farm which was just beyond our house.
Inquisitively ambling along, they gazed
From side to side to see what was happening.
Misty barked and the whole scene changed.
The cows stiffened up and the mood changed.
Everything stopped and Misty stiffened,
And there was a moment when
Everyone awaited the next step forward.

Vera found it comforting to remember the cows and her collie, Misty, and this helped her to connect with me. Another earlier very happy memory was Vera's wedding day, and she explored this in another poem.

The dress

It was 1945 and pure silk material was difficult to find
And I wanted to be married in pure fabric.
My friend Dorothy was very good at sourcing.
She located pure silk and it felt
Lovely and gossamer soft and was pale blue.
I could show it to you. I've got it somewhere.
I'm still the same size you know.

I couldn't find any silk stockings.
But my friend Dorothy had a source.
She must have posted them to me,
So, after the wedding, I washed the pair again
And carefully packed and posted them back.

On my wedding day I got into the church,
But at the door I didn't recognise my husband.
I hadn't seen him for six months and he looked different,
When I first saw him, he had a lot of fair hair.
He had gone bald. He was only twenty-nine.
He was still nice looking though.

Soon after my grandparents met, Grandpa was sent up to Scotland to work in a bank. My grandparents kept in touch by letter. Grandpa had been unable to fight in the war due to having a weak heart. During this time, Vera was working as a secretary in London. Dorothy was her oldest friend, as mentioned at the start of this chapter. In the above poem, Dorothy helps Vera to enjoy her wedding day by lending her the silk stockings. Dorothy herself never had the good fortune to find someone lovely to marry, and here in this poem Vera can connect enough to remember Dorothy's generosity, and how thrifty she was – as Vera said, 'she was very good at sourcing'. Vera appreciated Dorothy's friendship and took care to post back her stockings after her special day. Notably, Vera draws on old-fashioned words, such as 'gossamer soft', to describe the luxury of having a dress made of pure silk at the end of the war.

When writing poems got too much for Vera as the cognitive decline worsened, I thought of other ways to connect. Vera enjoyed war-time music, and I would play her songs like Vera Lynn's 'We'll Meet Again'. I took some wind-up plastic toys to the nursing home, and Vera and I had fun with the other residents, winding up caterpillars and ladybirds and racing them across the long coffee table in the lounge.

Some of Vera's great-grandchildren went to the nursing home with their mums to sing popular songs to Vera, and she enjoyed these visits. On her last birthday, all of her children and many of her grandchildren and great-grandchildren celebrated the special occasion with her.

I would like to finish with one of Vera's shorter poems, which reflects on her last birthday.

Birthdays in the nineties

For my birthday I had three cakes.
They were all nice.
One was chocolate, another was vanilla and strawberry,
And the third was lemon.
Everybody sang me 'Happy Birthday',
And it was such a jolly day.
I've had many birthdays,
But this one seemed to be everlasting.
I had lots of visitors and goodwill was everywhere.

Here, Vera appreciates the 'goodwill' of her visitors; indeed, she wants the party to be 'everlasting'. The environment of the nursing home, which might at other times have inhibited human flourishing, has been changed by her family and friends into one of a nurturing 'home', where cake and company are enjoyed, so that it is 'a jolly day'. Vera's wellbeing is paramount, and she is encouraged to connect with her children and grandchildren in a way where they can all celebrate her 94th birthday.

Human flourishing is very important in dementia care, as the emphasis is placed on maximising the potential for people living with dementia to thrive. All of the time that I knew Vera, she had a spiritual life, and even in the last two or so years of her life she still believed that she would go to a better place when she died. Perhaps Vera was able to relax in this environment when she was surrounded by family and friends because she was at peace with passing away. Chapter 8 explores the subject of spirituality and dementia, including the role that loved ones can take in supporting the person with dementia to express and connect with their own spirituality.

Fortunately, much can be done to improve the quality of life for people with dementia. The arts can do a great deal to ease their suffering, and to provide companionship. Vera and I enjoyed our cups of tea and slices of cake together and the time that we spent creating poems about her memories. The novelist E.M. Forster wrote in *Howards End* (2000), 'only connect'– and certainly the power of words and music do go a long way to making a connection with a loved one with dementia, when they are feeling lonely and confused.

Learning point 3

- Have you tried playing songs from the past to your relative or friend with dementia? Do they like to sing along?

- Have you played simple games, like racing wind-up cars? Games that help someone to live in the moment are particularly helpful.

- How have you involved the grandchildren of the person with dementia? Children often enjoy singing or playing musical instruments, as do people living with dementia. Music can join the different generations together. Grandchildren can also help their grannies or granddads to write a poem, and the process can be intergenerational and rewarding for all involved.

- If you can't be with them in person, I recommend using Zoom when assisting a person with dementia to write a poem, as then you can use puppets and song to help the writing process.

Reference

Forster, E.M. (2000). *Howards End*. Penguin Classics.

Further reading

Austin, R. (2019). Making, shaping and celebrating together. *The Journal of Dementia Care, 27*(Jan/Feb), 24–25.

Hayes, K. (Ed.). (2006). *The edges of everywhere: Poetry by people living with memory loss* (2006). City Chameleon.

Killick, J. (2008). *Dementia diary: Poems and prose*. Hawker Publications.

Killick, J. & Cordonnier, C. (2000). *Openings: Dementia poems and photographs*. Hawker Publications.

Knoll, E. (Ed.). (2022). *Sweet memories: Poetry by people living with dementia*. New Generation Publishing.

4   The practical realities of caring for a loved one with dementia

Marianne Talbot

In 1996, my 80-year-old father had a massive stroke, on a walk to the village. He lived another four years but never again managed a lucid conversation. Dad's stroke didn't kill him, so his will wasn't activated. But Dad didn't have what was then called an Enduring Power of Attorney (the precursor to the current Lasting Power of Attorney (LPA)). He had to be made a ward of the Court of Protection. I became his 'Receiver'. This meant gathering his income and distributing it for the benefit of him and my mother.

That sounds straightforward, doesn't it? It was anything but. I hope the Court of Protection has improved. But I wonder? I would apply for a Court Order and two months later it would come – but with the decimal point in the wrong place. I'd get £100 rather than the £1000 I needed (or vice versa). Every year I'd have to audit Dad's accounts and submit them to the Court, and I'd have to do his (and Mum's) tax returns. For someone whose financial training comprised discussing my overdraft with the bank manager, it was no fun.

> ### Learning point 1
>
> Do you have a Lasting Power of Attorney (LPA) for your loved one? Does your loved one still have decision-making capacity? If so, the conversation is worth having.
>
> - An LPA for financial decisions can be used while your loved one still has capacity or it can be activated when they no longer have capacity.
> - Your loved one can restrict or not restrict the types of decisions their attorney can make.
> - Your loved one can ask for details of how much is spent and how

much they have or arrange for such details to be sent to a solicitor or a family member.

- There is also an LPA covering health and welfare, which gives your loved one the powers to make decisions about your care and treatment, including end-of-life preferences.
- You need to register the LPA in advance, and you then activate it if/when the person loses capacity to make their own decisions.
- Having an LPA will save you a lot of money and stress.

A year before Dad died, Mum was diagnosed with Alzheimer's. She was 79. She sank into a depression from which she didn't emerge until her doctor persuaded her to take antidepressants. These might not work for everyone, but they worked for Mum. She was on them until her death 10 years later. As soon as they kicked in, Mum became again the charming, cheerful person she had always been.

Aware that Mum soon wouldn't be able to live alone, I started to look at care homes. Residential homes wouldn't look at Mum because of her diagnosis. This was more than 10 years ago. Later in the progression of her dementia, when her need for residential care became unavoidable, I was able to look with a different eye at homes for those with dementia. But at that point I had little personal experience of dementia (Dad was cared for by Mum). The nursing homes seemed to me like Bedlam. If I had relinquished Mum's care to such a home, I would have hated myself.

So began the process of wondering what to do about Mum that culminated in bringing her to live with me.

Learning point 2

Before you visit homes, familiarise yourself with what you think your loved one will need in terms of their care.[1] There is a wealth of information and advice on the internet.

- Check out the websites of relevant organisations and charities (for example Age UK[2] or the Alzheimer's Society[3]).
- Your local council may be able to help.
- Make a list of homes in the area where your loved one might live and visit them all.

1. Garton, D. (Undated). *A guide to finding the best care home.* Kindle. www.amazon.co.uk/Guide-Finding-Best-Care-Home-ebook/dp/B01N4I753G/ref=sr_1_20?dchild=1&keywords=dementia+and+respite+care&qid=1587032269&s=books&sr=1-20

2. For Age UK's advice on finding a suitable care home, go to www.ageuk.org.uk/information-advice/care/arranging-care/care-homes/help-finding-care-home

3. For advice from the Alzheimer's Society on finding a care home, go to www.alzheimers.org.uk/get-support/help-dementia-care/finding-care-home

- Before you visit, make a list of questions – features you'd like to see and those you *wouldn't* like to see.

A live-in elderly parent with dementia

I wouldn't dream of saying to anyone else that bringing their parent to live with them is the solution to a diagnosis of dementia. I lived alone and could make a unilateral decision. Mum's personality played a huge part in my decision: she was a very easy person.

I had heard stories of people with dementia getting aggressive. When I asked Mum's consultant, she told me that people with Alzheimer's tend to become more of whatever they were before. The only exception, she said, was when a person had been suppressing their real nature. Then the Alzheimer's would then reveal the underlying reality and shock everyone into thinking the person had 'changed'. I spent a morning wondering whether Mum had been suppressing a nasty side. I then dismissed it and invited Mum to live with me.

When she said 'Yes', I had to sell both our houses and buy a house that would suit the two of us. It took 18 months. Mum deteriorated and living on her own became hard for her. When I realised she wasn't eating, I ordered meals on wheels. Then I opened tabs at every shop in the village so she could take whatever she wanted without paying. This is the joy, of course, of a small village.

Mum's car became a bone of contention. Her driving was erratic and, I believed, dangerous. She disagreed. Thankfully, she crashed and wrote it off without hurting anyone. When I learned she was going to buy a new one, I shopped her to the DVLA and they took her licence away. She was incandescent with rage. But – here is one of the main advantages of Alzheimer's disease – she soon forgot about it!

Learning point 3

Expect resistance when you suggest that your loved one gives up driving – to them it may represent freedom and independence.

- You must, by law, inform the DVLA and your car insurer if you are given a diagnosis of dementia. This does not mean you have to stop driving but you may be asked to do an assessment to check you are still safe to drive.
- Ideally the doctor making the dementia diagnosis will inform the person if they are not safe to drive, which relieves their loved ones of the responsibility (and blame!).
- Be prepared to inform the DVLA if you think your loved one is unsafe to drive and they do not yet have a diagnosis.

By the time Mum moved, she was definitely ready to do so. Her friends had melted away and she was lonely. But then I realised that I had forgotten about her cat. Oh dear. My 10-year-old cat had to learn to live with another 10-year-old cat. Every time they met unexpectedly, the hissing and spitting would shock Mum to her core.

But Mum flourished and started to regain her social skills. She'd lean over and kiss me, saying, 'I *love* living with you.' I loved living with her too! I showed her off to my friends and even took her to work. She sat in the front row of my lectures, nodding and smiling and saying to everyone who'd listen, 'That's my daughter!'

I can hear you thinking, 'It won't last'

As Mum's mind fragmented, life got harder (Moller, 2019). It became difficult to entertain her. Books were the first casualty. She couldn't keep a story in her head. The newspaper lasted longer. But she'd read out the same piece over and over (and over) again. I learned that, if I responded in the same way every time, using the same tone of voice, she would think we were conversing. I could go on doing whatever I was doing almost as if uninterrupted.

Her embroidery then became difficult. She'd keep unpicking it, telling me over and over again that she was stupid. This distressed me enormously. As did her habit of asking me, every five minutes, to thread the needle. Eventually, I bundled up the embroidery and put it in the loft. That left her with *nothing* to do. Sometimes she'd sit happily, saying, if asked, 'I am thinking'. Other times she'd be at my side, asking what I was doing, if she could help, whether it wasn't time to be doing this, that or the other. It drove me batty, especially if I was working.

My intention had been to involve Mum in whatever I was doing. That worked for a while. She felt she was doing her bit and we worked companionably together. But then she started washing up by just passing the item under the cold tap. Drying up lasted a bit longer, as did setting the table and hanging up and taking in laundry. But, task by task, her competence atrophied.

So, Mum started going to day care three times a week. It was a boon for both of us. Again, her social skills improved dramatically. She enjoyed the games, liked meeting new people, and I was able to get some work done. A special transport bus collected her and dropped her off. Poor Mum had no idea where she was going or why. I could see a sort of learned helplessness setting in – as if Mum was having the joy sucked out of her. If I had my time again, I would certainly arrange to drop her off and collect her myself.

Learning point 4

Arrange day care before you are exhausted and while your loved one is still able to benefit from the social interaction it offers.

- As soon as you become (or realise you have become) a carer, you need to arrange for a carer's assessment from social services.

- Find out what is available in the way of day care (state or private), before you need it.
- Use the internet to do your research on how to benefit from day care.[4]

Respite care

Mum had lived with me for three years before I realised that I was entitled to six weeks' respite care annually. When I found out, I couldn't wait to book her in. I visited the home and everything seemed fine. I knew Mum wouldn't like being away from me. But I also knew that afterwards I would be better able to care for her. But our first – and last – respite week was a disaster.

When I got back, I was looking forward to seeing Mum. But the moment she saw me she burst into floods of tears. She sobbed and sobbed and kept repeating 'I'm a bad person'. She was frightened to go to bed and to have a bath; she didn't want to eat or even to leave my side.

I have no idea what happened, and never will. When I complained, the home staff said they were mystified. They explained the fact that she arrived home filthy and without her teeth or her bra by saying that she had refused to wear the teeth and the bra and that she must have dirtied herself on the bus, because she was fine when she left.

I tried an official complaint, but it was so difficult that I gave up, thereby guaranteeing it would happen to others. But I was too tired and beaten down to care. I paid for one week's respite care with five weeks of angst for both Mum and me.

Learning point 5

Prepare for respite care in such a way as to guarantee (as far as possible) that you and your loved one benefit from it.

- As soon as you become (or realise you have become) a carer, find out about local arrangements for respite care.
- Visit all the homes that might provide respite care, with a list of questions (and likes and dislikes).
- Take your loved one several times to visit the home where they will go for respite care, so they get to know the staff and it feels familiar to them.
- Consider using your first week as a 'dummy run', visit your loved one every day, and join in with whatever they do.

---

4. The government guide *Dementia, Social Services and the NHS* can be found at www.nhs.uk/conditions/dementia/social-services-and-the-nhs/

Direct Payments

After an assessment, social services then deemed I was eligible for Direct Payments.[5] I was delighted. This would give me the freedom to arrange and pay for the kind of care that I wanted for Mum. But it was the responsibilities that came with the Direct Payments that did for me.

I employed an agency who promised to provide a 'small team of trained carers'. But for every carer who did her best, there'd be another one who already had her coat on and couldn't get out fast enough as soon as I came through the door. I soon gave up with the agency and advertised and interviewed carers myself. But then I had to write contracts for everyone, construct rotas and calculate everyone's pay, including holiday pay, tax and national insurance. When my carefully constructed rota collapsed, I started crying and couldn't stop. A doctor was called, valium was dispensed and the machinery started to get Mum into a home.

Learning point 6

Do not take on responsibilities simply because they are the sort of thing you used to be able to do – remember, you are now running a three-legged race!

- Before agreeing to anything, stop and give it some real thought.
- Ask yourself exactly what you are planning to do and how, realistically, you are going to fit it into your life.
- If there is any question to which you cannot give a convincing answer, say 'no'!
- Just because whatever you have been asked to do is supposed to benefit informal carers, this does not mean it will benefit *you*.

Finally – a home

That Mum could not go on living with me was obvious to everyone. The family rallied round until a place could be found for her. This took about eight weeks of guilt, nightmares and spitting arguments with siblings. We had assessment after assessment and always there was the underlying worry about money – how were we *ever* going to afford to pay for residential care?

We were lucky. Mum was awarded 'continuing care' funding, which is covered by the NHS and therefore not means-tested.[6] This is often not the case with dementia, as people are deemed only to need social care, not nursing care.

---

5. For information about Direct Payments, see the Carers' UK website: www.carersuk.org/help-and-advice/practical-support/getting-care-and-support/direct-payments

6. For information about means-testing, see www.nhs.uk/conditions/social-care-and-support-guide/money-work-and-benefits/nhs-continuing-healthcare/

So they remain the responsibility of social services, and funding is means-tested.

Mum moved into her new home. She was allocated a sunny room, looking onto the garden. The moving day was agony for me, but Mum took it in her stride. I went to visit her the next day and found her tormenting a carer with a rubber toy and being teased in return. Such a relief.

Learning point 7

Recognise that you will need to find a residential care home for your loved one at some point. End-stage dementia is too much for family to cope with.

- Check out Learning Point 2 again.
- Find out whether your loved one is eligible for continuing care.[7]
- Find out exactly what evidence you have to submit and gather it in advance.

Institutionalisation

Mum quickly became institutionalised. She stopped spending her nights walking the corridors, settled in and started sleeping well. The chef took her coeliac disease as a challenge that he was determined to overcome, and she enjoyed the food. She ignored the things I did to make her feel at home. But she enjoyed the music therapy and liked to watch the ducks and doves in the garden. I'd take her outside in the wheelchair she was then using, and she'd insist I run – 'faster, *faster*, **faster**'!

But the weight was falling off her. I walked behind her once as a carer took her to the loo. My always-robust Mum was skin and bones. I asked them to bring a doctor in. Ominously, the doctor found a 'mass' in her tummy. This prompted much soul-searching – I really couldn't see Mum coping with being examined in hospital, far less having exploratory surgery.

A few days later, the phone startled me awake at midnight. Mum had been sick and the home thought I ought to come. When I got there, Mum was awake and clearly in pain. Unforgivably, they could give her only paediatric paracetamol. They put a mattress beside Mum's bed, but so long as she was in pain, I wasn't going to sleep, so I tried to soothe her. At 4am she fell into an uneasy sleep. At about 5am her breathing changed and somehow I knew this was the end. I held her and told her over and over that I loved her. Her breathing became more ragged and intermittent. At 5.30am, my lovely Mum died.

Luckily, I had completed an Advance Directive[8] with Mum while she retained capacity to do so. In it, she stated that she did not want to be hospitalised or

---

7. You can find out more about eligibility for NHS Continuing Care funding here: www.gov.uk/government/publications/nhs-continuing-healthcare-checklist

8. See www.nhs.uk/conditions/end-of-life-care/advance-decision-to-refuse-treatment/

resuscitated under various specific conditions, one of which was if she had dementia. I had given this to the care home when she first moved there. So Mum died in her own bed, with me beside her, instead of being forced back into a life that had lost its meaning for her.

I took her wedding ring from her finger and slipped it, still warm, onto mine. For three hours, I stayed with her, brushing her hair, washing her face and exchanging reminiscences with the carers who came to express their condolences. Then I left to make the phone calls that would send the news ricocheting around the family.

Learning point 8

- An Advance Directive (or Advance Decision to Refuse Treatment) is a statement that sets out any medical treatment you wish to refuse, should you lack capacity to communicate those preferences yourself. The medical authorities are legally required to follow your wishes if they are aware of the Directive. You need to get the statement witnessed and should give it to your GP and any other medical/health/care authorities involved in your care, so they know about it (see also Chapter 12).

The aftermath

It is 10 years since Mum died. It took me five years to fully shed my role as her carer. I have never regretted bringing her to live with me. I learned things I would never have learned any other way – in particular, that there is an army of people out there who devote their lives to honouring people whom society has written off. Recently Covid-19 forced us all to value properly the work carers do. May we never forget again.

Learning point 9

Although I had three siblings, I looked after Mum largely on my own. Try hard not to find yourself in this position:

- Call a family pow-wow at the first opportunity.
- Do not assume no one else will help (if you do, no one else *will* help you!).

Reference

Moller, M. (2019). *Alzheimer's through the stages: A caregiver's guide*. Althea Press.

5   The challenge of supporting an elderly parent with dementia

Gary Lockhart

I am the only child of my parents, Bill and Rosemary. In this chapter, I will share my experience of supporting my elderly mother with vascular dementia in Australia, where we both live. The ongoing task of care for my mother requires me to navigate the challenges involved in addressing her physical health issues and her practical needs, while ensuring that she can still maintain a connection to her life as she remembers it. By moving both of my parents interstate, their physical health improved, and they maintained a connection with their family, but unfortunately they lost social connections. I am originally from Melbourne, but I have lived in Sydney for more than 20 years and operate a youth service there. I will share some of the tough decisions that had to be made and some of the ways that I look after myself and maintain my independent life while caring for and sharing a home with my parents.

Background/story

My parents, Bill and Rosemary, are from Melbourne, Australia, and have spent their lives living and working in the suburbs there. They inherited their home from my grandmother and lived there for more than 50 years. Before retirement, Rosemary worked as a book-keeper, and Bill as a payroll officer. After retirement, Rosemary was active in the community, visiting elderly people in nursing homes and undertaking church-based volunteering. She was also a keen football fan and would go to the matches weekly. Bill was not particularly social, but he enjoyed swimming at the beach nearby, and he had a small group of friends there. Rosemary took on most of the household responsibilities, including the financial affairs. Neither of them had a plan of what to do in their old age; they were content in their day-to-day life and didn't seriously consider their future. As they grew older, I tried to encourage them to consider planning for their old age, which included them both having a session with a counsellor, which showed them that it was extremely likely that they would eventually need to move to another home. They verbally agreed with the planning and its logic in theory, but they were unwilling to put the plan into action.

In 2013, when Rosemary was aged 82 years, she started displaying signs of dementia in her behaviour. I noticed these behavioural changes in particular during one visit to my parents' home; Rosemary's memory loss was affecting her day-to-day function. She was forgetting things more often, and she had difficulty performing familiar tasks. For example, she had trouble remembering all of the steps involved in preparing a meal. She also got confused about the time and felt disorientated at times. On occasions, she found it difficult to choose the right words. *Dementia Australia* (2020) notes that these behaviours can be a warning sign of dementia.

My father had also noticed these changes in Rosemary's personality and behaviour. At times she exhibited rapid mood swings and she became inventive with finding different ways to conceal her poor memory by keeping hidden notes that reminded her about ordinary day-to-day activities that she needed to do. She also had standard answers that she would always give to questions and would use an assertive tone of voice to stop further questioning. I noticed these changes and spoke to her doctor, who said that she most probably had vascular dementia with mild cognitive impairment. Di Carli (2014) notes that vascular dementia includes symptoms of amnesia, which are regarded as common in older people.

I had mentioned this previously to my father, who didn't consider that it was a disease that would progress. Some years later, my father had a minor accident and needed to be hospitalised for a short period. During this time, I noticed that my mother couldn't remember the details of his accident or which hospital he was in. It became clear that Rosemary wasn't managing the finances properly and that the house was sliding into disrepair and becoming untidy.

Learning point 1

- Do these 'symptoms of dementia' sound familiar?
- Have you seen similar behaviour being displayed by a family member?
- What are some of the behaviours that you are noticing that your family member displays?
- Does that family member recognise the behaviours as being indications that they may be living with dementia? Can the issue be raised easily with family members, including the person with dementia, and their doctor?

I was still unable to motivate my parents to consider changing their situation, and it became clear that nothing would happen until it was absolutely necessary. This didn't occur until a number of years later, when my mother was exhibiting some disturbing physical symptoms that included breathlessness and dizziness.

Rosemary went for tests and she was diagnosed as having heart fibrillation and fluid on her lungs. She was admitted to hospital.

During this time, I stayed down in Melbourne with my father, who was unable to look after himself as he lacked the skills to cook or to undertake most basic household duties. During this period, medical staff explained to Bill that Rosemary was exhibiting clear signs of dementia, and Bill began to accept the diagnosis and the prognosis for her. The heart condition and other physical health problems could be controlled with medication; however, the dementia would remain. During Rosemary's stay in hospital, she slipped in the bathroom and fractured her pelvis. She had to remain in hospital for a number of months to recover from this and undergo rehabilitation.

Planning the move to Sydney

This period became the crucial decision-making period for my parents and for me. The choices made now would affect their future life situation. During this period, it was necessary to find a balanced life solution for the future. My mother's dementia had progressed to such an extent that she was unable to understand why she was in hospital or that she had a dementia. She could not comprehend her condition. The recommendation from her doctors and social workers was that she would not be able to return to living in the family home as it was, and she would most likely have to go into care. The planning for this would involve doctors, social workers, me and my parents, as there were no other close family members.

If my parents decided to stay in Melbourne, my mother would enter a care home and my father would remain in the family house. This option wasn't ideal for my father, as he would also need physical care and assistance in the house. He was assessed, and I was told that he did not require higher-level care in a nursing home placement. However, my mother would require a high level of care, as she would require supervision in a locked dementia ward, for her own safety. So, both of my parents entering care wasn't a great option, as they would most likely be separated.

The option that we eventually chose was for both of my parents to move to Sydney, where I could take on the role of primary carer and both organise and manage their care for them. So we sold the family house and found a new property for all three of us in a convenient location that was familiar to both of them. So my parents have been able to remain together in their own home for the past five years and have become physically healthier and more active due to the warmer climate.

Learning point 2

Moving house can be arduous and difficult for anyone, but when you are considering someone with dementia whose short-term memory is failing, it can be a traumatic experience, as they may not realise or understand why they have to move in the first place. Consider whether a move is really necessary. If a person is able to remain in their own home and in familiar surroundings, this may reduce the amount of stress that they experience.

- Weigh up the options of moving house for the person with dementia – they can't weigh up the decision in the way you are able to. What are the benefits of moving house for the person with dementia? What are the negative consequences of the move?
- Who else might be involved in making the decision as to whether or not the person with dementia moves house? What supports might be available to the person with dementia in their own house?
- Is it absolutely necessary for the person to leave their current property?

Latimer (2012, p.45) notes that familiar surroundings can help those who are ageing keep a sense of personal continuity. Therefore, familiar items, such as photo albums, favourite chairs or ornaments, can help a person to keep a sense of their own home. When relocating them, I ensured that my parents' original furniture was brought up to Sydney and my mother's room was recreated in the new property. This helped Rosemary to settle and to maintain a sense of identity. The property was also in a location that was familiar to both of my parents, as Bill had attended the local public school 80 years before, and both of my parents had stayed in the local hotel on several occasions when they were on holiday. With the assistance of a local home care service, the property was fitted out so that my parents could stay there safely. The apartment is ideally located, being close to shops, chemists, banks and medical services. The new apartment requires less cleaning and maintenance than the old house, and is on the ground floor, with easy access. It is also close to the local amenities, but still right next to a beach.

Learning point 3

When relocating an elderly relative to a new area, think about what amenities will be useful to them. How mobile are they? Do they shop for themselves? Do they drive a vehicle? Will they be able to continue to drive? What type of climate do they prefer?

1. Think about when you have moved house. What do you look for in an area? What types of things are important to you?
2. Now think about what amenities your relative uses now and consider whether they will be able to access these amenities in the future.

Access to friends

The aspect that was most difficult to manage was social contact. Most of my mother's friends were elderly and were not able to travel to Sydney. Phone calls don't replace face-to-face interaction. However, some of Rosemary's younger friends have come to visit her. She has enrolled in local weekly activity groups and enjoyed them. However, her poor memory has limited her ability to form any lasting friendships. There has been some consistency with her interactions with nursing care staff, so she is able to develop some familiarity with them.

Learning point 4

When relocating a person with dementia, try to maintain their long-term friendships if possible. An elderly person with dementia will find it hard to make new friendships due to their poor short-term memory. If the person doesn't have access to their friends, try to use technology (e.g. telephones, social media) where possible. Connect the person to local groups to facilitate human interaction. If the person with dementia is receiving care, try to keep the carers as consistent as possible.

- Consider how you felt on an occasion when you have been separated from your friends. How do you maintain these friendships?
- Think about periods in your life when you have tried to make new friends, perhaps when you have moved house, or started a new job. What did you do to develop new relationships?
- In the past, in what ways have you been helped to build friendships with others? How might you be able to facilitate someone with short-term memory problems to build friendships where they share similar interests and/or cultural backgrounds with others?

The ongoing process of care

Setting up a reliable home care service for my parents has enabled them to receive consistent quality care. O'Connor et al. (2020) note that setting up care for elderly people with dementia can be complex. My efforts at navigating the care system for the elderly has helped my mother to receive a high level of care that has enabled her to remain in her own home. In Australia, home care for older people is accessed through the Australian Government's 'My Aged Care' website,[1] and is well supported financially. To be eligible for services, a person must be seen by the Commonwealth Aged Care Assessment Team. This is commonly called an ACAT assessment. The care services are aimed at keeping people well and independent. They provide personal care nursing, such as showering, self-care, hygiene, grooming, wound management and help with medicines.

Health and therapy services, such as podiatry, physiotherapy and occupational therapy, are also available, as well as specialised support for particular conditions,

---

1. www.myagedcare.gov.au

such as dementia, and assistance with meal preparation, feeding and household chores. Services also include assistance to fit safety equipment, such as rails, and mobility aids, such as walking frames and wheelchairs. The care packages also facilitate services that keep people connected to their community, such as transport and enrolment in community group activities (Commonwealth of Australia, 2020).

Home care is delivered as a package by registered home care providers, and recipients have a case manager. Our local care-provider has put in place several carers who are able to visit my parents on a regular basis, so that my parents can have consistency in their care, and build supportive, ongoing relationships with their carers.

Learning point 5

Try to familiarise yourself with the care system for older people in your local area.

- Are there assessments?
- Are there waiting lists?

A family member overseeing the management of home care can greatly improve the situation for older people, as they can manage communication issues and ensure autonomy in their decisions.

My parents have been able to develop ongoing relationships with their care providers. Since our apartment is located close to coffee shops and amenities, my parents are able to walk there with the staff and get daily exercise. My mother often feels well and is able to enjoy her time in the community and have a wider focus beyond the home. I take my parents out weekly to the local shopping centre to have fish and chips for lunch. My mother and father both celebrated their 90th birthdays in the past few years. Family and friends came to these celebrations.

Self-care

Self-care is important for someone in my position, or I won't remain effective in my role as a carer for my parents. It is well noted that family members who are caregivers experience elevated levels of stress, and often experience depression, anxiety and a sense of burden (Mitrani et al., 2005). The government-assisted home care service available here in Australia has greatly helped me to maintain an independent life alongside looking after my parents. While I have lived with my parents, I have ensured that I have space to myself and have maintained relationships outside of the home, and also engaged in activities in the community. Gagliano (2014) notes that taking care of someone else is a difficult task and requires a lot of effort if you are to maintain your sense of self and identity. Fortunately, where I have placed my parents has a beautiful swimming beach, and I ensure that I am able to continue my social life and engage in the local music scene. Stepping back from doing everything to assist my parents has also been a way to give myself time, and this has also helped my father and mother to thrive and maintain some independence. Leaving some tasks for my father, Bill, such as shopping for bread, milk and other household items, has kept him physically and mentally active. I have found that Bill will step back from taking responsibility if possible. Yet, he is competent to complete many household tasks successfully, if shown how to do so.

Learning point 6

- Think about the different ways that you take time out for yourself when you are at work or going about your daily life. How do you ensure that you have time to relax?
- When you feel overwhelmed, do you find it easy to say 'no'?
- Think about activities that you enjoy doing. How can you incorporate these activities into your life, while still being a carer?

Maintaining the balance between ensuring that my mother stays physically healthy while at the same time keeping her feeling positive has been an ongoing and arduous task. Maintaining aspects of an independent life apart from caregiving has enabled me to remain mentally well and physically up to the task. The difficult decision to move both of my parents interstate was, in some respects, a gamble. However, they have been able to remain relatively well mentally and physically for the past five years, which allows me to think that the move has been a success. Considering my parents' very advanced ages and my mother's level of dementia, it is a wonderful result for them to be able to walk along to a coffee shop every day. This provides me with great happiness and a sense of satisfaction that I am supporting them in the best possible way. My mother's wish at her 90th birthday was for 'everybody to have a happy life'. I hope that discussing my experience here will provide the reader with a platform for ideas and inspiration for their future endeavours in caring for someone with dementia.

References

Commonwealth of Australia. (2020). *Help at home.* www.myagedcare.gov.au/

Dementia Australia. (2020). *Warning signs of dementia.* www.dementia.org.au/information/about-dementia/how-can-i-find-out-more/warning-signs-of-dementia

Di Carli, C. (2014). Vascular cognitive impairment. In B. Dickerson & A. Atri (Eds.), *Dementia: Comprehensive principles and practices* (pp.260–273). Oxford University Press.

Gagliano, J. (2014). *The Australian ageing generation handbook.* Jane Curry Publishing.

Latimer, J. (2012). Home care and frail older people: relational extension and the art of dwelling. In C. Ceci, K. Bjornsdottir & M. Ellen Purkis (Eds), *Perspectives on care at home for older people* (pp.35–61). Routledge.

Mitrani, V.B., Feaster, D.J., McCabe. B.E., Czaja, S.J. & Szapocznik, J. (2005). Adapting the structural family systems rating to assess the patterns of interaction in families of dementia caregivers. *The Gerontologist, 45*(4), 445–455.

O'Connor, C.M.C., Gresham, M., Poulos, R.G., Clemson, L., Mc Gilton K.S., Cameron, I.D., Hudson, W., Radoslovich, H., Jackman, J. & Poulos C.J. (2020) Understanding in the Australian aged care sector of reablement interventions for people living with dementia: A qualitative content analysis. *BMC Health Services Research, 20*, 140. https://doi.org/10.1186/s12913-020-4977-1

6   The difficulties and triumphs of the single carer

Peter Hemsley

First signs: The family doctor

Six years ago, my wife and I went to our local GP for a routine visit. At the end of the consultation, he pressed my wife's neck, and thought something was wrong. It transpired that she needed cardio-vascular surgery to clear obstructions in her artery. The surgery went ahead at a hospital 30 miles away, and we were asked to be there at 7.30am. The operation took place six hours later, which caused my wife much agitation. An overnight stay after the operation added to the trauma. The return home brought her relief.

Though this may not be connected with the onset of dementia, it did have an adverse and unsettling effect. Might the fact that my wife became irrational and difficult soon after be merely coincidental?

She smoked and wore high-heeled shoes. Initially I let her carry on, but gradually realised that the situation was worsening. At first, I thought that I was well able to cope with this. I was in denial of the situation.

I was made redundant at the age of 63 and applied for more than 200 jobs during the following year. However, I was becoming scared to leave my wife for any length of time and was leading a very insular life. I felt that I could cope, but the bad days were getting worse. I tried to see our GP, but he had retired early through burn-out. My new GP could not see me for six weeks. Our previous GP had always shown us a caring attitude, but this had now changed. The new GP told me I should have seen her earlier, which seemed unfair, after having waited so long for an appointment. That my trusty GP and confidant was no longer there to support us was bitterly frustrating and life was steadily becoming more stressful. He had been our GP for 30 years, had witnessed my wife losing her first husband with cancer at 40, and had also seen her son, who was quadriplegic, pass away aged 20. He had empathy with both of us.

The onset and living with dementia

Dementia was affecting my wife's sleeping habits and she developed day-night syndrome. The situation was worsening. Most nights she went to sleep in bed but after a few hours would get up thinking it was morning. She would open the curtains when it was pitch black, make a cup of tea, light a cigarette and perform her normal morning routine, and then go back to sleep again on the settee. Initially I would let her get on with it. I was worried about what she might do if I did not watch her, so I bought an air bed and slept on the floor next to her. Now I had to protect her from herself. She would try to light cigarettes, which could not only cause fires but also harm her. She would try to make cups of tea and I had to restrain her. Even when, usually with my help, she managed to fill the cup, she was liable to try to stir the tea with an unlit cigarette. She would get up several times in the night.

A further consultation with the GP took place, which took 23 days to arrange. One morning, my wife woke at five, giddy and disorientated. She was screaming, as she was anxious. This was a once-only occasion. I called the paramedics and they diagnosed labyrinthitis. They calmed her down, gave me the paperwork to take to the health centre and told me that the GP would be in touch. I heard nothing.

Two weeks later, we were in A&E with my wife suffering terrible head spinning and disorientation. After consultation, which proved negative, we arrived back home at 3.00am. I went to the GP 14 days later to find no correspondence had been received from either visit. When I asked why not, I was told that reports from hospitals take ages to be actioned. I phoned the hospital and they faxed over the details and the conclusion immediately. I saw the GP as a matter of urgency, and she recognised a vitamin B12 deficiency. A course of six injections were prescribed, to be administered every other day. These went well, but my wife's recognition of the exact time of the appointment was a major issue, as she got ready four or five hours before appointments. She was impatient to get there. I tried to placate her by driving her to the health centre to show that it was too early.

The GP said that my wife would be referred to the memory clinic. It took seven weeks to arrange. As part of the consultation, my wife was given a memory test. This was a one-to-one experience with the nurse. I was not allowed into the test for fear of influencing her.

The consultant was excellent and proposed a change of drugs. My wife realised that he was nice and would help her. She was now making involuntary mouth movements. I was told that this could be a dentistry problem. I tried to arrange an appointment with a dentist who specialises in dementia. The GP practice could not help, so I went to my private dentist, who recommended one. This was a spectacular success as my wife enjoyed the experience!

She had a heavy fall in the bathroom at 3.00am one morning, I took her to A&E for a thorough check-over. This was not her first fall. I had dealt with previous falls myself as best as I could, but this was by far the most serious. The consultant called me in at 5.00am for a one-to-one, and I was told in no uncertain terms that

I needed help. He said he would write to my GP about my health. Whether he did, I don't know, as I did not hear anything.

I was frustrated and annoyed by the standard of care we both received. Our previous GP showed empathy and compassion, but the new NHS does not seem to deal in this.

I was advised to see our family solicitor to get our affairs in order. I took my wife and her son. The solicitor could see that the dementia had taken hold and advised me to seek a Court of Protection order. She recognised that time was important because of the illness's quick development. Nearly two months later, she phoned to say she had not received the signed paperwork, marked urgent (the CoP order) from our doctor. I was asked to go and try to hurry things up. At reception I was told, 'We are doctors, not form fillers'. To my surprise, I learned that our new doctor was part time and worked only two days a week. For the previous two weeks she had been on holiday and was away for the next week, so the form would not be signed until her return. I found this unacceptable and demanded to see the practice manager. I explained my frustration, and was told the practice only had part-time doctors, which included our GP. A next-day appointment was arranged with the duty doctor. I sat with her to help with the form filling.

I was unhappy with the NHS, and with the practice in particular. I composed a letter to our MP complaining about the state of the NHS in a small market town and how dementia patients and carers were not supported. The MP sent and received correspondence from the local community health council, but he deemed the reply unsatisfactory and redirected my initial letter to the Health Minister, who duly replied.

Learning point 1

Before you read any further, you may like to consider these questions. They are hard to answer, even to come to terms with, but nevertheless they all have to be taken into consideration because they are typical experiences for many single carers.

- Might it be possible to pinpoint a specific event that could mark the onset of dementia? Even if this is groundless, can you see how it might be actually helpful to you psychologically?

- Single carers are often looking after a loved one with whom they have an emotional relationship as well as complete responsibility for them. How can you reconcile this with adverse circumstances that may occur in other areas of your life (e.g. redundancy or bereavement), especially when help from outside agencies such as social services and the NHS is, in present circumstances, not always forthcoming?

- What other agencies besides the NHS and social services might offer help?

The memory clinic

The second meeting with the memory clinic was reassuring to both of us. They really supported us with a full diagnosis of her condition, which I photocopied and produced regularly when visiting hospital specialists. This made life so much easier. We were allocated a social worker, who was tolerant, helpful and put our fears to rest. She came to our home at regular intervals to talk through and review the situation. One of her recommendations was for us to employ an agency to provide activity. This was a godsend as it broke up my wife's day and provided stimulation. My wife enjoyed the variation in routine – they would look through old photo albums with her and talk about old times. This was wonderful. Old experiences and feelings were rekindled and the effect was profound, as my wife showed great pride in her life. The agency worker was an exceptional person. My wife realised she had a friend.

However, life at home was getting worse. She was now getting up four or five times each night. I always tried to get up with her and this led to my fatigue. My aim was to stop her coming to harm. She was tired and slept for hours during the day, while I attempted to stay awake and watch her at night. She was becoming irrational and I was increasingly tired and jaded. The memory clinic sent a nurse to spend an hour a week with her, to allow monitoring to take place. Trips out with the nurse were arranged and time was spent in coffee shops and ladies' fashion shops. This really was a godsend, because my wife had found another friend and I received sound advice about how to cope.

Then came another unexpected boost. In the middle of summer, I was cutting the back lawn when I was interrupted by the cleaner who worked for my neighbour, who was a casual friend to both of us. The cleaner enquired how my wife was and I explained the situation. She came round after finishing work. I never thought that this would be the start of a relationship that would see our lives change for the better. We had a great talk and a giggle over a cup of tea. My wife lightened up and joined in. It was refreshing for both of us. Our new friend said she would come back the next day, to have a girlie morning with my wife, while I went out for an hour or two. She made up my wife's face, manicured her nails, and they drank copious amounts of tea. When I returned, they were all grins and giggles. Her character, kindness and understanding lifted us both. No airs and graces – a real 'rough diamond'.

Learning point 2

- Peter Hemsley managed to get help from the memory clinic (part of the NHS) and a private agency. But the help offered by concerned friends was in the end the most decisive. Does this seem reasonable to you, or do you think carer-patient situations should remain private, confidential and entirely the carer's business?

- It is noteworthy that the memory clinic, the social worker sent by the agency and the cleaner from next door provided activities that activated memories, increased involvement and engendered intellectual and emotional activity that, until relatively recently, was not seen as possible for people living with dementia. In all cases, the effect on Peter Hemsley's wife was electrifying. How important do you feel such activities are?

- Who would you turn to for help in this? In fact, could *you* do it? Just remember that people living with dementia have the right to see themselves as the stars and centres of attention.

A realisation dawns

The mental health team was beginning to express concerns. I ignored them, feeling that most of the problems were figments of my imagination and the situation would improve. After a few months, while I was still in denial, I had a telephone call to say that two nurses were coming to see me and they would arrive in a few hours. It was obvious they were now serious, telling me to get things sorted. The words still ring in my ears: 'We have one patient now and the way you are behaving we shall have two.' I was told to go and visit three care homes and decide which would be suitable. They left quickly, with no niceties. I was shocked and tearful, as it appeared now there was only one outcome. I sought advice regarding the three homes I should consider. The residential home in my own town was not included, due to poor CQC ratings.

I made appointments to visit two sites, and duly went and had tours of inspection. The third offered a home visit and sent two agents. They parked their minibus right outside our bungalow, with the name of the home plastered all over it. My wife went to the window and asked who they were. They came in and they assessed her. She was twice asked if she would like to go on holiday with them. She said no both times. The third time was too much. She swore and told them to get out. I was surprised by this action, but I had a sense of pride that she made her feelings known forcibly. My own thoughts were by now completely scrambled.

The weekend that followed was the worst of my life. On Friday she went to bed at 9.00pm but was up at 10.15pm. She was wandering around, overbalanced and fell on the gas fire, smashing her head on it. I examined her and found a big bump developing on her forehead. The after-hours doctor would not arrive for at least six hours. I panicked and drove to A&E. Twelve hours later we left, with a walking frame. I had had no sleep and was struggling to keep awake.

The next night she got up while I was asleep. There was an almighty crash, and I found my wife lying on our glass-topped table with shattered display glasses all around. She could have severed her wrist. This convinced me that the time was up.

An amazing conclusion

On the Monday, I phoned around the three care homes to explain my problem. No one had a vacancy. Our friend came and I explained the situation to her. She told me in no uncertain terms to contact the local home, which I had been advised not to do because of its poor CQC rating. Our friend got really angry, stating that she would do it for me if I did not. I phoned the manager and told her of my plight, and she was sympathetic. She said she needed to make an assessment, so my heart sank. I told her that I lived in the same town, and she asked when I would like the care to start. I replied 'As soon as possible.' I was amazed that she came to the bungalow within an hour. The assessment was done, the manager went back to the home, and she phoned me within 20 minutes to ask me to bring my wife to the home.

I drove my wife to the home and parked outside. She would not get out of the car. 'This place is for silly people,' she said. No amount of enticement could persuade her. For more than an hour she refused to budge. I came back home to fetch one of her favourite toy dogs, in the hope that it might help her change her mind. But when I returned, she was walking in, pushing her frame, encouraged by our friend and the staff. I followed behind as she went into the day room, where five dolls were arranged on the settee. She was transfixed and could not keep her eyes off them. A doll was passed over to her and she sat embracing it for a long time.

This one small action seemed to end all the trauma. The dolls are the key to this story. She immediately took ownership of them and treated them like her own children, talking to them, cajoling them and chiding them. She cultivated an amazing friendship with them, and they sustained her during the transition. I was told not to see her for a few days but had to drop off some clothes the next day. The manager saw me and beckoned me over, and I looked through the window. My wife was sitting on front of a mirror, having her hair done and being pampered. But the marvellous thing was that she was smiling.

Things settled down, but for some time she was not sure of this new environment. She was grossly underweight and not at ease with her situation. I feared the worst as she became unresponsive and I thought she was losing the will to live and would only see out a matter of weeks. However, with the encouragement of all the staff, she began to eat more and gradually became more responsive. Nevertheless, I still felt that she would never accept her life there. A spell of six days in hospital with suspected sepsis saw her will to live bounce back. I feared for her return to the care home. I walked behind her while she was wheeled in. The staff came out to greet her. She smiled and smiled, and I knew then that the right decision had been made.

Conclusion

I cannot believe what has happened in these last three years. I battled long and hard for my wife, and at times became very frustrated and angry with the care she received. The NHS is overstretched, and the old and frail are cast aside due to cost and the inability of society to care. I have been exceptionally fortunate to come through this unscathed. We both have a better quality of life. I am 10 years younger than my wife, and I feel that I have the ability to fight her corner. I visit every day; she now has the best quality of life she can have. I have absolute trust in the home and its staff. They have given me my life back and I am determined to make the most of it. The care industry is under overwhelming pressure, but this residential home has defied all perceived logic and come up trumps for both of us.

Learning point 3

- Peter Hemsley's story ends happily, both for him and for his wife. He had been advised not to approach the care home in the same town because it had received adverse CQC reports. Was disregarding this advice a risky, even irresponsible thing to do, in view of the reports? Is taking a chance in such fraught situations justifiable?

- Peter's friend insisted his wife moving to the home was the best thing for her, and she was right. The proof of the pudding is in the eating, so is it reasonable always to accept official verdicts? Would you think to question the criteria by which such verdicts are arrived at? (It is noteworthy that the home in question has received another adverse report.)

Part two

Caring for people with dementia

7 Dementia and living at home: What can your general practitioner do for you?

Marieke Perry

As people grow older, they tend to become more forgetful. People react differently to these memory changes: some worry immediately, whereas others start denying these changes or argue that they are normal for their age. But are they normal? How does dementia actually differ from memory loss? These are questions that preoccupy not only people with memory complaints and their informal caregivers but also general practitioners (GPs). To them, dementia is a complex condition. It is a 'syndrome', based on clinical criteria (McKhann et al., 2011). This means that there is currently no single test that can tell whether a person has dementia or not; instead, the diagnosis is mainly based on a person's story.

The most important instrument for a doctor making a diagnosis is taking the patient's history, which will explore any changes in memory, other cognitive functions and their behaviour. A dementia diagnosis can be made when such changes are so severe that they start to influence a person's daily functioning. Because of GPs' gatekeeping role and longstanding relationships with both patients and carers, they are in an ideal position to observe and interpret those changes in cognition or function. However, GPs usually apply watchful waiting strategies, driven by barriers such as a lack of knowledge, lack of valid diagnostic instruments and fear of diagnostic disclosure (Foley et al., 2017). This leads to significant under-diagnosis of dementia of some 50% in many Western countries (Lang et al., 2017).

The complexity of dementia comes across not only in the diagnostic trajectory but also in post-diagnostic care. Once a dementia diagnosis is given, GPs generally feel there is not much that they can do, as there are no treatment options for dementia. They wonder how and if patients would benefit from available medication (Hansen et al., 2008). Moreover, the clinical picture of dementia is very heterogenous and it leads to a large variety of multiple memory and executive functions. Consequently, people with dementia and their informal caregivers have a similar variety of care needs. This often requires the involvement of multiple primary care professionals, and they often do not align their services. As a result, primary dementia care is often fragmented, which leads to poor quality of care and dissatisfaction among patients and informal caregivers. An example could be that professionals give contradicting advice to caregivers as to how to handle challenging behaviour. However, GPs can help to overcome these barriers, as the strong involvement of GPs in local professional networks seems to facilitate interprofessional collaboration and this improves the quality of dementia care (Richters et al., 2018).

When first consulting your GP

People with dementia lack insight into their condition. This is a symptom of the disease. Therefore, it may be difficult to convince them to consult their GP as they usually think there is nothing wrong with them. Moreover, it is understandable that people would want to avoid receiving a diagnosis as severe as dementia, as it has major consequences. On the other hand, it is important for everyone to know what causes the memory loss and behavioural changes. Reversible causes can be treated, and in the case of dementia, adequate care can be arranged. The following suggestions and strategies may help you to draw the GP's attention to your concerns regarding the 'symptoms' of your loved one. The strategy that you choose depends on your own preferences, and on what you think works best with your loved one.

- First, talk to the GP alone to express your worries. It may be difficult to discuss the symptoms of your loved one in full detail with them present without hurting his/her feelings. Sometimes GPs do not want to discuss your worries with you, because of privacy issues. You can overcome this barrier by saying that you do not expect any information from the GP concerning your loved one, and that you are just looking for advice as to how to handle the situation.

- If the GP agrees you may have reason for concern, try to convince your loved one to consult the GP – say it will reassure you, as you are worried about their health.

- Tell your loved one that any symptoms they are experiencing may be reversible, as they may be caused by vitamin deficiencies or a thyroid gland problem, for example. Also mention that a simple blood test administered by the GP may be needed to clarify this, so that they can start treatment if needed.

- Combine the GP consultation with a check-up for hypertension or diabetes. Ask for a double appointment and inform the GP in advance about your worries.

- Ask the GP or practice nurse to invite your loved one for a general geriatric screening. This kind of screening is becoming more and more common in primary care. This may help to reveal any cognitive problems.

- Many people with dementia want everything to stay as normal as possible, so that they can live independently in their own homes. They unconsciously think that denying the diagnosis is the best way to achieve that situation. Discuss with your loved one that the opposite is more likely to be true: with a clear diagnosis, adequate care can be arranged and problems can be anticipated, instead of letting the problems pile up so that they lead to a crisis.

Learning point 1

- Do not be afraid to consult your GP if you are concerned about your own or your loved-one's cognitive functioning. It is better to get a timely diagnosis and be prepared than to hide from the reality.

What information will your GP need to know?

As mentioned above, dementia is a clinical diagnosis. This means that a diagnosis is mainly based on a person's story and how he or she has changed over time. Therefore, it is very important to provide the GP with a number of examples of the changes. GPs can do a memory test to see whether this confirms the person's story. The memory test that is most commonly used worldwide is the Mini Mental State Examination (MMSE) (Folstein et al., 1975). However sometimes people get good scores on memory tests but fail terribly when you give them a complex task, such as going to the supermarket for grocery shopping. You can then ask for an MRI scan of the brain, which will show any damage to the brain, but it will not tell you how they are functioning. Moreover, when people become older, there is sometimes little difference between the brain of a healthy person and the brain of a person with dementia (Bloudek et al., 2011). Hence, a person's story provides the key information for a dementia diagnosis.

With the following questions, you can prepare your stories for your consultation with the GP. Try to capture what has changed in comparison with the situation one year ago. Try to clarify why these changes are disturbing and worrying to you:

- Give examples of your/your loved one's declining memory.
- Are you/is your loved one capable of joining a conversation?
- Do you/does your loved one constantly repeat yourself/himself?
- Are you/is your loved one capable of expressing yourself/themself and speaking clearly?
- Do you/does your loved one show strange behaviour (for example, putting money in the refrigerator)?
- Are holidays different from the way they used to be?
- Are you/is your loved one capable of performing ordinary daily tasks (for example, self-care, running a household, managing finances, medication management)?

- Do you/does your loved one get lost easily?
- Have you/has your loved one developed a different sleeping pattern?
- Does your/your loved one's personality seem to have changed?

For informal caregivers of people with cognitive problems, the IQCODE is a questionnaire that asks you to go back to the situation of your loved one 10 years ago and compare that with the situation of today. It addresses issues such as memory, complex daily tasks and learning new things. It can help to structure your thoughts and stories and identify what exactly has changed in your loved one's cognition and behaviour (Jorm, 1994).

Learning point 2

- The GP will base much of their diagnosis on your or your loved-one's behaviour and daily functioning and how it differs from previously. Go prepared to give this information.

How can medication for dementia help, if at all?

Unfortunately, there is no effective cure for dementia (Livingston et al., 2020). In many Western countries, drugs known as cholinesterase inhibitors are prescribed for people with Alzheimer's disease, Parkinson's disease or Lewy body dementia. They include rivastigmine, galantamine, donepezil and memantine. But these drugs are not effective with other types of dementia. It is widely thought that these drugs slow down disease progression, but in fact they simply temporarily decrease dementia symptoms. Effects that were found in clinical studies were small, and studies did not last longer than six months, so it is unclear whether it is wise to keep using the drugs after this period. Only a few people respond to these drugs. Unfortunately, it is not possible to predict who is going to be a responder. When the drugs were developed, the hypothesis was that the drugs were more effective if started earlier in the disease trajectory. Research has not confirmed this (Birks et al., 2015; Birks & Harvey, 2018; Matsunaga et al., 2015, 2016; McShane et al., 2019). Moreover, the drugs are very likely to cause side effects. People experience weight loss and gastro-intestinal complaints, such as diarrhoea and dyspepsia. In approximately one third of people taking them, the side effects are so severe that the person needs to stop (Ali et al., 2015).

Even though the effects of the drugs are limited, and in some cases the benefits do not outweigh the side effects, these drugs are regularly prescribed in memory clinics. The controversy around the medication can be seen very clearly in the Netherlands, where, based on the same evidence, the dementia guideline for GPs advises against the use of medication (NHG, 2020), whereas specialist guidelines recommend that drug treatment is included in individual care plans (NVKG,

2020). The advice you get on medication is likely to depend on who you ask. What or who should you believe? These conflicting recommendations at least show us that these drugs are definitely not miracle pills.

Because of the lack of effective medications, integrative complementary treatments such as ginkgo biloba, curcuma, vitamins, green tea, fish oil and coconut oil have been tried with people with memory complaints or dementia and their informal caregivers. None of these treatments has been found to prevent the development or progression of dementia (Burckhardt et al., 2016; Yang et al., 2014).

Learning point 3

- There is no medical cure for dementia. Some medications decrease the symptoms but only temporarily. Research has disproved much of the early optimism about these drugs delaying progression.

How can medication for other symptoms help, if at all?

Sadness, restlessness, anxiety and delusions are common 'symptoms' that negatively influence the quality of life of people with dementia and their informal caregivers. Therefore, their management is important, but it is complex. Often multidisciplinary professional expertise and support is needed (Zwijsen et al., 2014).

According to guidelines (NHG, 2020; NVKG, 2020), behavioural problems in dementia can be divided into five categories:

- psychotic behaviour (delusions and hallucinations)
- depressed behaviour (listlessness)
- anxious behaviour
- agitated behaviour (restlessness, listlessness, irritable, aggression), calling, nightly disturbance and sexual disinhibition
- apathetic behaviour (no initiative, inactive).

Before medication is introduced to attempt to decrease behavioural problems, it is important to look for factors that are causing these problems. Our behaviour is influenced by biological, psychological and social factors, and this is even more profound in people with dementia. This means that, in the case of behavioural problems, a person may be in pain or their attempts at communication are not understood; they may be feeling lonely, or they may be trying to do things they used to do (like go to work), for example. All of these underlying causes may respond better to a non-pharmacological treatment or approach.

Research showed that the effectiveness of pharmacological treatment in the case of behavioural problems is limited (Livingston et al., 2020). Side effects can be serious, as detailed below. Therefore, psychopharmaceuticals (medication that can influence a person's behaviour) should only be prescribed when all of the other treatment options have failed. When starting psychopharmaceuticals, it should always be the intention to use the drugs for a limited amount of time (Pan et al., 2014; Declercq et al., 2013). Three different types of psychopharmaceuticals can be considered to treat behavioural problems:

1. Tranquillisers or anxiolytic/antipsychotic medication – these drugs can be prescribed in the cases of aggression, agitation, anxiety and wandering (nightly disturbance). Side effects are often drowsiness and listlessness. When this medication is used on a long-term basis, the risk of cardiac diseases increases. Guidelines advise a gradual withdrawal attempt at least after three months. Only in exceptional cases, when withdrawal leads to a severe relapse of behavioural problems, should antipsychotic treatment be restarted. Long-term use of antipsychotic drugs is only advised when all other interventions and two withdrawal attempts have failed.

2. Antidepressants – these should only be prescribed in the case of severe depression, when all other interventions have failed. All antidepressants have their own typical side effects, which are usually present most profoundly during the first few weeks of use, and then slowly decrease. A noticeable change will only begin to emerge after a few weeks.

3. Hypnotics – adequate sleep is important to everyone. Nightly disturbance is not only a burden to the person living with dementia; it also affects their informal caregivers. Again, in this situation, it is important to try non-pharmacological interventions first before starting the use of sleeping pills. Sleeping pills can cause drowsiness during the day and consequently increase the risk of falls. After two weeks of use, people tend to get increasingly dependent on and addicted to sleeping pills. This means that they need to increase the dose to achieve the same effects. When they attempt to stop taking sleeping pills, they will experience withdrawal symptoms, which can be severe.

Side effects

Older people have increased chances of developing side effects when using drugs. When your loved one starts psychopharmaceuticals, it is advised that you help with monitoring effects and side effects. You know your loved one well, and you will be better able to spot any subtle changes in their behaviour or mood. You can help to determine whether the medication causes the desired effects or if the benefits outweigh the side effects. This information may also help the doctor select the right dosage for your loved one.

> **Learning point 4**
> - Drug treatments for other symptoms, such as insomnia, depression, agitation and restlessness, generally have significant side effects and do not address the causes of these behaviours. The more effective and less risky approach is to try to understand the causes of the behaviour. Some complementary therapies may be helpful.

Conclusion

Dementia diagnosis is complex as there is no single test available to establish the diagnosis. It differs from normal forgetfulness because it negatively influences daily functioning. The patient's history with regard to how the cognitive changes are affecting daily functioning is the most powerful test. The history can be supplemented with memory tests, blood tests and, in hospital, a scan of the brain. Some GPs diagnose dementia in primary care; others refer their patients with memory problems to memory clinics.

There is no medical treatment for dementia. Some medications may relieve symptoms for a while, but a cure does not exist. Drug treatment for challenging behaviour has also proved disappointing. However, non-medical approaches are often effective – in particular those that seek and find a likely cause for the behaviour and enable the person to be better understood. Integrated and well co-ordinated care is the most effective support for both the person with dementia and their families/carers and can enable people to live a good life longer with the disease.

References

Ali, T.B., Schleret, T.R., Reilly, B.M., Chen, W.Y. & Abagyan, R. (2015). Adverse effects of cholinesterase inhibitors in dementia, according to the pharmacovigilance databases of the United States and Canada. *Plos One, 10*(12), e0144337.

Birks, J.S., Chong, L.Y. & Evans, J.G. (2015). Rivastigmine for Alzheimer's disease. *Cochrane Database of Systematic Reviews, 9*(9), CD001191.

Birks, J.S. & Harvey, R.J. (2018). Donepezil for dementia due to Alzheimer's disease. *Cochrane Database of Systematic Reviews, 6*(6):CD001190.

Bloudek, L.M., Spackman, D.E., Blankenburg, M. & Sullivan, S.D. (2011). Review and meta-analysis of biomarkers and diagnostic imaging in Alzheimer's disease. *Journal of Alzheimer's Disease, 26*(4), 627–645.

Burckhardt, M., Herke, M., Wustmann, T., Watzke, S., Langer, G. & Fink, A. (2016). Omega-3 fatty acids for the treatment of dementia. *Cochrane Database of Systematic Reviews, 4*(4), CD009002.

Declercq, T., Petrovic, M., Azermai, M., Vander Stichele, R., De Sutter A.M., van Driel, M.L. & Christiaens, T. (2013). Withdrawal versus continuation of chronic antipsychotic drugs for behavioural and psychological symptoms in older people with dementia. *Cochrane Database of Systematic Reviews, 3*(3), CD007726.

Foley, T., Boyle, S., Jennings, A. & Smithson, W.H. (2017). 'We're certainly not in our comfort zone': A qualitative study of GPs' dementia-care educational needs. *BMC Primary Care, 66.*

Folstein, M.F., Folstein, S.E. & McHugh, P.R. (1975). 'Mini-mental state': A practical method for grading the cognitive state of patients for the clinician. *Journal of Psychiatric Research, 12*(3), 189–198.

Hansen, E.C., Hughes, C., Routley, G. & Robinson, A.L. (2008). General practitioners' experiences and understandings of diagnosing dementia: Factors impacting on early diagnosis. *Social Science and Medicine, 67*(11), 1776–1783.

Jorm, A.F. (1994). A short form of the Informant Questionnaire on Cognitive Decline in the Elderly (IQCODE): Development and cross-validation. *Psychological Medicine, 24*(1), 145–153.

Lang, L., Clifford, A., Wei, L., Zhang, D., Leung, D., Augustine, G., Danat, I., Zhou, W., Copeland, J., Anstey, K. & Chen, R. (2017). Prevalence and determinants of undetected dementia in the community: A systematic literature review and a meta-analysis. *BMJ Open, 7*(2): e011146.

Livingston, G., Huntley, J., Sommerlad, A., Ames, D., Ballard, C., Banerjee, S., Brayne, C., Burns, A., Cohen-Mansfield, J., Cooper, C., Costafreda, S.G., Dias, A., Fox, N., Gitlin, L.N., Howard, R., Kales, H.C., Kivimäki, M., Larson, E.B., Ogunniyi, A., Orgeta, V., Ritchie, K., Rockwood, K., Sampson, E.L… & Mukadam N. (2020). Dementia prevention, intervention, and care: Report of the Lancet Commission. *The Lancet, 396*(10248), 413–446.

Matsunaga, S., Kishi, T. & Iwata, N. (2015). Memantine for Lewy Body disorders: Systematic review and meta-analysis. *American Journal of Geriaric Psychiatry, 23*(4), 373–383.

Matsunaga, S., Kishi, T., Yasue, I. & Iwata, N. (2016). Cholinesterase inhibitors for Lewy Body disorders: A meta-analysis. *Interntional Journal of Neuropsychopharmacology, 19*(2).

McKhann, G.M., Knopman, D.S., Chertkow, H., Hyman, B.T., Jack, C.R. Jr., Kawas, C.H., Klunk, W.E., Koroshetz, W.J., Manly, J.J., Mayeux, R., Mohs, R.C., Morris, J.C., Rossor, M.N., Scheltens, P., Carrillo, M.C., Thies, B., Weintraub, S. & Phelps, C.H. (2011). The diagnosis of dementia due to Alzheimer's disease: Recommendations from the National Institute on Aging- Alzheimer's Association workgroups on diagnostic guidelines for Alzheimer's disease. *Alzheimers & Dementia, 7*(3), 263–269.

McShane, R., Westby, M.J., Roberts, E., Minakaran, N., Schneider, L., Farrimond, L.E., Maayan, N., Ware J. & Debarros, J. (2019). Memantine for dementia. *Cochrane Database of Systematic Reviews, 3*(3), CD003154.

NHG. (2020). *Standaard dementie.* Utrecht: Nederlands Huisartsengenootschap.

NVKG. (2020). *Richtlijn diagnostiek en behandeling van dementie.* Nederlandse Vereniging voor Klinische Geriatrie.

Pan, Y.J., Wu, C.S., Gau, S.S.F., Chan, H.Y. & Banerjee, S. (2014). Antipsychotic discontinuation in patients with dementia: A systematic review and meta-analysis of published randomized controlled studies. *Dementia and Geriatric Cognitive Disorders, 37*(3–4), 125–140.

Richters, A., Nieuwboer, M.S., Rikkert, M.G.M.O., Melis, R.J.F., Perry, M. & van der Marck, M.A. (2018). Longitudinal multiple case study on effectiveness of network-based dementia care towards more integration, quality of care, and collaboration in primary care. *Plos One, 13*(6).

Yang, M.M., Xu, D.D., Zhang, Y., Liu, X.Y., Hoeven, R. & Cho, W.C.S. (2014). A systematic review on natural medicines for the prevention and treatment of Alzheimer's disease with meta-analyses of intervention effect of ginkgo. *American Journal of Chinese Medicine, 42*(3), 505–521.

Zwijsen, S.A., Smalbrugge, M., Eefsting, J.A., Twisk, J.W.R., Gerritsen, D.L., Pot, A.M. & Hertogh, C.M.P.M. (2014). Coming to grips with challenging behavior: A cluster randomized controlled trial on the effects of a multidisciplinary care program for challenging behavior in dementia. Journal of the American Medical Directors Association, 15(7), 531.e1-531.e10.

8   Providing person-centred spiritual care for people living with dementia

Kathy Fogg Berry

This chapter will first delineate why spiritual care is an essential part of holistically caring for people living with dementia. It will explore the differences between spirituality and religion and the importance of nurturing the spirit through spiritual and spiritually religious practices. An assessment tool is introduced to assist with discerning a person's spiritual and/or religious needs. Then attention is given to presenting creative ideas and effective ways in which person-centred spiritual care can be provided for people in various stages of dementia. Family and professional caregivers, as well as communities of faith, are encouraged to apply these ideas as they seek to care for people with dementia.

For the past 22 years, I've been a spiritual care provider/chaplain with people experiencing dementia and their caregivers in hospital, hospice and long-term elder-care settings, including the past 12 years at Westminster Canterbury Richmond in Richmond, Virginia, USA – a 960-bed continuing care retirement community. This chapter is based on my experiences in those settings, where, after discerning residents' spiritual needs, I used a variety of approaches and practices. These included music, art, prayer, worship, meditation, nature walks and service projects to enhance each resident's spiritual wellbeing and provide holistic care. A primary goal was encouraging residents to use their spiritual strengths to help them face the challenges of dementia, such as short-term memory loss.

Why is spiritual care an essential aspect of caring for people with dementia?

Although statistics vary from country to country, a significant percentage of elders say religion is important to them (Pew Research Center, 2018). In the US, more than 70% of people aged 75 and older consider their faith to be important and almost 80% say they attend religious services/activities regularly (Pew

Research Center, 2014, 2015). Given that a third of people aged 85 years and older have Alzheimer's disease and nearly half have some other form of dementia (Alzheimer's Association, 2020), these figures suggest that the majority of people experiencing dementia are likely also to be spiritually religious. Unfortunately, as their dementia progresses, they become increasingly unable to participate in religious organisations or initiate faith practices that comfort, connect and uplift them. Thus, family and professional caregivers and others need to assist people experiencing dementia in practising their faith and nurturing needed connections to enhance their overall wellbeing.

Providing holistic care for people living with dementia and their caregivers requires more than addressing their physical, psychological, emotional and social needs, which are normally the main focus. We are all spiritual beings. Each of us has a soul, an essence that longs for meaning, love and connection throughout life.

Learning point 1

- 'The key point is this: the neurology of dementia doesn't destroy the self.' (Swinton, 2012, p.59)

When grappling with spirituality and striving to answer life's existential questions – who am I, why am I here, what does my life mean, does some higher power exist? – many people connect with a particular religion or faith expression. They may join with others of like-minded belief to follow a particular faith tradition – Judaism, Christianity, Islam, Hinduism, Buddhism, or one of many others. Some people are born into a family system that professes and practises a particular faith tradition. As they age, they may remain within their family's faith tradition or, through self-searching and spiritual questioning, change to embrace a new faith or non-religious spiritual expression. Some people never resonate with a particular faith group or belief in a divine being but continue to express their spirituality in non-religious ways, such as reverencing nature or practising various meditative styles. Regardless of whether we are spiritual or spiritually religious, our inner being needs nurturing to maintain holistic health and wellbeing.

Life is not what we 'have' or even what we do, connected as these may be; we are what and how and who we are, and be-ing is a real activity. Like 'love', spirituality is a way that we 'be'. The way of be-ing defies definition and delineation; we cannot tie it up or in any way package or enclose it. Elusive in the sense that it cannot be pinned down, spirituality slips under and soars above efforts to capture it, to fence it in with words. Centuries of thought confirm that mere words can never induce the experience of spirituality (Kurtz & Ketcham, 2002, pp.15–16).

People sometimes hesitate to talk about spirituality because it is so personal and hard to articulate. When we take time to truly listen to and accept one another for who we are, we can build trusting relationships as we begin to see, understand and accept each other's essence/spirit. People experiencing dementia, and all of us, have the spiritual need for unconditional love, reassurance, support, encouragement, trust, acceptance, inclusion and hope.

Discerning spiritual needs

When a person first visits a physician's office, a nurse soon arrives with a set of questions and does a physical assessment. The nurse seeks to discover why the patient requires treatment and what may be contributing to the problem. Similarly, a visit to a psychiatrist, psychologist or social worker necessitates a psychological assessment to discern what's going on psychologically/emotionally. Both physical and psychological assessments usually involve finding out about a person's family background with regard to physical and psychological health. These assessments enable the care provider to offer person-centred care to meet the specific needs of each person. A spiritual assessment seeks the same goal.

Learning point 2

- Along with physical and psycho-social assessments, a spiritual assessment is needed for people experiencing dementia to ensure holistic care is provided. These assessments can benefit caregivers and, in fact, each of us.

- The box below outlines a spiritual assessment tool to aid this process.

Spiritual assessment tool
- What gives you hope, purpose, peace, joy?
- Where nurtures your spirit?
- Where/when do you feel the closest to God?*
    - Examples include with family and friends or your faith community, in nature, listening to or playing music, observing or creating artwork, visiting with or caring for pets, acts of service for other people…
- What spiritual/religious practices or symbols bring you comfort and/or help you feel closest to God?
    - Examples include meditation, prayer, being in nature, movement, a worship experience, reading sacred scripture, praying, being in a worship centre, hearing or making music, enjoying artwork, seeing religious icons, a menorah, hearing Buddhist chimes, smelling incense…

*Whether someone adheres to a particular faith tradition usually surfaces in response to the first question. Successive questions can then reflect that information.

If possible, conduct a spiritual assessment through conversation as a relationship evolves. If you arrive with a clipboard or computer screen full of questions, it may be daunting for someone experiencing dementia who is having increased difficulty articulating herself. People sometimes hesitate to share deep aspects of themselves unless they trust the 'interviewer'. Each person is different with regard to their comfort levels and ability to share personal information.

Sometimes sharing from your own experience first can help others feel comfortable sharing. For example, I might say: 'When I'm feeling stressed or overwhelmed by life, I need to get outside. Walking in the woods, planting and caring for flowers or watching a beautiful sunrise gives me hope for a new day with new possibilities. How about you? What brings you comfort and hope?'

In the early stages of dementia, most people should be able to articulate their thoughts, if allowed enough time. If someone has progressed in their dementia disease process beyond the ability to process or articulate responses, talking with their caregivers can provide answers. Caregivers can also benefit from spiritual assessment of their needs and benefit from addressing them. Tapping into their spiritual and/or religious traditions can help them cope with the burdens of caregiving.

Once the spiritual assessment is complete, you will know how to provide effective person-centred care. This completed tool can then guide you in providing spiritual care throughout the course of the person's life. When the person can no longer articulate what they need, you will know what and how to continue to offer spiritual care that is valuable to them.

Learning point 3

- Providing person-centred spiritual care is essential because dementia affects each person differently and each person has unique spiritual needs and life situations.

Providing spiritual care through different stages of dementia

Each person experiences dementia differently and no one's dementia progresses in the same way or to the same time schedule. There are, however, commonalities that demarcate stages of dementia for explanation – early, middle and late. The following ideas for providing spiritual care can be achieved at home between caregiver and loved one, in a faith community or in an institutional care residence.

Spiritual care in the early stages

As people begin experiencing memory loss and other aspects of dementia in their lives, a variety of feelings, emotions and spiritual needs emerges. Some people are able to take it in their stride, saying things like, 'Oh well, it is what it is.' But most people experience a range of what may be quite disabling emotions and feelings, such as fear, confusion, frustration, anger, anxiety and depression. These emotions understandably surface as people start to forget things they always knew, miss appointments, find they cannot complete familiar tasks, have difficulty expressing themselves, repeat questions or stories and experience other challenges signifying mental changes.

Having someone who will listen non-judgementally and in confidence to their concerns is essential. Being a compassionate listener is one of the greatest gifts we can give. They, and their caregivers, need people who will walk beside them during often scary and overwhelming times. Keeping in mind the emotions, feelings and spiritual needs of people experiencing dementia enables us to respond compassionately as we foster or build relationships with them. As they feel our care and concern, staying engaged and involved in life may become easier and the temptation to withdraw and self-isolate may lessen.

With the spiritual information you glean over time, you'll be able to encourage and assist the person living with dementia to continue to practise their faith and nurture their spirit. This will bring them added strength and skills to cope with the life changes they're facing.

Other ways of providing spiritual care in the early stages include:

- providing frequent presence and conversation
- spiritual reminiscence – encouraging them to share their spiritual or religious background and development. Ask them to reflect on how their spirituality/faith helped them cope with past challenges, and how it could help them now
- providing them with uplifting devotional literature
- individually and collectively assisting them in doing purposeful activities that bring fulfilment and joy
- helping them stay engaged with religious services/activities and social activities that provide purpose, encouragement, comfort and peace.

Agnes loved working with her hands and doing things for other people. She was an avid knitter, but since the onset of dementia had not made anything for herself or others. She seemed sad and directionless. Agnes could no longer initiate doing the things she enjoyed. She couldn't figure out what supplies she needed in order to knit or where to get them. When someone helped her get the equipment and wools she needed and gently guided her in starting the process, Agnes' memories kicked in, and she was able to knit dozens of baby caps for a local hospital. Her joy and sense of accomplishment shone out from her.

Spiritual care in the middle stages

While continuing to provide the spiritual support started in the early stages, add some further offerings. People in the middle stages of dementia may need increased guidance and direction. As language and memory become more compromised, confusion and anxiety levels may heighten. Once familiar people and activities may become unknowns. Patient, respectful care nurtures and calms the spirit:

- Visit frequently to build up trust and familiarity.
- Offer familiar spiritual/religious services and provide familiar religious symbols to prompt memories and provide comfort.
- Be a calming presence as a favourite activity is enjoyed.
- Provide narrative rather than dialogical conversation – since the person's language skills are becoming more compromised, plan activities where you carry the conversation and don't lean heavily on question-and-answer expectations.
- Appeal to the senses to prompt memories:
  - music – almost everyone enjoys some form of music, and most religious traditions contain musical expression
  - touch – stuffed animals, sand, shells, flowers, hand tools, fabric…
  - visuals – picture books, calendars, computer generated scenery, strolls outside, drawing, painting
  - aromas – cinnamon, cloves, citrus, nutmeg, anise, lavender. As they smell each scent, ask if it prompts a memory, or suggest one
  - food – challah bread might remind someone of Jewish faith of a Seder, decorated sugar cookies might recall Christmas, oranges prompt memories of a fun trip to Florida…
- invite faith representatives to celebrate their religious holy days and ceremonies. Plan solstice celebrations and other significant calendar events in alternative belief systems.

Jim had trouble sitting still. A 70-year-old man with Alzheimer's disease, he often anxiously paced the house as if looking for something. Each day at 3.00pm, his wife, Alice, prepared a plate of his favourite cookies and a glass of milk. Together, they'd sit down to enjoy the treat, then Alice would open the family's Bible and read a familiar scripture. Often Jim, who was no longer speaking in complete sentences, recited the scripture with her. Alice then sang a few of the songs they knew from the church they'd grown up in. Jim remained in his chair, singing along. After reciting The Lord's Prayer together, Alice would kiss Jim's cheek and remind him of God's love.

He might soon be up pacing again, but this daily ritual nurtured both of their spirits. It connected them to one another and to the God they worshipped. For several years, they'd been unable to attend church because of Jim's pacing and sometimes impulsive shouting out. They both missed their community of faith where Jim used to sing in the choir and Alice taught the children. But tapping into their faith at home brought moments of joy and much-needed connection.

> **Learning point 4**
>
> - Tapping into the senses ignites memories and enhances spiritual experiences: holding a rosary, singing a hymn, blowing a shofar, burning some incense, lighting a candle:
>
>   People may not be able to access certain memories via the normal processes. It may be that music, art, prayer, and so forth act as keys which allow aspects of the memory to be unlocked and accessed even if that access is only temporary and sporadic... when a person is caught up in a familiar prayer or hymn, or when they simply clap their hands to the rhythm of a song, they may well be remembering, cognitively or bodily, experiences they have had with God – or they may be having an experience with God at that very moment. (Swinton, 2012, p.251)

Spiritual care in the late stages

A person in the late stages of dementia may be barely communicative, non-ambulatory, in need of total care and transitioning toward death. Communication requires attention to mostly non-verbal cues and expressions. Making connection is still possible through careful attention and calming presence. At this stage you will need to apply the person-centred spiritual assessment information you gathered earlier in the person's life to help you know what is most important to them. Continue to value the person for who they are, not what they can do.

Dr Sultan Lakhani, a geriatric psychiatrist in Richmond, Virginia, is a life-long Shia Muslim. He says:

> Muslims learn prayers when they are very young, and they are not forgotten by most people, even in the end stages of dementia. The prayers, which come from the Quran, keep them calmer. (Personal communication)

He adds that hearing the Quran read and prayers recited may spur the memory of a Muslim living with dementia and enable him to practise his faith (Biggar et al., 2019, pp.114–115).

Other suggestions include:

- Provide a calming, listening presence – words aren't necessary. Become comfortable in the silence, listening to the rhythm of their breathing and focused on their spirit.
- Provide gentle touch on the hand or arm, if it is comforting to the person.
- Offer experiences that appeal to the senses:

- · soft fabric touching the skin
- · lavender scent in a diffuser
- · sounds of waves lapping
- · the taste of their favourite treat
- · nature scenes or family photos positioned in their line of vision
- · quiet, familiar music playing.
- Read sacred scriptures or prayers from prayer books. Play chants or meditative suggestions.
- Offer verbal blessings and words of thanks for their life. Honour them.

Spiritual care and faith community

Faith communities can play a vital role in the spiritual care of people living with dementia and their caregivers. As statistics have shown, the majority of elders are connected to a congregation and their faith is important to them. The need for understanding, acceptance, encouragement and inclusion within their faith community is crucial and too often overlooked. Thankfully, this is changing as more faith communities are working hard to become dementia-friendly congregations.

Some ways to reach out include:[1]

- Educate your faith community about dementia and how it affects people's lives. Focus on communication, acceptance and unconditional love.
- Pay close attention to congregants so no one slips through the cracks. When caregivers and their loved ones experiencing dementia feel they can no longer attend services, they are too often forgotten.
- Create a safe and friendly environment. Seek advice from local Alzheimer's and dementia care organisations to educate the congregation on safety measures to take and ways to be encouraging, caring and inclusive.
- Collect and lend medical equipment and resources.
- Get involved in finding a cure:
  - · join a walk to end dementia
  - · encourage people to join clinical studies then support them as they go through the process.
- Form volunteer teams to assist caregivers with needed tasks. gardening, grocery shopping, lifts to medical appointments, friendly home visits and so forth.

---

1. These ideas for spiritual care throughout the different stages of dementia and faith community involvement come from the book *When Words Fail* (Berry, 2018). You can find many more ideas on providing spiritual care and demonstration videos at www.whenwordsfail.com

- Encourage and assist families to obtain help with legal planning.
- Open your church to support groups for people living with dementia and their caregivers. Start a support group or attend a support group with a friend you're supporting.
- Start a dementia-friendly choir, band, acting troupe, movement or art class for congregation and community members experiencing dementia.
- Invite affected families to participate in congregational life.
- Decide how to serve, then organise the effort.
- Pray… act.

Conclusion

Each person is a precious gift. Cognitive impairment presents many challenges but doesn't negate a person's value and worth. As we acknowledge each person's essence and provide compassionate spiritual care, we strengthen the essential bonds of humanity and create a better world.

References

Alzheimer's Association. (2020). 2020 Alzheimer's disease facts and figures. *Alzheimer's and Dementia 16*(3), 391–460.

Berry, K. (2018). *When words fail: Practical ministry to people with dementia and their caregivers.* Kregel Publications.

Biggar, V., Everman, L. & Glazer, S.M. (2019). *Dementia-friendly worship: A multifaith handbook for chaplains, clergy, and faith communities.* Jessica Kingsley Publishers.

Kurtz, E. & Ketcham, K. (2002). *The spirituality of imperfection: Storytelling and the search for meaning.* Bantam Books.

Pew Research Center. (2014). *Religious landscape study: Age distribution.* Pew Research Center. www.pewresearch.org/religion/religious-landscape-study/age-distribution/

Pew Research Center. (2015, January 22). *Importance of religion in one's life among evangelical churches.* Pew Research Center. www.pewforum.org/religious-landscape- study/importance-of-religion-in-ones-life

Pew Research Center. (2018). *The age gap in religions around the world.* Pew Research Center. www.pewresearch.org/religion/2018/06/13/the-age-gap-in-religion-around-the-world/

Swinton, J. (2012). *Dementia: Living in the memories of God.* Eerdmans.

9 Early onset dementia

Anthea Innes, John O'Doherty and Helen Rochford-Brennan

In the UK, around 42,000 people living with dementia (that is, some 5%) are diagnosed at a younger age (under 65) and therefore receive the diagnosis of what has been termed 'early onset', 'young onset' or 'working life' dementia (Alzheimer's Society, 2014). If you develop dementia while still working and have school-age or dependent children, the impact can be very different than if you are diagnosed with dementia after you have retired (Rabanal et al., 2018). So too can be the ripple effects on relationships with a spouse or partner and other family members and friends. There are now a growing number of personal accounts written by younger people living with dementia that document their struggles and successes in learning to live with the symptoms and challenges dementia brings, the reactions of others and the value of supportive relationships. The books by Keith Oliver (2019) Christine Bryden (2018) and Kate Swaffer (2016) may all provide insights and, most importantly, hope – not just for the person diagnosed with young onset dementia but for their family members too.

Learning point 1

- Consider the world you might inhabit as a 55-year-old, approaching retirement perhaps, but most likely still working, having achieved a career goal, maybe still providing support and care to older and/or younger relatives. You notice something is impacting on your cognitive abilities and you go to the GP. After investigations you are told you have dementia. What might this mean for your day-to-day life?

In this chapter we consider the impact of receiving a diagnosis of young onset dementia. John and Helen share some of their experiences of the impact of receiving a diagnosis of dementia at a younger age. John lives in an urban area in the north-west of England and was diagnosed with dementia at age 56. Helen lives in a small rural town in the west of the Republic of Ireland and was diagnosed at age 57.

Work experiences

Employers may not be equipped to support someone who receives a diagnosis of dementia – for example, you may have to learn how to ensure your employer makes what are known as 'reasonable adjustments' (see Chapter 21). If you are self-employed, the challenges may be far greater, as there is a lack of organisational support, and the buck stops with the self-employed individual.

Helen and John's experiences (described below) demonstrate that, despite holding valued roles, they were unable to continue working. Both took early retirement due to the perceived lack of support and understanding from colleagues and employers. Their working lives changed dramatically, leading to feelings of inadequacy and fear of judgement from others. The fact that they stopped working had an impact on the structure of their day-to-day lives, their families' financial position and their sense of self.

Helen's experience

I wanted to continue to work as I loved my job fighting for the rights of people with limited mobility. I had a great team. I also needed to work, as my husband had to retire early, so my financial income was important. I was having difficulty remembering meetings and was stopping mid-sentence, wondering what I was about to say. I never seemed to get my in-tray emptied, and this was causing me great anxiety.

I was very aware of employee rights, but I was too embarrassed to tell anyone about my problem. I chose early retirement, which looking back on it was wrong. How I wish I had asked for support or a less demanding role. For me, work kept me active, and it was good for me emotionally. I had seen clinicians prior to my decision, as I had a head injury and was informed I might have Alzheimer's. I was afraid to mention this to my employer or colleagues, due to the stigma, which I was very aware of. I could have asked for reasonable adjustments, as this was my right. I did not want to be dismissed and I was full of fear that this would happen.

I chose early retirement as I felt I was not doing my job to my full potential. I missed my colleagues and the disability platforms I worked on; it was such a lonely time. The loss of income was a great challenge.

Today I encourage others to talk to their employer as they may be able to offer support to enable them to carry on working for as long as they can.

I am still in touch with some of my colleagues. We meet for lunch and chat often. It's so rewarding to reminisce, and it was a great support during lockdown.

John's experience

Throughout my working life, I was employed in the public sector, latterly in a senior role for a local authority. For a number of years, I performed my role to a high standard, collectively with colleagues. I was responsible for sums in excess of £90 million, therefore I had to work effectively and with great precision. Such was my responsibility that, if I made mistakes, it would impact on the revenues of the authority and it would influence the amount of money attributed by central government, which in turn would affect the amount the local population would have to pay in council tax.

Within my working environment, I enjoyed a good relationship with colleagues. My advice was regularly sought and considered both factual and informative. I was known to be affable, with a keen sense of humour, and could be relied upon to be caring and sensitive to colleagues who, for a variety of reasons, might not be working to their normal effectiveness.

Progressively, I found myself to be less effective in my role. I was working to a slower pace and found myself making significant mistakes. For example, on one occasion I created a cheque to be paid from 7th January 1959, this date being my birthday. Fortunately, because of the huge amount on the cheque, it was not issued.

Increasingly I was making more and more mistakes; I could not remember how to perform simple actions, and my advice was considered to be ineffective and unreliable. Progressively, I became the person asking questions, as opposed to the person answering them.

My personality began to change. I was becoming increasingly agitated and morose. I would easily lose my temper with colleagues, to the extent that people began to avoid me at all costs. Invitations to functions were no longer extended to me.

Such was the deterioration in my relationship with colleagues that I was invited to attend meetings about my performance and attitude with senior management. Indeed, I was demoted twice, and was now principally dealing with post and scanning documents – a role that I still found to be increasingly problematic.

During this time, I was becoming more and more depressed. My memory was getting worse and I could no longer even remember the names of people I had worked with for more than 15 years. Even the process of writing letters was problematic. I was getting information wrong – for example, sending letters to incorrect addresses. I was unable to perform the simplest of tasks.

I was by now having regular consultations with my doctor and, after a period of time, was eventually diagnosed with vascular dementia. This to me was like an awakening. I knew now why the difficulties I was experiencing in work were happening. As a result of this diagnosis, I came to the realisation that I could no longer work effectively. Regretfully, and with great reluctance and sadness, I made the decision to take retirement on grounds of ill health. While my employer did everything they could to support me and stay within the requirements of the Disability Discrimination Act, I had already been reduced twice in my employment status. My role at this stage involved photocopying documents, opening the post and mailing letters. I began to experience difficulties with even these tasks, and the fact was, there was no other role I could perform in any department.

In fairness to my former employer, I must express gratitude for the support that they did offer me, but the reality was they had exhausted all means available to provide me with further support.

Family experiences

Receiving a diagnosis of any long-term condition that has implications for the way you live your life is a lot to take in and deal with, both for the person diagnosed and for close family members (Svanberg et al., 2011). John and Helen's experiences of how different family members reacted to their diagnosis demonstrates the shock, fear and general unpreparedness of families to adapt to the person having dementia and the process of learning and change required for all concerned.

Everyone reacts differently to dementia, but the person who receives a diagnosis perhaps needs their friends and family even more after they are first diagnosed and as symptoms emerge that are difficult for both the person living with dementia and their family members to come to terms with and adapt to. Navigating the support and services that may be available to them is not always easy (Millenaar et al., 2016).

John's experience

Since my diagnosis of dementia, my relationship with family members has deteriorated greatly. I have become increasingly isolated. I find it difficult to communicate and play with my grandchildren. Prior to my diagnosis, I babysat my grandchildren. Now I am no longer trusted with this responsibility. I no longer have the patience to look after them and, sadly, I have been told by members of my family I cannot be relied on to look after them safely. It is a painful fact that I agree with them.

I rarely leave my home and therefore visits to my family are essentially non-existent. My family now rarely visit, and I have come to terms with the fact that when they do, it is to see my wife and not me.

Christmas is now no longer something I look forward to. I am unable to cope with what is a large number of children being excited about playing with their presents; I have to leave the room and go upstairs. This has caused a number of arguments between me and my sons. I have tried to explain my dementia and how it affects me and the limitations it presents, but my sons and their partners cannot understand that I cannot help who I have become and that I cannot help the way dementia has affected me.

Helen's experience

When I was diagnosed, it took a long time to tell all my family (I am one of nine). Telling my family was so overwhelming: some cried, others, in true Irish fashion, joked and said I always had a problem, and some did not believe me. It was the beginning of lots of different emotions. We experienced lots of frustration, anger and fear for the future.

My husband and son were heartbroken. They were so sad for a life we would never have. They went into carer mode, which was the last thing I needed. Very soon, they realised I needed support to carry on with my life and encouragement to get out and about and stay the person I was before my diagnosis. I was still the same Helen, but I needed not just their love and support but also support from the rest of my family.

Speaking to all my family was so important because we have all adjusted to my brain disorder. We have lots of WhatsApp meetups, which are full of fun. I need lots of laughter. The illness does not define me.

Learning point 2

- What support do you think family members need to enable them to support the person living with dementia? What do you think is needed to enable a greater understanding of dementia to underpin future family relationships?

Other health issues

Dementia does not occur in a vacuum and is often accompanied by other health conditions or care responsibilities, as John and Helen's experiences demonstrate.

Helen had to learn to live with dementia while providing and receiving support from her husband, Sean, who had his own long-term chronic health conditions (and is now deceased).

John has had not only dementia to deal with but also cancer.

Helen's experience

Sean was diagnosed many years ago with heart failure, COPD and diabetes. My life has always been about trying to support Sean, as he supported me with my short-term memory. We were there for one another.

During Covid lockdowns in Ireland, we faced many challenges – mainly with getting homecare support. I kept forgetting to give Sean his medicines and this became a health issue. It also impacted on my anxiety, as I lay awake at night feeling guilty when I realised I forgot, and got up in the middle of the night to give him his medications when I did remember. Then we were both awake, and I knew how much Sean needed his sleep. We eventually got some extra help.

In late 2020, I supported Sean by sitting with him every day for the 12 weeks of treatment for cancer, until he passed away, 65 miles from home. It was a joy to be with him as he had been supporting me for so long. There was no support for me during this time. I tried to carry on with some advocacy and attend my working group meetings to help me through this difficult time.

Chronic illnesses have a major impact on our lives. They can limit lifestyle. I also have heart stents. I would love to participate more in outdoor pursuits but that is no longer possible.

John's experience

Initially I experienced a reluctance of health professionals to tell me anything about their concerns before my cancer was diagnosed. The GP, consultant urologist and Macmillan nurse all directed their concerns and then explanations to my wife, rather than me.

I was told many times about the procedures I would undergo, but I could neither absorb nor compute the explanation, because of my dementia. This meant that the time before the procedure was spent in a state of worry, concern and projection as to how the treatment would affect me.

I was alone in the treatment room, and I found the experience extremely frightening, to the extent that I kept pressing the panic button.

I eventually completed my treatment and was in a state of euphoria as I thought my cancer was now gone. It was later explained to me that the treatment did not cure my cancer, merely slowed it down. No matter how many times this is explained to me, I do not understand it. I see an oncologist to have regular tests to determine my cancer progression. I know I have cancer but still cannot understand the way it will affect me as it progresses.

I now live my life in a state of worry. The reality of my life is that I can be in a room full of people and still feel like the loneliest man in the world.

Support from the wider community

The support of wider community members can be crucial to the positive, or otherwise, experiences of adapting to life with dementia.

Dementia-friendly community policies (e.g. Department of Health, 2012, 2015) provide the structure and directives for including people living with dementia in social life. But how this can be implemented remains an active challenge (Local Government Association, 2015). Yet people living with dementia have much to offer, as Helen and John illustrate. Both John and Helen are advocates for others living with dementia. John has worked with the Alzheimer's Society's 3 Nations Dementia Working Group in the UK,[1] Helen with the Alzheimer Society of Ireland Irish Dementia Working Group[2] and the Alzheimer Europe European Working Group of People with Dementia.[3] Their dedication and passion for supporting others (established in their working lives and their roles in their communities and families) remains strong and true. They have battled with the adversity dementia has brought and provide powerful reminders of the contribution people living with dementia can make to others living with dementia.

John's experience

My only friends now are those who I would describe as members of the dementia community. Prior to my diagnosis, I had a wide circle of friends. I immersed myself in community activities, performing a range of voluntarily work. I had a strong reputation and was considered highly reliable. At the point of my diagnosis, things changed rapidly.

I became unreliable and my personality began to change. I no longer had patience

---

1. https://www.alzheimers.org.uk/get-involved/engagement-participation/three-nations-dementia-working-group

2. https://alzheimer.ie/creating-change/self-advocacy-groups/irish-dementia-working-group-3/

3. https://www.alzheimer-europe.org/about-us/european-working-group-people-dementia

or the capacity to understand things. People began to lose patience with me, and I came to the conclusion that not only was I no longer fit enough to perform paid work; I was no longer capable of even performing unpaid work.

While working, I was a trade union representative. I supported people not only in their day-to-day work but also when they found themselves in difficulties with employment issues. Since my diagnosis and retirement, I have not heard a single word from any former colleagues! I had established strong friendships, but following my diagnosis, these friendships ceased.

This means that, if I did not work within the dementia community, I would be totally isolated.

Helen's experience

I am truly blessed with my neighbours; never more so than in lockdown, and they have shown such kindness since Sean, my husband, passed away in December. They know my challenges and have adjusted to my lapses of memory. After my diagnosis became public, they were hesitant to chat with me as they did not understand the illness; they were only aware of it at a later stage. But now, they have no problem giving me a prompt; they all watch out for me.

My friends were very sad and upset when I was diagnosed. It was hard to explain as, like me, they knew nothing about the illness. Time and awareness have educated them about early onset dementia. They can see I still drive, shop and do most of what I did prior to diagnosis. We have enjoyed many years of fun, and I hope, when the lockdown is over [this was written in 2021, during the height of the Covid-19 restrictions on movement], *we can meet again, if only to go for a walk and have a coffee. We all miss the human connection. I know they are only a phone call away.*

Every day I try to bring meaning and a sense of purpose to my life. In my advocacy work, I encourage communities and the newly diagnosed to forget the myths and misconceptions and look at the person, not the illness – we still have so much to contribute. We need to stay engaged in the community (e.g. go to a match or concert). I want to be connected and be as independent as possible. By speaking out, I hope I am creating more awareness and influencing change in government and community policy.

Learning point 3

- What could you do to support those living with early onset dementia in your community? What have you noticed in your community buildings, streets or open public spaces that may pose challenges for those living with dementia?

Conclusion

There is much to adapt to when diagnosed with dementia at a younger age. The experience is influenced not only by the personalities, mental strength and resilience of the person diagnosed, but also by the reactions of others, their ability to change and challenge when required, and the social resources within a community. Personal accounts of young onset dementia, from Helen and John in this chapter but also from others in published books, demonstrate the challenges and change that are required, not only of the person diagnosed but of families, communities and policy, to help ensure that future generations of younger people diagnosed with dementia have a more supported experience of life with dementia.

References

Alzheimer's Society. (2014). *Dementia UK: Overview* (2nd ed.). Alzheimer's Society.

Bryden, C. (2018). *Dancing with dementia*. Jessica Kingsley

Department of Health. (2012). *Prime Minister's challenge on dementia: Delivering major improvements in dementia care and research by 2015*. Department of Health. https://assets.publishing.service.gov.uk/government/uploads/system/uploads/attachment_data/file/215101/dh_133176.pdf

Department of Health. (2015). *Prime Minister's challenge on dementia 2020*. Department of Health. www.gov.uk/government/publications/prime-ministers-challenge-on-dementia-2020

Local Government Association (LGA). (2015). *Dementia friendly communities: Guidance for councils*. LGA. www.local.gov.uk/sites/default/files/documents/dementia-friendly-communi-8f1.pdf

Millenaar, J., Bakker, C., Koopmans, R., Verhey, F., Kurz, A.D. & Vugt, M. (2016). The care needs and experiences with the use of services of people with young-onset dementia and their caregivers: A systematic review. *International Journal of Geriatric Psychiatry, 31*(12), 1261–1276. DOI: 101002/gps.4502

Oliver, K. (2019). *Dear Alzheimer's – A diary of living with dementia*. Jessica Kingsley.

Rabanal, L.I., Chatwin, J., Walker, A., O'Sullivan, M. & Williamson, T. (2018). Understanding the needs and experiences of people with young onset dementia: A qualitative study. *BMJ Open, 8*, e021166. doi:10.1136/bmjopen-2017-021166

Svanberg, E., Spector, A. & Stott, J. (2011). The impact of young onset dementia on the family: A literature review. *International Psychogeriatrics, 23*(3), 356–371.

Swaffer, K. (2016). *What the hell happened to my brain?* Jessica Kingsley.

10 Open Dialogue: A social network perspective in dementia care

Amy Jebreel, Rachel Butterfield and Robert Freudenthal

Reports from Western Lapland suggest that the Open Dialogue approach has contributed to significant changes in mental health care practice and outcomes for adults over the past four decades (Seikkula et al., 2006, 2011). As a result, there has been a keen interest in implementing the approach in other countries and healthcare systems, including in the UK (e.g. Razzaque & Stockman, 2016; Burbach et al., 2015; Hendy et al., 2015). Additionally, the broad principles of Open Dialogue tend to be appealing to clinicians as well as to service users and their families (Razzaque, 2019).

Open Dialogue originated in services for people experiencing a first episode of psychosis (Seikkula et al., 2006). The majority of the published work exploring its application within other settings has still broadly been within services for early intervention and crisis response in adult mental health (e.g. Freeman et al., 2019).

Why Open Dialogue?

As we work in mental health services for older people, and particularly those with dementia, we were struck by the absence in Open Dialogue of conversations about older people and, in particular, dementia. There is much about the approach that seems to speak to some of the central concerns in dementia care, such as how best to work with families and social networks to reduce the social isolation, stigma and disempowerment that can come with a diagnosis.

So, what does the literature tell us? Are there others who have tried to bring Open Dialogue or dialogical ways of working to the mental health care of older people and those with a diagnosis of dementia, and if so, with what results?

The short answer to the question above is that, to date, the literature has very little to tell us about Open Dialogue and dementia. We could find no account of the direct implementation of this approach in older people's services or dementia care.

We were inspired by accounts from other healthcare systems internationally, as well as our colleagues' early experiences of a peer-supported Open Dialogue research trial in adult services in the UK (Kinane et al., 2021), to think how we might develop dialogical practice or a form of adapted Open Dialogue in community mental health services for older people, particularly thinking about people with dementia and their families and carers. We strongly believe that this approach has the potential to transform the way services interact both around and with the person with dementia and that it has much to offer their wider community, including family, friends and carers.

What is Open Dialogue?

Open Dialogue can be understood as an approach to mental health care that encompasses both the way in which services are organised and the type of therapeutic conversations that take place. Seven principles underlie the approach, intertwined with the core values of openness, authenticity and unconditional warmth. A service organised around the Open Dialogue model would be structured in a way that allows for the responsiveness, flexibility and continuity of involvement that is central to the approach. We recognise that this may require some radical changes to the way health and social care services are currently organised. However, the core principles and values can also guide clinical practice within existing services and enrich the way we all think about and approach dementia care.

The first five of these principles describe the operational aspects: in other words, how the service works. The final two relate to the practice of Open Dialogue that occurs mainly within *network meetings*, which are meetings where the patient, key people in their life, and the health professionals come together to respond to any of the difficulties that may be arising.

The seven principles of Open Dialogue

1. Immediate help – It is recognised that the timing of a crisis for a person and their family is significant. When a person in crisis or their family makes contact with the service, or a referral is made, the service should respond within a day or at most within a few days.

2. Social network perspective – The important people in the patient's life are invited to participate as partners in the process of care. The 'social network', as defined by the patient or their family, is invited to join network meetings, in which discussions evolve about the current situation, their care and any other significant matters. Where possible, attempts are made to bring together and remain closely in communication with the different parts of the system engaged in that person's care, guided by the patient's preferences about who should be involved.

Learning point 1
- What is helpful about having family members and other significant

others involved in the network meetings? Could any challenges arise from this? Sometimes a person with dementia may not be able to choose who they would like to invite to the network meeting. How could a network meeting be arranged in this situation that still keeps the person with dementia at the centre of concern?

- What 'non-medical' aspects of care may it be helpful for professionals with dementia services to be involved with?

3. *Flexibility and mobility* – The service is patient-centred and non-directive. Care is tailored to the needs of each network. For example, the service user and their network decide where and when to hold network meetings, with meetings often taking place in the service user's home, or other non-clinical settings. There is an openness to all suggestions of care that arise from the dialogue, with a move away from focusing only on traditional notions of healthcare.

4. *Responsibility* – Those professionals who are involved at the start of care take on the responsibility to organise care with and for the network throughout their care episode, regardless of which other teams may become involved with care. The aim is to avoid continually passing patients on to different services and to make a commitment to work with the patient through the duration of their difficulties or episode of care.

5. *Psychological continuity* – There is a commitment to maintain continuity of care, with the same clinicians involved from the start continuing with the network throughout the episode of care. Where possible, any subsequent referrals are made back to the service.

6. *Tolerance of uncertainty* – The fundamental attitude required of clinicians is to facilitate dialogue and maintain an open space throughout and to avoid making premature conclusions or decisions. The continuity and ongoing relationships between the team and network create a safe setting in which there is room for contradictory or conflicting perspectives to be heard.

Learning point 2

- In dementia there are frequently areas of uncertainty – for example, often it is not known which interventions will be helpful for a person with dementia and their family.
- How might it feel for a patient or their family if professionals in a dementia service were uncertain about their management plans?

7. Dialogue – The essence of the therapeutic conversations is to enable each participant in the meeting (the person, the network and helpers) to be heard so that new understandings and ways of being with one another emerge. The participants work toward creating a space for each voice. This includes 'bringing forth the voices of those who are silent, less vocal, hesitant, bewildered or difficult to understand' (Olson et al., 2014, p.5). There is an emphasis on discovering the multiplicity of views present in the room ('polyphony') and meeting each of these with openness and deep respect, acknowledging the value of each. When practised skilfully, this can lead to a shift in agency from the traditionally assigned experts in the room (professionals – in particular, doctors) to a shared decision-making about the treatment plan that can hold contradictory and conflicting perspectives within the social network of the patient.

Learning point 3

- How might this be approached in a family where the members may have opposing views? For example, one member of the family might feel that their relative with dementia should move into a care home, while another member of the family disagrees.

Working with power dynamics

Open Dialogue explicitly recognises the inherent process of disempowerment when patients and their families access traditional medical services. There is an understanding that there are multiple experts in the room, and that each voice brings an important and valid contribution, not just the voices of the professionals. This includes the emphasis on peer practitioners (people with lived experience of mental health difficulties) playing a central role in Open Dialogue services in the NHS. For example, in a dementia service, the peer practitioner may be a carer for someone with dementia or have had experience of being a carer for someone with dementia in the past.

Learning point 4

- What power dynamics may be in play for a person with dementia accessing support from health services?

Traditional services rely heavily on having conversations and making decisions when the service user is not in the room: for example, in team meetings and in supervision between professionals. In Open Dialogue, the emphasis is on decisions being made in the network meetings. The decisions emerge from the discussions with the person and their network and are not made by professionals talking elsewhere. Team meetings are used for professionals to reflect on their own responses to working with different networks.

Intervision

Team meetings would also be held using the 'intervision' dialogical format, which allows team members to share their uncertainties and to reflect on their own feelings about working with a particular network. Enabling clinicians to understand and reflect on their own responses can lead to more open and honest communication, which may in turn reduce the risk of burnout. The goal of team meetings would not be to come to a specific plan with regards to diagnostic considerations or medication plans (although these could be considered) but rather to create a supportive framework for the team members such that these considerations could then be explored directly with the person with dementia and their family.

As well as ensuring that different people's perspectives are understood, it is also important to place particular emphasis on all the communication made by the person with dementia and their network as significant and meaningful. For example, the person with dementia may talk about concerns or show feelings that don't appear to have a connection with the reality, as it is seen by others. Attention is given to all forms of communication, including sounds, actions and utterances. The Open Dialogue team considers such communications to be meaningful, regardless of the level of cognitive impairment.

Learning point 5

- What can be understood or learned from the communications of someone with dementia that may not appear to be connected to the reality of what is happening around them?

Open Dialogue as a 'natural fit' for dementia services

Open Dialogue has mainly been used in adult services, typically where service users are presenting with a psychotic episode, usually at an earlier time in life than the people we see in dementia services. There are specific additional challenges and opportunities that using Open Dialogue in a dementia service may bring.

Many aspects of the Open Dialogue approach may already be familiar to clinicians working in a dementia service. For example, it is increasingly recognised that behaviour in dementia is meaningful. Interpreting what is being communicated through behaviour is central to providing high quality care when the person with dementia can no longer express themselves coherently with words. Families and carers who know the person well can often share essential insights, and most dementia services already have a practice of involving family members and carers in formulating treatment plans and making decisions. There is also a widespread acknowledgement that psychosocial interventions that take a much broader view of the person, their context and their personal history should be explored in relation to the psychological and behavioural changes that may be involved in a crisis situation, rather than just prescribing psychotropic medication.

There may, however, also be particular challenges. Individuals with a severe cognitive impairment may not be able to decide which carers and family members they would like to be included in network meetings. If, as a result of this, it is a carer that is identifying people to be included, the perspective of the person with dementia should explicitly be mentioned – for example, 'Who do you think is most important in the person with dementia's life? Who do you think they would like to include in the network meeting?' The person with dementia may not understand what the meeting is about and may not want to be present, so decisions may need to be made with the network about how best to proceed in the person's absence. The aim would be to try to keep the person with dementia's perspective in the room, even if they cannot be physically present. One common way of doing this in a network meeting is to ask the question, 'What would [the patient] say in this situation?', and to invite all those present to comment, bringing a richness that may capture something of the patient's wishes.

The Open Dialogue approach encourages us to reflect on power dynamics in relation to clinical interactions. These power dynamics can be particularly stark in the situation where an individual has an advanced cognitive impairment, and particular care needs to be taken to keep their wishes central to any decision-making that may take place.

The Open Dialogue approach also encourages clinicians to be flexible about what is considered to be a 'treatment' and what can be included in treatment plans. Health and social care services may be situated in separate departments and locations and the responsibility that is central to the Open Dialogue approach may mean clinicians staying involved where they might otherwise have passed the case on to a new team. Remaining involved keeps a degree of continuity for the individual and their network and helps to ensure that the understanding of the person's needs that has evolved through the work is not lost in the transition to a different service.

In dementia, there is frequently diagnostic uncertainty regarding whether an individual has a diagnosis of dementia, what sub-type it might be, and how quickly the dementia may progress. Open Dialogue allows the professionals to be explicit about this uncertainty with the individual and their family, while also providing information about specific forms of dementia and potential challenges that may arise. It is common for people with dementia and their carers to ask about what the future will hold, and the professionals can feel under pressure to provide answers when they cannot be sure. An Open Dialogue approach would support the professionals to be frank about what is unknown and would offer them space, through intervision, to explore the personal impact of working with these concerns.

A person with a diagnosis of dementia may, at different stages, face a number of challenges, including a threat to their identity, reduced interconnectedness and diminished agency. The network meetings, with their emphasis on dialogue, meaning making and the strengthening of relational bonds, may reduce isolation and enable the person with dementia to feel heard and validated.

Limitations of the approach

The implementation of Open Dialogue as a treatment system in dementia care would require significant cultural and structural change to existing mental health practice (Razzaque, 2019). However, a more modest move towards dialogical practice may be achievable within existing systems.

We anticipate that, to adopt an Open Dialogue approach, dementia services would need to support professionals to work beyond their current professional boundaries, taking responsibility for the care of individuals who have a progressive condition and may have ongoing needs. The expectation of a rapid discharge of patients once the immediate crisis is over is not compatible with Open Dialogue. There are unique challenges in considering how peer workers could be involved. There is also much to consider in relation to the creation of a culture that allows professionals to maintain uncertainty in a system where concerns such as mental capacity, best-interests decisions and safeguarding processes may appear to demand clarity and certainty about what is the right thing to do.

Conclusion

Open Dialogue is a social network approach to mental health care that was developed in Finland in the 1980s. Over recent years, the model has been adopted across a number of settings worldwide, mainly in adult mental health services. Beyond this, the approach offers guiding principles at both the therapeutic and service levels that lend themselves to addressing many of the specific challenges faced by people diagnosed with dementia and their carers.

At a service level, the priorities include flexible, responsive care delivered by the same treating team and throughout the service-user journey. All treatment decisions are made collaboratively within network meetings. These meetings offer an opportunity for the person with dementia, family members, carers, clinicians and others to unearth the multiple narratives present in the room and to come to a deeper understanding of each person's perspective. A person with a diagnosis of dementia may, at different stages, face a number of challenges, including a threat to identity, reduced interconnectedness and diminished agency. The network meetings, with their emphasis on dialogue, meaning making and the strengthening of relational bonds, reduce isolation and enable the person with dementia to feel heard and validated.

There is little published work on the effectiveness of an Open Dialogue approach in managing difficulties associated with dementia. Nevertheless, many aspects of Open Dialogue can be usefully adapted to dementia services, and other aspects (particularly related to involving families and carers in decision-making) are already a key part of the care provided by dementia services.

References

Burbach, F., Sheldrake, C. & Rapsey, E. (2015). Open Dialogue in Somerset. *Context*, *138*, 17–19.

Freeman, A.M., Tribe, R.H., Stott, J.C. & Pilling, S. (2019). Open Dialogue: A review of the evidence. *Psychiatric Services*, *70*(1), 46–59.

Hendy, C., Wright, D., Sutherland, L. & Shutt, J. (2015). Becoming dialogical in Nottingham. *Context*, *138*, 20–21.

Kinane, C., Osborn, J., Ishaq, Y., Colman, M., & MacInnes, D. (2021). Peer-supported Open Dialogue in the National Health Service: Implementing and evaluating a new approach to mental health care. *BMC Psychiatry*, *22*, 138. https://doi.org/10.1186/s12888-022-03731-7

Olson, M., Seikkula, J. & Ziedonis, D. (2014). *The key elements of dialogic practice in Open Dialogue: Fidelity criteria.* The University of Massachusetts Medical School.

Razzaque, R. (2019). *Dialogical psychiatry: A handbook for the teaching and practice of Open Dialogue.* Omni House Press.

Razzaque, R. & Stockmann, T. (2016). An introduction to peer-supported Open Dialogue in mental healthcare. *BJPsych Advances*, *22*(5), 348–356.

Seikkula, J., Aaltonen, J., Alakare, B., Haarakangas, K., Keränen, J. & Lehtinen, K. (2006). Five-year experience of first-episode nonaffective psychosis in Open-Dialogue approach: Treatment principles, follow-up outcomes, and two case studies. *Psychotherapy Research*, *16*(02), 214–228.

Seikkula, J., Alakare, B. & Aaltonen, J. (2011). The comprehensive Open-Dialogue approach in Western Lapland: II. Long-term stability of acute psychosis outcomes in advanced community care. *Psychosis*, *3*(3), 192–204.

11 Values-based practice in dementia care

Toby Williamson

This chapter is about values and dementia. Yet facts seem to dominate everyday dementia care. There are the observable effects of dementia: memory loss; difficulty in understanding, communication and decision-making; marked changes in behaviour, agitation and distress. Technology allows us to see the physical damage done to the brain by illnesses causing dementia, such as Alzheimer's disease. There is the stress and despair of many family carers. There is currently no cure, and the evidence base for effective treatments is still very limited. With facts like these, who needs values?

But values are important in dementia care precisely because of these facts. Limitations of current treatments mean that facts alone are not enough to inform decision-making about care and treatment. Quality of life, rights, what's important to the person and their family, all come into play, and all involve values. The impact that dementia has on people's lives, identity, understanding of the world and ability to communicate and make decisions go beyond just facts and raise profound issues involving values.

Words like 'independence', 'dignity' and 'respect' are frequently referred to as key values in dementia care. Sure, these are values, but they are a rather narrow way of understanding values. In everyday situations they may be of limited use and there may be tensions or conflict about which are the 'right' values for care and treatment decisions. Values include these concepts but much more besides.

This chapter explains the importance of values in dementia care. It describes a practical approach to working with values – 'values-based practice' (VBP). The chapter explains how VBP can work in partnership with other important approaches in dementia care, such as evidence-based practice and a rights-based approach.[1]

---

1. For a more detailed explanation of VBP, evidence-based practice, a rights-based approach and other ideas in this chapter, see Hughes & Williamson, 2019.

Values

Values can be thought of simply as the words that come up on a screensaver or are stuck on the office wall as a laminated poster listing 'This organisation's values'. These are often ignored or deemed to be of little relevance in everyday dementia care. This is an unhelpful way of defining values.

Learning point 1

Values are difficult to define. People have different definitions of values, but this doesn't mean they aren't all values. Write your answers to the question below. Then ask some colleagues to do the same. Compare your answers.

- 'What words or phrases come to mind when you hear the word "values"?'

It is likely that you and your colleagues will generate quite a long list of words and phrases in answer to the question in the Learning Point. You may have listed words such as 'beliefs', 'ethics', 'principles', 'respect', 'honesty', 'fairness', 'right and wrong', 'morals' and 'rules for behaviour'. There are likely to be similarities and differences in your lists. So which ones are values and which aren't?

Probably they are all examples of values. Values can be defined very broadly and vary from person to person, and with time and place. But values are not random; they can be understood in terms of what's important to a person (or an organisation), or 'action-guiding words'.

Where can one find values?

Now think about where you might find examples of values in a professional or work setting. They could be in a professional code of conduct, organisational policies or the law. Values are expressed in ethical frameworks for providing care, including dementia care (Nuffield Council on Bioethics, 2009).

Values are personal, held by individuals with dementia, family carers, and practitioners. Values are also expressed collectively through social norms or the media. All of these may influence everyday dementia care. But remember, although values may not be consistent, they are coherent. Values are like an extended family – they may not all get on with each other, but they are all related!

Values and dementia

Understanding values as described above enables us to see that dementia is as full of values as it is of facts. Here are some examples.

- The way a person describes their dementia or shows signs of dementia may be underpinned by values, albeit ones that are difficult to understand. They may insist there's nothing wrong with them, despite showing cognitive or other impairments. They may express an unusual belief in their situation, such as believing that they are in a previous life phase ('time-shifting'), not recognising family members or friends or believing they are imposters, or seeing things that aren't there. The person may believe their values are 'right', even if what they are based on is 'wrong'.

- Historically, mainstream values in society about dementia have been negative ones, based on fear, ignorance and stigma. Dementia was 'under-valued' as a health priority, often seen (incorrectly) as an inevitable part of ageing, and not diagnosed, or the diagnosis was not disclosed. People with dementia were seen at best as objects of pity who lacked any decision-making ability or agency ('value-less'), and family carers were ignored. More recently, the increasing numbers of people being diagnosed at an earlier stage of their dementia, who are able to express their views and values, have helped change attitudes (Mitchell, 2019; Oliver, 2019; Williamson, 2012).

- The work of Tom Kitwood and others has been fundamental in refocusing dementia care onto the person, not just the disease, and towards concepts of personhood and person-centred care (Kitwood, 1997; Kitwood & Brooker, 2019). These approaches require an understanding of the person's values. Kitwood's concept of 'malignant social psychology' showed the damaging impact that negative values about dementia have on people.

- The evidence base for effective biopsychosocial treatments and interventions for dementia is limited, and there are currently no cures. Decisions about caring and supporting people affected by dementia will therefore involve values because there is no one 'right' solution.

- The impairments caused by dementia mean that it can also be defined and understood as a disability. This draws attention to the important values underpinning quality of life, inclusion, citizenship, and rights (Mental Health Foundation, 2015; Hare, 2016; APPG on Dementia, 2019).

Values crop up in many areas of dementia care. They can make things complex, but not recognising or ignoring them is likely to make things more difficult and lead to unhelpful disagreements and conflict. So, it's important to have an effective way of working with values.

Values-based practice

The range and diversity of values in health and social care is a key theme of 'values-based practice' (VBP). VBP was developed to enhance professional practice in mental health and psychiatry (Woodbridge & Fulford, 2004). VBP works alongside evidence-based practice (EBP) but highlights the limitations and disputes about what works in mental health, especially where service users reject service interventions. VBP has subsequently expanded into other areas of health and social care, including dementia (Fulford et al., 2012; Hughes & Williamson, 2019).

Recognising differences in values and the disagreements these can cause is at the heart of VBP. The 'right' values for one person may not be the 'right' values for another. Here are a couple of examples involving people with dementia.

- Mr Iqbal is in hospital following a fall. He is ready to be discharged. The doctor and his family think Mr Iqbal isn't safe to return home and should go into a care home (key values – risk and protection). Mr Iqbal and a social worker disagree and think Mr Iqbal should return to his own home (key values – Mr Iqbal's autonomy and respecting his wishes).

- Mrs Smith lives in a care home. She keeps on tearfully asking to see her husband (who died several years ago) and trying to leave the care home, saying that she 'wants to go home'. Mrs Smith's family tell her that her husband will visit later, and she can go home tomorrow, which calms Mrs Smith down (key value – wellbeing). Staff don't want to say this because they don't want to lie to Mrs Smith (key value – being honest).

In the examples above, the different values are fairly *explicit*. But VBP also points out that values are often not stated (*implicit*), and this can lead to further problems. For example, an explicit healthcare value is 'non-maleficence' – do no harm. Most people would say that lying is harmful, but sometimes practitioners may base their response on an implicit value of not telling the truth to someone with dementia because it would cause the person distress.[2] In situations where there is tension between implicit and explicit values, VBP emphasises the importance of being open and honest about both sets of values.

Learning point 2

Dementia poses unique challenges involving values, in understanding the condition and in the provision of care. Values-based practice enables practitioners to work with diverse values, including those of the person with dementia, family carers and colleagues, even if their values may be in conflict and not made explicit.

- Re-read the examples of Mr Iqbal and Mrs Smith.
- What would your values be in these situations?
- How would you be explicit about your values?
- What would you do if your values differed from other people's?

---

2. For a more detailed discussion of truth-telling and dementia, the Mental Health Foundation has published a report (including practical guidance) on *What is Truth? An inquiry about truth and lying in dementia care* (2016). The report can be accessed at www.bl.uk/collection-items/what-is-truth-an-inquiry-about-truth-and-lying-in-dementia-care

Using values-based practice to help with decision-making in dementia care

The point of VBP is to support balanced decision-making within a framework of shared values based on mutual respect for differences in values (the *premise* of VBP). VBP is therefore especially helpful where there is a disagreement involving a person with dementia, their carers and practitioners over outcomes: whose values are 'right'? VBP focuses on process, not outcome. If the process for deciding on a course of action is one where all the different values 'in play' – as well as evidence – are considered, then the chances of a positive outcome are greatly increased and the likelihood of unhelpful conflict is reduced.

But not all values have to be respected equally. Values that exclude or discriminate, such as racist values, may sometimes have to be considered. But they must not dominate decision-making as they are intolerant of diversity and therefore violate VBP's premise of mutual respect.

VBP emphasises that the service user's values should be the starting point, but they will not always be the ones that determine decisions and action alone; other values must also be considered.

In some situations, there may be a clear evidence base or consensus for a particular course of action and VBP may be unnecessary. But if the person with dementia has capacity, for example, and refuses that particular course of action, their views (and values) must be respected. This is where VBP also comes in useful.

At a practice level, VBP involves 10 key elements of 'good process'. They do not have to be followed sequentially, but they are the key ingredients that need to be in the VBP 'pot' to make for a good 'stew' – i.e. a good outcome! They are divided into four categories, described below with prompt questions and examples relevant to dementia care.

Clinical/practice skills

Below are some fundamental skills that are helpful when bringing values to encounters with people with dementia, their carers and other practitioners:

1. Awareness – of the values present in any given situation. Listen to the language people use.

2. Knowledge – understand the values and facts relevant to the situation.
    - What's the person with dementia saying that is important to them?
    - If they can't communicate this, are there other ways of finding out about their values?
    - What's important to family carers and other practitioners involved?
    - Are some values not being openly expressed?
    - Are there different values?

3. Reasoning – consider issues and consequences where values affect decisions and actions.

- What are the possible outcomes if the values of the person with dementia are followed?
- What are the possible outcomes if other values prevail?
- What's the best possible outcome that can be achieved, incorporating as many values as possible, especially for the person with dementia?
- If a decision is reached that excludes some key values, can this be justified in terms of the person's wellbeing, best interests, values or wishes they have expressed at some other time, or because of absolute necessity (e.g. not respecting the person's wishes to return home, or truth-telling)?

4. Communication – use good communication skills to come to a balanced decision and resolve conflicts where there is a diversity in values.

- Is the person with dementia being listened to and given support to participate in decisions?
- Are family carers, other people who know the person and other staff being listened to (e.g. care home staff)?
- Is there a clear and open conversation involving everyone that explains the decision that's been reached and acknowledges differences in opinion?

Professional relationships

These approaches will help practitioners engage positively with everyone's values in their interactions:

5. Person-centred practice – the first (but not the only) source of information on values is the person with dementia.

- Is everyone clear what's important to the person with dementia?
- If the person can't express this, has someone who knows them been asked, or an advocate?
- If family are involved, what's important to them?

6. Multidisciplinary – make positive use of diverse values in teams, across disciplines and with other services and organisations.

- Are there suitable meetings, forums or processes where values held by different teams, disciplines or organisations can be expressed, understood and respected?

Links with evidence-based practice

Use EBP where relevant. Practitioners need to think facts *and* values:

7. The 'two feet' principle – all decisions are made with 'two feet on the ground' – i.e. considering values and facts (or evidence).

- Are we taking into account evidence of relevant interventions (eg. the NICE dementia guidelines (2018)?
- Are the values consistent with the facts (e.g. someone believing a deceased relative is still alive)?

8. The 'squeaky wheel' principle – like a squeaky wheel on a car, we only notice values when there is a problem. If there's a consensus about values and what action to take, there's probably no need to discuss values.

- Are differences in values causing difficulties?
- Could differences in values cause difficulties in the future (e.g. avoiding being truthful to someone with dementia because it might upset them)?

9. Science and values – new knowledge creates more choices in care and treatment, therefore involving more values.

- Am I open to new knowledge about dementia and interventions?
- How does this affect my values?

Partnership-based

10. Partnership – decisions are taken together, by the person with dementia, carers and practitioners. Aim for consensus, but there may be differences of opinion (*dissensus*). This does not mean deciding between 'right' and 'wrong' values. 'Dissensus' simply means 'agreeing to disagree' and keeping all values 'in play'. Different values can continue to be referred to, and followed, depending on how things develop.

- Can a consensus be reached about what to do?
- If there are still differences in values, can we still come to a balanced decision and successfully negotiate this with everyone (reach 'dissensus')?
- Are we ensuring that we avoid talking about 'right' and 'wrong' values?

Final word: VBP and rights-based approaches

There is growing awareness about the importance of legal frameworks and human rights for people with dementia. This is because of the growth in legislation, such as mental capacity and social care laws, and greater awareness of how equalities and disability rights affect people with dementia.

Laws are expressions of values considered important by society and, because of their legal status, stand somewhat separately from other expressions of values. Rights expressed in law cannot be treated in quite the same way as other values. Although laws can change (or be inconsistent), VBP must also work in partnership with a rights-based approach to dementia care (Hughes & Williamson, 2019). This creates an 11th component to VBP's 'good process'.

A rights-based approach

11. A rights-based approach – in partnership with VBP. Ensure relevant legal frameworks are considered. Try to apply them in the most helpful way, consistent with the values identified through VBP.

    · What legal frameworks apply to the situation?

    · If different legal frameworks have conflicting values, can VBP (or legal processes) be used to resolve these conflicts (eg. best interests)?

Learning point 3

VBP provides a process for resolving difficulties in dementia care involving values. It can be used in conjunction with evidence-based practice and a rights-based approach. Think of a situation that you have experienced in dementia care where there have been conflicting values:

- Which parts of VBP's process could be helpful?

- How would you use VBP's 'good process'?

Conclusion

Values are everywhere in dementia. Understanding values provides a crucial way of understanding the person with dementia: their identity, experiences, relationships, their place in society, their decisions and their actions. Values also help us to reflect on ourselves and our relationships with people with dementia. Values help us to understand the condition more, not just as a disease but also as a disability and an aspect of what it is to be human.

The values of personhood, humanity and disability are crucial for understanding dementia, but may not provide practical solutions when complex situations arise in dementia care and values are divergent or in conflict. VBP, in partnership with other approaches, provides a good way of dealing with these situations.

References

All Party Parliamentary Group (APPG) on Dementia. (2019). *Hidden no more: Dementia and disability.* Alzheimer's Society. www.alzheimers.org.uk/about-us/policy-and-influencing/2019-appg-report

Fulford, K.W.M., Peile, E. & Carroll, H. (2012). *Essential values-based practice.* Cambridge University Press.

Hare, P. (2016). *Our dementia, our rights.* The Dementia Policy Think Tank and Innovations in Dementia CIC. www.innovationsindementia.org.uk/resources/our-publications/

Hughes, J.C. & Williamson, T. (2019). *The dementia manifesto: Putting values-based practice to work.* Cambridge University Press.

Kitwood, T. (1997). *Dementia reconsidered: The person comes first.* Open University Press.

Kitwood, T. & Brooker, D. (Eds.). (2019). *Dementia reconsidered, revisited: The person still comes first.* Open University Press.

Mental Health Foundation. (2015). *Dementia, rights and the social model of disability.* Mental Health Foundation.

Mental Health Foundation. (2016). *What is truth? An inquiry about truth and lying in dementia care.* Mental Health Foundation.

Mitchell, W. (2019). *Somebody I used to know.* Bloomsbury Publishing.

National Institute for Health and Care Excellence (NICE). (2018). *Dementia: Assessment, management and support for people living with dementia and their carers (NG 97).* NICE. www.nice.org.uk/guidance/ng97

Nuffield Council on Bioethics. (2009). *Dementia: Ethical issues.* Nuffield Foundation. www.nuffieldbioethics.org/publications/dementia

Oliver, K. (2019). *Dear Alzheimer's: A diary of living with dementia.* Jessica Kingsley Publishers.

Williamson, T. (2012). *A stronger collective voice for people with dementia.* Joseph Rowntree Foundation. www.jrf.org.uk/report/stronger-collective-voice-people-dementia

Woodbridge, K. & Fulford, K.W.M. (2004). *Whose values? A workbook for values-based practice in mental health care.* The Sainsbury Centre for Mental Health.

12   Advance care planning for people with dementia

Dylan Harris

The thing is, once you've spoken about these things (as hard as it might be), you can put them away and focus on enjoying things.

(National Council for Palliative Care, 2011, p.4)

In its advanced stages, dementia affects the ability of the brain to process thoughts and make decisions. At that point, those close to the person with dementia may need to make decisions for them, alongside health and social care professionals (Harris, 2006).

It is, however, possible for someone with early dementia to think about some of the decisions that may need to be made in the future and their thoughts and preferences about them. This is often termed 'advance care planning' (sometimes shorted to ACP), or future care planning, and can greatly help those caring for them to make the best decisions for them when they are no longer able to do so themselves.

Some of these things can be difficult to contemplate, but equally there can be a sense of relief that they have been thought about and the person with dementia has been able to express their wishes and preferences.

There are multiple terms and phrases used around advance care planning. Terms like 'advance directive', 'living will', 'advance decision to refuse treatment' and 'power of attorney' all relate to aspects of advance care planning. 'Living will', for example, is an outdated term that was previously used to describe what we now call an advance care plan.

Why is advance care planning important in dementia?

'In understanding that dementia could ultimately deny her the capacity to decide… our attempt at advance care planning alleviated some of her

concerns and allowed her to make some decisions about the end of her life.
(NHS England, 2018, p.7)

Advance care planning is a process of dialogue between a person with dementia and those close to them, relating to their preferences and values when it comes to future treatment and care, including end-of-life care (Piers et al., 2018).

No one is obliged to carry out advance care planning (it is a voluntary process) and you don't need to consider and plan everything in one go:

You can always revisit things, but because you've done that first step it's a bit easier. (National Council for Palliative Care, 2011, p.15)

What are the challenges and barriers to advance care planning for people with dementia?

I think the client [person with dementia] would have been quite open to the discussion, but the daughter was quiet, that wasn't somewhere that she wanted to go... so we didn't. (Poppe et al., 2013, p.4)

Because dementia is a condition affecting memory and decision-making, it is important to think about having advance care planning discussions earlier, while the person themselves is still able to do so. But there are a number of reasons why this may not always be the case. These may include, for example (Harris, 2006; Harrison Dening et al., 2011; Poppe et al., 2013):

- procrastination (waiting to do it later)
- lack of knowledge or awareness of advance care planning
- difficulty talking about or raising the subject (either from the point of view of the person with dementia or their family/carers or healthcare professionals)
- fear of 'signing my life away' or not being treated
- not thinking about dementia as being a progressive, life-limiting condition and therefore not thinking advance care planning is relevant (either from the point of view of the person with dementia, or their family/carers, or their healthcare professionals)
- the unpredictable disease trajectory makes it difficult to prompt discussions (from the perspective of healthcare professionals).

It is also important to recognise that it is hard to fully predict the future in its whole context. While some decisions can be followed (e.g. specific wishes for aspects of medical treatment that the person has decided they would *not* want, such as resuscitation), it can be challenging to always fulfil preferences that the person *did* want (e.g. to always remain in their own home). However, at least if these are known, they will always be taken into consideration.

> **Learning point 1**
>
> Advance care planning is a process of reflection and dialogue between a person with dementia and those close to them, relating to their preferences and values when it comes to future treatment and care, including end-of-life care:
>
> - Have you ever thought about what you may or may not want for your future treatment and care?
> - If you have thought about these issues before, have you spoken to anyone about them: friends, family, healthcare professionals?

Advance care planning and mental capacity

> Dementia is a terminal illness, you don't recover from it... to make choices about their care, it has to be done early before loss of capacity occurs. (NHS England, 2018, p.6)

Mental capacity is a legal term relating to the Mental Capacity Act 2005. To have mental capacity, a person needs to understand the information about a decision they are making; retain that information; balance up the options, and then communicate their decision. Mental capacity is decision specific – a person with some memory impairment may be able to make straightforward decisions, such as which clothes they want to wear on a particular day, but not be able to make more complicated ones around managing their finances.

Where someone doesn't have mental capacity, the health and social care professionals caring for them, along with their family and carers, will need to decide what to do for the best (termed 'best interests') in situations such as when the person develops a serious illness, like severe pneumonia. Professionals are required to take into account the views of those close to the person (family, for example). They must also take into account anything the person themself has said or written down before (such as an advance care planning document).

What might prompt conversations about advance care planning?

> I suppose really it was the wisest thing to do because there is no use leaving things like that too long before things are going to get worse... I would rather know what I am doing, so that's why I decided to make arrangements and things, so if anything happens now, they all know. (Poppe et al., 2013, p.3)

Ideally, advance care planning should be thought about early for a person diagnosed with dementia and discussed on several occasions. The person with dementia may choose to talk to their family, friends and health and social care professionals (either separately or all together). Those professionals may be their GP, district nurse or staff at a memory clinic, for example, or an Admiral nurse/ specialist dementia nurse, palliative care nurse or social worker.

There are several things that may in particular trigger these conversations: for example, around the time of diagnosis; when changes occur in the person's health/place of residence/financial situation, or when coming into contact/ referred to support services (e.g. palliative care, Alzheimer's Society) (Piers et al., 2018; Poppe et al., 2013). These sorts of broad, open questions can also help start a conversation:

- Your health is quite good now, but have you thought about what should happen when it's not so good in the future?
- What things would you want to know more about in relation to how your condition is likely to change over time and what is likely to lie ahead?
- Are there any types of medical intervention that you would not wish to have (such as resuscitation)?
- Is there anyone in particular (family, carer, friend) that you would want to be consulted about your care, or to look after your finances when you are no longer able to do so?

Aspects of advance care planning: what to talk about

'I knew she would have liked to have had the previous Methodist minister [at her funeral]… I rang her and asked her if she would, and she said yes. (Vries & Drury-Ruddlesden, 2019, p.2028)

Advance care planning may be considered as comprising three parts or components (Social Care Institute for Excellence, 2015):

1. Making statements about future wishes and preferences – for example, if in the future personal care needs could not be met in their own home, would they have any preferences where they would want to be cared for? Have they written a will? Do they have any preferences or wishes for their funeral?
2. Thinking about any types of medical/clinical care they would not want in the future ('advance decisions to refuse treatment') – for example, if they have decided that they do not wish to be resuscitated.
3. Thinking about whether there is someone particular who they would want to look after their finances or healthcare decisions in the future (a Lasting Power of Attorney).

A person may therefore consider part or all of these issues when starting to think and talk about advance care planning and may do them at different times.

Making a will is probably the most common form of planning for the end of life. If you die without making a will, your money and belongings ('estate') will be divided according to legal rules, and the process can be more time consuming (and costly) than if you have made your wishes clear in a will. Some people may also have specific thoughts about their funeral that they want to share – for example, what flowers, music, readings, whether they wish to be buried or cremated, and so forth.

Advance decisions to refuse treatment and Lasting Power of Attorney are explained below. These are the legal terms used in England and Wales; in Scotland and Northern Ireland, some of the terminology is slightly different, but the principles are the same.

Learning point 2

Advance care planning may be considered as three parts or components: making statements about future wishes and preferences; making any advance decisions to refuse treatment, and making a Lasting Power of Attorney. A person may consider part or all of these areas when starting to think and talk about advance care planning:

- Have you made a will? If you haven't, do you know what will happen to your property/belongings, by law? Is this what you want?

- What would you want your funeral to be like? Have you told anyone your wishes, or written them down where they can easily be found?

Lasting Power of Attorney

It's important to think seriously about whether they're [the person who will be the LPA] going to be alive over the whole prognosis. For example, Dad was older than Mum, so may not have been the right person [to be her Lasting Power of Attorney]. (National Council for Palliative Care, 2011, p.5)

A Lasting Power of Attorney (LPA) is a legal way of giving another named person(s) the power to make specific decisions on your behalf when you are unable to do so yourself. There are two types of LPA: one for property/finances and one for health/welfare. You can appoint an LPA for either or both.

The LPA for property and financial affairs allows you to choose someone to make decisions about how to spend your money and manage your property and affairs when you no longer have the capacity to do so for yourself. If this isn't in place, there may be no one who can access your bank account to pay bills, for example (the only option may then be to go to the Court of Protection for someone to be appointed who can do this, which is a more expensive, lengthy and complicated process). An LPA needs to be registered with the Office of the Public Guardian, ready to be activated when the person loses capacity, or if the person requests this, even though they still have capacity (the person may want someone else to take on the burden of paying bills) (Social Care Institute for Excellence, 2015).

The LPA for health and welfare allows you to choose someone to make decisions about your healthcare and welfare. This includes decisions to consent to or refuse clinical/medical treatment on your behalf. But it also includes such simple things as having your hair washed and cut. It only applies when the person no longer has mental capacity to make those decisions.

There are specific forms to complete for both types of LPA, which are available from the Office of the Public Guardian. Once they have been completed, signed and witnessed, they then have to be returned to the Office of the Public Guardian to register them. There is a fee to register each form (the Office of the Public Guardian website has more details).[1]

Advance decisions to refuse treatment (ADRTs)

> We'd had the opportunity to talk... before his dementia got too bad to know that he didn't want to be resuscitated. (Vries & Drury-Ruddlesden, 2019, p.3027)

Advance decisions to refuse treatment (ADRTs) allow people to decline certain types of clinical or medical care if they feel it is unlikely to improve their quality of life. To be legally binding, an ADRT must be written down, signed and witnessed. In addition, if the treatment the person is declining is a potential lifesaving treatment (for example, a feeding tube or resuscitation), they need to include in their ADRT statement that they understand that their decision to refuse those treatments would apply 'even if my life is at risk'.

The most common ADRT that people with dementia may relate to is not wanting to be resuscitated or to have artificial feeding.

Advanced dementia is associated with very poor likelihood of success of being resuscitated (cardiopulmonary resuscitation), and, even where successful, may result in significant further brain damage (Ebell & Afonso, 2011).

In the advanced stages, dementia also affects the person's ability to swallow safely. When this occurs, consideration is sometimes given as to whether they should have a feeding tube put into their stomach (this is called a percutaneous endoscopic gastrostomy, or PEG), or a tube that goes through their nose and down into their stomach (a nasogastric tube). A number of research studies have been conducted to see if there are any measurable benefits from doing this. Unfortunately, the studies have not, overall, shown a benefit in terms of things like prognosis, or the person's overall nutrition. Therefore, the current recommendation is that tube feeding should not normally be used for people living with severe dementia (Ijaopo & Ijaopo, 2019).

It is, however, something that has to be considered for each person individually, balancing any possible benefits against risks, as the procedure and the tube itself

---

1. www.gov.uk/government/organisations/office-of-the-public-guardian

have risks and possible complications. Some people with early dementia may feel strongly that they would not want a feeding tube later on and discuss this with their family and healthcare professionals. When swallowing problems do arise, alternatives to a feeding tube may be to modify the types and consistencies of food to make it easier for the person to swallow (e.g. having softer foods and thickened fluids) (see Chapter 15).

Learning point 3

A Lasting Power of Attorney is a legal way of giving another named person(s) the power to make specific decisions on your behalf when the time comes that you are unable to do so yourself:

- Is there somebody in particular that you would want to be involved in making decisions on your behalf at a point in the future when you are no longer able to do so?

Advance care planning: Where and how to record my wishes?

Advance care planning may take a variety of forms: from informal discussions with family through to specific documentation to appoint an LPA or make a will or an ADRT.

Your GP or hospital team may have a specific advance care planning pro forma that they can use to record your future wishes/preferences and file it electronically in your health record. They may also be able to allow that information to be shared between different health and social care professionals (e.g. the GP, hospital and ambulance services).

A number of online resources also have template documents you can download and either write or type onto. You can then make multiple copies and share the document with your family, and health and social care professionals.[2]

Summary

Advance care planning is a continuous process between a person with dementia, those close to them and relevant healthcare professionals concerning the person's preference and wishes when it comes to future treatment and care, including end-of-life care. It can involve any or all of the following: making statements about future wishes and preferences; making an ADRT and appointing a Lasting Power of Attorney. The topic can be difficult to raise, but people often feel relieved that they have told others about their preferences for future care and how they want their finances to be managed, and they feel empowered by doing so, which allows them to get on with enjoying living now.

---

2. For example, Dementia UK has an advance care planning template that is free to download from www.dementiauk.org/get-support/legal-and-financial-information/advance-care-planning/

References

Ebell, M.H. & Afonso, A. (2011). Pre-arrest predictors of failure to survive after in-hospital cardiopulmonary resuscitation: a meta-analysis. *Family Practice, 28*(5), 505–515.

Harris, D. (2006). Forget me not: Palliative care for people with dementia. *Postgraduate Medical Journal, 83*, 362–366.

Harrison Dening, K., Jones, L. & Sampson, E. (2011). Advance care planning for people with dementia: A review. *International Psychogeriatrics, 23*(10), 1535–1551.

Ijaopo, E.O. & Ijaopo, R.O. (2019, December 19). Tube feeding in individuals with advanced dementia: A review of its burdens and perceived benefits.[Online.] *Journal of Aging Research,* 7272067. doi: 10.1155/2019/7272067.

National Council for Palliative Care (NCPC). (2011). *Difficult conversations: Making it easier to talk to people with dementia about the end of life.* National Council for Palliative Care.

NHS England. (2018). *My future wishes: Advance care planning (ACP) for people with dementia in all care settings.* NHS England. www.england.nhs.uk/wp-content/uploads/2018/04/my-future-wishes-advance-care-planning-for-people-with-dementia.pdf

Piers, R., Albers, G., De Lepeleire, J, Steyaert, J., Van Mechelen, W., Steeman, E., Dillen, L., Vanden Berghe, P. & Van den Block, L. (2018). Advance care planning in dementia: Recommendations for healthcare professionals. *BMC Palliative Care, 17*(88): doi.org/10.1186/s12904-018-0332-2.

Poppe, M., Burleigh, S. & Banerjee, S. (2013). Qualitative evaluation of advanced care planning in early dementia (ACP-ED). *PLoS ONE, 8*(4), e60412.

Social Care Institute for Excellence (SCIE). (2015). *Advance care planning in dementia.* SCIE. www.scie.org.uk/dementia/supporting-people-with-dementia/decisions/advance-care-planning.asp

Vries, K. & Drury-Ruddlesden, J. (2019). Advance care planning for people with dementia: ordinary everyday conversations. *Dementia, 18*(7–8), 3023–3035.

13 Palliative and end-of-life care in dementia: What would good care look like?

Karen Harrison Dening

More people are living longer into old age, with a number of them reaching the oldest ages of 85 years and above. The changes to the age structure of the population influence both the prevalence and incidence of age-related conditions such as dementia, thus increasing the numbers of people who will die with or from this disease. Projections of annual deaths from dementia in England and Wales suggest they will rise by more than 25% by the end of 2040 (Etkind et al., 2017). Despite this demography, there is much evidence that people with dementia have inequitable access to good end-of-life care, and experience various barriers to services adequately meeting their needs (Sampson & Harrison Dening, 2020).

People with dementia are among the greatest users of health and social care as they move towards the end of their lives (Kulmala et al., 2014). Despite this, dementia is still not always recognised as a terminal or life-limiting condition (Sampson & Harrison Dening, 2020). A seminal study of care staff and physicians found they perceived slightly more than one per cent of residents to have a life expectancy of less than six months at the point of admission to a nursing home. However, more than 70% of those residents actually died within that period of time (Mitchell et al., 2004). Better understanding of the effects of dementia at the advanced stages would improve confidence in end-of-life care and reduce uncertainty in health-related decision-making for family carers and health care professionals alike (Kupeli et al., 2019).

Learning point 1

Before you read any further, think of a person with dementia (and/or their family members) who is in your care and nearing the end of life:

- What leads you to suspect that the person with dementia is nearing the end of their life?
- What signs and symptoms does the person with dementia display?
- Are there any difficulties for you in being able to deliver high quality end-of-life care?

We will now discuss some of these issues in more detail.

Nearing the end of life

Dementia is a progressive, irreversible neurodegenerative condition that is now considered to be life limiting or terminal (Xie et al., 2008), with a reported median survival time of 4.5 years from symptom onset to death. One in three people (30%) will die with or from dementia (Xie et al., 2008). Added to this, dementia has become the most common cause of death in both men and women over the age of 80 (ONS, 2021). Despite this, there is still widespread evidence that people with dementia have inequitable access to good palliative and end-of-life care (Sampson, 2010; Lloyd-Williams et al., 2017). This may in part be due to a failure to recognise when a person stops *living* with dementia and starts to *die* with dementia.

Palliative care versus person-centred care

The European Association of Palliative Care (EAPC) White Paper (van der Steen et al., 2013) provides a comprehensive description of optimal palliative care for older people with dementia, built around an 11-domain framework to provide guidance for clinical practice, policy and research. The EAPC White Paper argues that palliative dementia care, as with person-centred care (The Health Foundation, 2016), should be continuous and proactive and ensure timely recognition of the dying phase while providing comfort and psychosocial and spiritual support and avoiding unnecessary, burdensome treatments. The principles of each approach are not in competition with each other but have an inherent synergy in dementia care, as both value the person and their family. This means that it is important to treat the person with dementia as an individual and take their perspective into account when planning and providing care. This includes providing a positive social environment where the person can experience relative wellbeing, even in the dying phase.

The World Health Organization (WHO) defines palliative care as an approach that improves the quality of life of patients and their families facing the problems associated with life-threatening illness, including dementia, through the prevention and relief of suffering by means of early identification and impeccable assessment and treatment of pain and other problems, which could be physical, psychosocial or spiritual.[1] However, there is widespread evidence that good palliative and end-of-

---

1. www.who.int/cancer/palliative/definition/en/

life care for people with dementia is not widespread, despite a palliative approach to care being recognised as essential in UK practice guidance. This recommends that, from diagnosis, people living with dementia should be offered flexible, needs-based palliative care that takes into account how unpredictable dementia progression can be (NICE, 2018). However, there are still wide gaps in care in the dementia pathway, which are largely due to fragmented commissioning (Harrison Dening et al., 2018).

Recognising when someone is dying with dementia

There have been many attempts to identify prognostic indicators or indices (indications that someone is dying from dementia) to guide health care professionals to make a transition in their care to a more palliative approach, but these tools seem to be more reliable at identifying people with dementia at *low* risk of dying, rather than those at higher risk of death (van der Steen et al., 2005). Clinical judgement, discussion with families and carers, and taking the opportunity to reassess or shift the goals of care towards those of palliative care at times of additional illness or transition may be a more practical and reliable approach (Brown et al., 2013). For this to happen, a greater understanding of the potential symptom burden for people dying with or from dementia is essential.

Pain

One of the most common symptoms a person with dementia will experience is pain, especially towards the end of their life. However, pain is often poorly recognised and under-treated in dementia. Pain is a very personal thing – it is widely accepted in pain management that it is a subjective experience; it is what the *person* says 'hurts'. No other person can experience the pain of another or know what it feels like or how it really affects them physically and emotionally.

Learning point 2

Consider the following questions in relation to your own experience of pain:

- Think of a time recently when you experienced pain, such as a headache. Can you describe your pain?
- In what way might it be difficult to express your pain to someone if you did not have the ability to communicate verbally or in writing?
- Now think how you might respond if you were a person with dementia experiencing a headache.

People with dementia are mostly older, and the causes of pain will be the same for them as for all older people, such as osteoarthritis, dental pain, pressure sores and skin tears, leg ulcers, stiffening of joints, muscle rigidity or constipation. People with dementia may experience pain when being moved – for example, when they are being helped to turn in bed or dress and undress, or when a wound is being cleaned and dressed. However, as the person's dementia advances, they may lose the ability to recognise that the unpleasant sensation they are experiencing is due to pain, or, more commonly, they are unable to communicate their pain to others. These two factors combined often lead to the person with dementia displaying their pain through distress behaviours: for example, calling out repeatedly, pacing, and becoming angry when care is attempted. Due to such presenting behaviours, carers and care staff may not recognise when a person is in pain or may not know how to help.

The gold standard in assessing pain is to ask the person directly. Many people with moderate or even advanced dementia may still be able to let you know that they are in pain. However, asking a person with dementia to describe or locate the pain requires a high level of judgement and problem-solving. You may need to use other words to describe pain, such as 'sore', 'hurt' or 'ache'. Also, be aware that the person with dementia has poor short-term memory, so may only be able to say if they are in pain at that moment, although earlier pain may have left them with a feeling of unexplained emotional distress. When a person with dementia can no longer communicate their pain and discomfort, there is a range of observational pain assessment tools that can be used: for example, the Abbey Pain Scale[2] and PAINAD.[3] It is important that the tool covers situations where the person is both physically active and inactive, as some pain may only be experienced on movement, and other pain is present all the time. Pain observational tools are not 100% accurate in assessing pain and may require training and experience in their use.

Learning point 3

Consider the following case study:

Emily is a 78-year-old woman who is in the advanced stages of Alzheimer's disease. She has osteoarthritis and is doubly incontinent. She is not able to walk and needs help whenever she moves. Emily still manages to eat independently, with some assistance from care staff.

Usually, Emily is easy going and sociable. She is quite a happy woman, who sits and smiles at people around her. Today, when you enter Emily's bedroom with the aim of helping her to wash and dress for the day, Emily is sitting on her bed, which she has stripped completely. She has started to shred her night incontinence pad and is throwing it around the room. She is very restless, and on seeing you, she becomes more distressed and starts to shout at you. Emily appears very agitated and unhappy; she does not smile at you like she usually does. As you approach her, she holds her arms close to her chest. When you try to move her arms, she shouts 'No!'

---

2. www.wales.nhs.uk/sitesplus/documents/862/foi-286f-13.pdf

3. http://dementiapathways.ie/_filecache/04a/ddd/98-painad.pdf

> *You decide to leave her in her nightdress and help her to the dining room for breakfast.*
>
> *When breakfast is served, Emily normally just needs a little prompting to eat the first couple of mouthfuls and then carries on eating independently. But today you notice that this does not work. She appears to be unable to lift the spoon to her mouth, and she seems more restless and agitated in the company of others at the table.*
>
> - How has Emily's behaviour changed?
> - What are the possible reasons for each of the changes in Emily's behaviour?
> - Use the PAINAD tool (see previous page) to assess if Emily is in pain.

Other symptoms experienced at end of life in dementia

McCarthy and colleagues (1997) undertook a retrospective study comparing symptoms experienced in the last year of life (n=170) of people with dementia compared with people with cancer (n=1513). Findings showed that the symptom burden between the two groups was comparable: in particular, 64% of dementia patients experienced pain and 57% had loss of appetite. The healthcare needs of both groups were also similar. The careful management of these specific symptoms is vital in providing a holistic approach to end-of-life care for people with dementia. Other symptoms that are common towards the end of life in dementia include pressure sores (Romero Alonso, 2006), agitation,[4] difficulty with swallowing[5] and loss of appetite.[6] (There is not enough space to discuss these further here, but the references and Chapters 15 and 16 provide further reading.) What is important is that, if the person with dementia is engaged early enough after their diagnosis, when communication and mental capacity are intact, advance care planning can be undertaken to plan ahead and record their wishes and preferences for care in the event that they experience such symptoms (see Chapter 12).

Acute physical illnesses superimposed on dementia

The immediate response to acute physical illnesses (in addition to advanced dementia), like urinary tract infection or pneumonia, is often to admit the person to an acute hospital for active treatments. Towards the end of life in dementia, this may be inappropriate, because such intercurrent illnesses may be indicators of imminent death (van der Steen et al., 2012). Such a response may mean that people with advanced dementia nearing the end of life receive inappropriate, futile and painful investigations and procedures, such as arterial blood gas sampling.

---

4. www.palliativecareguidelines.scot.nhs.uk/guidelines/symptom-control/Delirium.aspx

5. www.scie.org.uk/dementia/advanced-dementia-and-end-of-life-care/end-of-life-care/eating-drinking.asp

6. www.verywellhealth.com/eating-appetite-changes-and-weight-loss-in-dementia-98582

End-of-life care guidance in dementia can be lacking. Following the withdrawal of the controversial Liverpool Care Pathway (LCP) end-of-life care guidelines in England in 2014,[7] researchers at University College London developed decision-making algorithms – 'rules of thumb' to offer an alternative to the LCP (Davies et al., 2016).[8]

Learning point 4

Think about someone you have supported or cared for with advanced dementia who has presented with agitated behaviours. Download the guide, *After the Liverpool Care Pathway Study: Rules of thumb for end-of-life care for people with dementia,*[8] and turn to page eight, where it discusses agitation and restlessness:

- Follow the decision-making algorithm when considering the person's presenting behaviours.

- What might be the underlying causes for their agitation or restlessness? Make a list of the possible causes.

- Are there any recent changes in their behaviour that might lead you to consider there may be a physical health problem? Make a list of the possible causes.

- Who else might you need to discuss your concerns with?

Conclusion

Delivering the best possible palliative and end-of-life care in dementia should be no different to how we might care for anyone who is dying. However, what is different is that frequently the person with dementia requires us to be more proactive in recognising the signs and symptoms, and especially as they near the end of life. This demands that we be more proactive earlier on in the course of the disease to encourage them to consider and record their wishes and preferences for their care and treatment, before they lose the ability to communicate and articulate how they feel and what they do or do not wish to happen to them.

---

7. The Liverpool Care Pathway guidance was intended to ensure all people in the final days or hours of life received high-quality care in hospitals. It was withdrawn by the NHS in England in 2014 after public outcry that it was being used inappropriately to terminate the lives of people who were not approaching end of life.

8. www.ucl.ac.uk/psychiatry/sites/psychiatry/files/rules_of_thumb_davies_iliffec.pdf

References

Brown, M.A., Sampson, E.L., Jones, L. & Barron, A.M. (2013). Prognostic indicators of 6-month mortality in elderly people with advanced dementia: A systematic review. *Palliative Medicine, 27*(5), 389–400.

Davies, N., Mathew, R., Wilcock, J., Manthorpe, J., Sampson, E.L., Lamahewa, K. & Iliffe, S. (2016). A co-design process developing heuristics for practitioners providing end of life care for people with dementia. *BMC Palliative Care, 15,* 68.

Etkind, S.N., Bone, A.E., Gomes, B., Lovell, N., Evans, C.J., Higginson, I.J. & Murtugh, F.E.M. (2017). How many people will need palliative care in 2040? Past trends, future projections and implications for services. *BMC Medicine, 15,* 102.

Harrison Dening, K., Scates, C. & Lloyd-Williams, M. (2018). Palliative care in dementia: A fragmented pathway? *International Journal of Palliative Nursing, 24*(1), 112–122.

The Health Foundation (2016). *Person-centred care made simple: What everyone should know about person-centred care.* The Health Foundation. www.health.org.uk/sites/default/files/PersonCentredCareMadeSimple.pdf

Kulmala, J., Nykanen, I., Manty, M. & Hartikainen, S. (2014). Association between frailty and dementia: A population-based study. *Gerontology, 60*(1), 16–21.

Kupeli, N., Sampson, E.L., Leavey, G., Harrington, J., Davis, S., Candy, B., King, M., Nazareth, I., Jones, L. & Moore, K. (2019). Context, mechanisms and outcomes in end-of-life care for people with advanced dementia: Family carers perspective. *BMC Palliative Care, 18*(1), 87.

Lloyd-Williams, M., Harrison Dening, K.H. & Crowther, J. (2017). Dying with dementia: How can we improve the care and support of patients and their families? *Annals of Palliative Medicine, 6,* 306–309.

McCarthy, M., Addington-Hall, J. & Altmann, D. (1997). The experience of dying with dementia: A retrospective study. *International Journal of Geriatric Psychiatry, 12,* 404–409.

Mitchell, S.L., Kiely, D.K. & Hamel, M.B. (2004). Dying with advanced dementia in the nursing home. *Archives of Internal Medicine, 164*(3), 321–326.

NICE. (2018). *Dementia: Assessment, management and support for people living with dementia and their carers.* NG97. NICE.

Office for National Statistics (ONS). (2021). *Deaths registered in England and Wales: 2020.* www.ons.gov.uk/peoplepopulationandcommunity/birthsdeathsandmarriages/deaths/bulletins/deathsregistrationsummarytables/2020

Romero Alonso, A. (2006). Rapid response: Pressure ulcers in advanced dementia may need a different approach. *British Medical Journal, 332,* 472.

Sampson, E.L. (2010). Palliative care for people with dementia. *British Medical Bulletin, 96*(1), 159–174.

Sampson, E.L. & Harrison Dening, K. (2020). Palliative and end-of-life care. In Dening, T., Thomas A., Stewart, R. & Taylor, J.-P. (Eds.). *Oxford textbook of old age psychiatry* (pp.395–408). Oxford University Press.

van der Steen, J.T., Lane, P., Kowall, N.W., Knol, D.L. & Volicer, L. (2012). Antibiotics and mortality in patients with lower respiratory infection and advanced dementia. *Journal of the American Medical Directors Association, 13*(2), 156–161.

van der Steen, J.T., Ooms, M.E., van der Wal, G. & Ribbe, M.W. (2005). Withholding or starting antibiotic treatment in patients with dementia and pneumonia: Prediction of mortality with physicians' judgment of illness severity and with specific prognostic models. *Medical Decision Making, 25,* 210–221.

van der Steen, J.T., Radbruch, L., Hertogh, C.M.P.M., de Boer, M.E., Hughes, J.C., Larkin, P., Francke, A.L., Jünger, S., Gove, D., Firth, P., Koopmans, R.T.C.M. & Volicer, L., on behalf of the European Association for Palliative Care (EAPC). (2013). White Paper defining optimal palliative care in older people with dementia: A Delphi study and recommendations from the European Association for Palliative Care. *Palliative Medicine, 28*(3), 197–209.

Xie, J., Brayne, C. & Matthews, F.E. (2008). Survival times in people with dementia: Analysis from population-based cohort study with 14-year follow-up. *British Medical Journal, 336*, 258–262.

14   Palliative care options in dementia

Sascha R. Bolt, Judith M.M. Meijers and Jenny T. van der Steen

The term 'palliative care' originates from the Latin word *pallium*, which means cloak. In palliative care, we aim to cloak symptoms, regardless of whether we can treat the underlying disease. It also means that we put a cloak around people with incurable conditions to provide them with warmth, comfort and a sense of safety.

The purpose of palliative care is to optimise the quality of life of people with a life-limiting illness and their families. Palliative care is holistic, which means that it focuses on the entire person by recognising physical, psychological, social and spiritual needs. Nowadays, more than 100 countries worldwide provide palliative care services. Yet, despite growing efforts, the rising needs for high-quality palliative care are still unmet in many parts of the world (World Health Organization, 2020).

Although it eventually incorporates terminal care, contemporary palliative care is much broader. Palliative care could refer to specialised services such as a palliative care team, specialised dementia nurses or specialised treatments. However, palliative care also refers to a general philosophy and approach to care (Sawatzky et al., 2016). Essentially, this is generalist care, and every healthcare professional should be able to apply palliative care principles.

People with any type of life-limiting condition should ideally benefit from this approach. Palliative care may be provided at any place and is not limited to the hospice. It is not restricted by time and may cover weeks, months or even years. Moreover, palliative care may be provided alongside treatments that prolong life or modify the (course of the) disease. In other words, applying a palliative care approach does not mean putting an end to all other (curative) care and treatment.

Dementia and palliative care

> Mrs Fiona Scott is 83 years old, and she has dementia of the Alzheimer's type. Fiona lives at home with her husband, Paul, 78 years old. Paul has undergone several treatments for cancer and calls himself 'a very bright man with some physical defects'. Although they argue at times, Paul thinks that he and Fiona make a great team together. Their daughter Millie visits them regularly.

Today, there is no cure for dementia, which implies that it persists until the end of life. In most forms of dementia, disease progression is inevitable and impairments increase over time. Our societies do not always recognise dementia as a terminal condition, and someone like Fiona is less likely to receive palliative care services than are people with other terminal conditions (Broady et al., 2018). However, an integrated palliative care approach is a vital element of high-quality dementia care.

A central characteristic of dementia is that it affects functions of the brain, such as memory, language and planning. This means that, over time, Fiona may lose her ability to think or talk about her wishes. Eventually Fiona may also lose her ability to walk, eat and drink by herself. A palliative approach to care recognises this decline and involves people with dementia and their families in conversations to enable shared decision-making and care planning at an early stage. Goals of care focused on comfort and symptom relief may be particularly important in the later stages of dementia. Nonetheless, we need to be aware of the life-shortening and terminal nature of dementia to prepare for problems that may arise in the future. Early anticipation supports the adequate provision of future palliative care and recognises individual needs (van der Steen et al., 2014).[1]

Palliative care for people with dementia is person centred, which means that it dynamically shapes itself according to the needs and journey of an individual, such as Fiona. Moreover, informal carers such as Paul and Millie should be involved in early palliative care, for there is a good chance that they will have to make decisions on behalf of Fiona some day. A palliative approach to care for families can start immediately after a relative is diagnosed with an incurable illness, and extends beyond bereavement. Families or other informal caregivers provide substantial care for people with dementia and their important role continues up to the end of life. Family involvement, too, depends on the specific situation and requires a person- and family-centred approach.

> Fiona thinks it is unfair that she has dementia, and she often asks Paul and Millie why this has happened to her. 'What is the meaning of this?' she asks them, in despair.

---

1. Experts from 23 countries around the world worked together on this White Paper, which sets out recommendations for palliative care in dementia.

Palliative care is holistic, and it responds to complex care needs that may be physical, psychological, social or spiritual in nature. For instance, Fiona sometimes struggles with questions about the meaning of life. Care on the spiritual domain pays attention to such sensitive questions. Holistic care also means that a variety of caregivers may be involved, which underlines the importance of continuity of care. Palliative care aims to contribute to the quality of life and, eventually, the quality of dying. Fiona, like anyone else, deserves a peaceful death and a worthy farewell. In this chapter, we describe some of the most important aspects of palliative dementia care in more detail.

Learning point 1

Before you read any further, you may like to consider the following questions:

- Looking at your own situation, how do you or how could you integrate a palliative care approach in your daily life or daily practice?
- How could a palliative approach to care improve the quality of life for people with dementia and their formal and informal carers?

Advance care planning and place of care

Fiona notices increasing difficulties in making decisions and expressing herself clearly. Fiona once signed a form stating that she does not want to be resuscitated. 'There is no need for all that fuss,' she told Millie and her family doctor at the time. 'If my time here is up, so be it.'

Advance care planning (ACP) is a communication process in which healthcare professionals discuss goals of care and wishes for future care with the person with dementia and their informal caregivers. Planning ahead may help reduce stress for Paul and Millie, who may at some point take over decision-making. People with dementia need timely opportunities to discuss goals of care while they are still capable of weighing up preferences and sharing their thoughts (Harrison Dening et al., 2019). This way, wishes for future care can be heard and respected. Advance care planning is further explained in Chapter 12 of this book.

In the context of palliative care, healthcare professionals have an important role in informing people like Fiona, Paul and their daughter on the prognosis of dementia and the potential benefits of advance care planning at an early stage. They need thoughtful guidance towards accepting the inevitable decline associated with dementia to facilitate their conversations about future wishes. As with any other aspect of palliative care, advance care planning should be tailored to the individual. Even if she does not want to talk about the end of life explicitly, professionals can still explore with Fiona her view on life and what 'a good life' means to her. Moreover, the willingness to talk about the end of life may change over time and Fiona should still have the opportunity to discuss topics that she previously preferred to avoid. Fiona's wishes regarding care and treatment may change over time. Therefore, advance care planning requires regular updating.

Advance care planning enables shared decision-making about palliative care options and may include the documentation of wishes in advance directives. Documented wishes should be up to date and accessible to all the care professionals involved. Thinking through certain scenarios beforehand and discussing desirable actions may provide peace of mind for Fiona, Paul and Millie.

> Fiona enjoys strolling in the woods. Although she prefers not to think about this, she might slip or fall and risk a fracture. Fiona has already told Paul and Millie several times that she does not want to go into hospital.

Shared decision-making about the place of care can be challenging, as people generally prefer to stay in their own, familiar environment. Feelings of guilt, shame or loss, but also relief, are common among family members after a relative's transition to residential care (Graneheim et al., 2014).

> Paul sometimes worries about caring for Fiona if the dementia gets worse. It may become difficult for Fiona to stay at home when her needs grow beyond Paul's capacities. Paul thinks it would feel like 'giving up' if Fiona moved to a nursing home.

Residential care organisations should recognise family members as important partners in care, which may facilitate them to get used to the new situation and their new caring role. Families and professional caregivers both benefit from openly discussing their expectations and wishes and from investing in trustful care relationships. Families experiencing shame or guilt may find support from speaking with others who share the experience of relinquishing care for a relative with dementia.

Learning point 2

Before you read any further, you may like to consider the following questions:

- When is a good time to start talking about the future and about the end of life (with people with dementia), and why?
- Who should be involved in these conversations, and why?
- Do you ever discuss *your* end of life with others? If yes, why? If no, why not?
- How do you feel about discussing the end of life?

Person-centred palliative care

Palliative care is person centred. The perspective of the person with dementia is central to caregiving throughout the dementia journey. A key figure in describing person-centred care for people with dementia was Professor Tom Kitwood. In his theory, he stressed the importance of social bonds (Kitwood, 1997, p.8). According to Kitwood, healthcare professionals should invest in trustful and respectful relationships with people with dementia to preserve personhood and to promote wellbeing. Western societies tend to emphasise cognitive abilities as central to human beings' functioning as individuals. Dementia is characterised by cognitive decline, which is why Fiona experiences difficulties with memory, language and planning. Nonetheless, Fiona's personhood should not be denied or undermined. The individual life story is central to the delivery of care throughout Fiona's and Paul's journey. The accents and focus of care may shift, following their specific needs each step of the way.

> For Fiona, quality of life relates to a feeling that she 'matters and belongs'. She is a worthy human being and wants to be treated that way. Fiona finds meaning and joy in painting. Millie has arranged for a creative therapist to visit Fiona every week for a painting session. During these sessions, Fiona sometimes gets emotional, and she talks about her thoughts and feelings.

Psychosocial interventions such as creative therapy, reminiscence therapy and life-story work emphasise personhood and help to establish interpersonal connections and meaningful relationships between people with dementia and their caregivers. Even in advanced dementia, tailored psychosocial approaches (such as Namaste Care[2]) may help to build social and emotional connections. Trustful care relationships that recognise the person with dementia as a worthy individual foster warm and dignified care in the last phase of life. Ideally, person-centred care relationships should be established in the early stages to stimulate conversations about personal values when people with dementia are still able to express themselves. Longstanding care relationships have advantages for both the person with dementia and the professional caregiver. For people like Fiona, it is important to have trusted and familiar caregivers. Being aware of Fiona's history, her interests and her particular wishes may help (future) healthcare professionals to tailor palliative care to her needs, until the end of life.

Learning point 3

Before you read any further, you may like to consider the following questions:

- How can you build a trustful care relationship? What do you need

---

2. See https://namastecare.com

to know about the other person? What does the other person need to know about you?

- How would you approach someone if you wanted to acknowledge their personhood? And how would you do this with someone who is nearing the end of life?

Organising continuous and interprofessional care

Paul feels they have seen many, perhaps too many, different healthcare professionals since Fiona was diagnosed five years ago. First, there was Fiona's family doctor, then another doctor they had not met before, and a psychologist at the memory clinic. Later, a dementia nurse visited Fiona and Paul at home. The creative therapist joined after a few months, followed by an occupational therapist. Around three years ago, 'the girls from home care' arrived. Paul is glad that the dust has settled and that he and Fiona are now familiar with the professional caregivers. He says, 'Some are really lovely.'

Holistic palliative care requires an interprofessional approach. When care professionals from different disciplines and family are involved, interprofessional collaboration is essential to ensure continuity. Continuity of care involves communication, co-ordination and transferring information among the involved parties. It is important that different disciplines and family are working together as a team with a shared goal and vision. It may be beneficial to appoint one member of the healthcare team, such as the dementia nurse, as the central contact for people such as Fiona, Paul and Millie and the other involved healthcare professionals.

Well-co-ordinated interprofessional care may help postpone or prevent admissions to a nursing home or hospital. Nonetheless, in many Western countries, most people with dementia live in a residential facility at the end of life. This means that a transition from one place of care to another is common. To avoid fragmented care and to promote continuity of care after transitions, former professionals should communicate care plans to new professionals, involving the person with dementia and their family (van der Steen et al., 2014). Information transfers in transitions of care should also involve personal information about the person with dementia, to facilitate a warm and personal welcome in a new and unfamiliar setting. Admission to acute care is a concern in palliative dementia care. The hospital may be a threatening and confusing environment for people with dementia. Drawbacks of hospitalisation include the presence of unfamiliar caregivers, a higher risk of complications such as delirium (acute confusion) or pressure sores and overall functional and cognitive decline. The appropriateness of hospitalisation should be weighed carefully.

Interprofessional healthcare teams must work together to promote person-centred, safe and smooth transitions of care (Hirschman & Hodgson, 2018).

Eventually, Fiona moves to a nursing home in her own, familiar neighbourhood. Although a warm welcome awaits, Fiona misses Paul and her former home. Paul feels guilty at first. One afternoon, in the nursing home, Fiona suddenly turns to Paul and says: 'I am happy that this is my home.' Paul feels a flurry of relief and smiles carefully.

A good end of life with dementia

Fiona is now 88 years old and settled in her nursing home, where she has been for the past 15 months. Paul, now 83 years old, still says he is 'a bright fellow'. Paul visits Fiona daily and Millie visits them weekly. The nurses and nurse assistants are kind and caring with Fiona. Over the past weeks, Fiona has become nearly completely dependent on others: she cannot get out of bed or eat without help. Paul and Millie feel that they have an important role in voicing Fiona's needs now that her end of life is nearing.

Fiona's end of life is approaching and goals of care focus mainly on comfort, which has become more important than prolonging her life. The family's perspective is valuable to professional caregivers when trying to hear and understand the voice of the person with dementia at the end of life. The nursing staff have a key role, and their longstanding care relationship makes it easier for them to recognise and manage Fiona's discomfort and respond to her needs.

Palliative care for people with dementia at the end of life attempts to fulfil care needs in all domains, adopting a person-centred approach (Perrar et al., 2015). In Chapter 13 of this book, Karen Harrison Dening explores how people with dementia experience pain and how pain is managed. Although physical care is indispensable to ensure Fiona is free of pain, we must not forget the psychological, social and spiritual aspects. The nursing staff should pay attention to emotions such as fear, anger or resistance, and they should invest in warm, trustful and respectful relationships to foster social and spiritual connectedness. Care for families is an important part of palliative care. Witnessing Fiona approaching the end of her life brings along feelings of loss and grief for Paul and Millie. Families need support throughout the care trajectory and up to the end of life to help them deal with multiple losses and anticipatory grief. Their need for support, preferably from familiar professionals, continues after bereavement (Broady et al., 2018).

Palliative care should contribute to a good end of life and, eventually, a good death. Although the meaning of a 'good death' is debatable, people generally wish to die peacefully and comfortably. This is the same for Fiona. Being at peace at the end of life involves a sense of tranquillity, inner harmony, wellbeing and closeness to one's family. Humane and compassionate care, reflected in sincere attention to a person nearing the end of life, may foster peaceful dying.

For Paul and Millie, being able to say goodbye to Fiona and experiencing her death as peaceful may allow them to deal with grief and to accept their loss.

Conclusion

The ultimate goal of palliative care is to optimise quality of life until the end of life. A palliative care approach promotes care for people with dementia and their families that is comprehensive, person-centred and continuous. A palliative care approach can be flexibly adapted to the changing needs of a person and his or her family throughout the dementia journey. An early adoption of a palliative approach to care enables people with dementia to express their wishes and preferences for current and future care. Healthcare professionals and especially nursing staff are vital in guiding people with dementia and their families during their journey to the end of life.

In the words of the founder of the UK hospice movement, Dame Cicely Saunders:

> You matter because you are you, and you matter to the end of your life. We will do all we can not only to help you die peacefully, but also to live until you die.[3]

In loving memory of Irene Geertruida (Rien) Bolt-de Klerk.

References

Broady, T. R., Saich, F. & Hinton, T. (2018). Caring for a family member or friend with dementia at the end of life: A scoping review and implications for palliative care practice. *Palliative Medicine, 32*(3), 643–656.

Graneheim, U.-H., Johansson, A. & Lindgren, B.-M. (2014). Family caregivers' experiences of relinquishing the care of a person with dementia to a nursing home: Insights from a meta-ethnographic study. *Scandinavian Journal of Caring Sciences, 28*(2), 215–224.

Harrison Dening, K., Sampson, E.L. & De Vries, K. (2019). Advance care planning in dementia: Recommendations for healthcare professionals. *Palliative Care: Research and Treatment, 12,* 1178224219826579.

Hirschman, K.B. & Hodgson, N.A. (2018). Evidence-based interventions for transitions in care for individuals living with dementia. *The Gerontologist, 58*(suppl 1), S129–S140.

Kitwood, T. (1997). *Dementia reconsidered: The person comes first.* Open University Press.

Perrar, K.M., Schmidt, H., Eisenmann, Y., Cremer, B. & Voltz, R. (2015). Needs of people with severe dementia at the end-of-life: A systematic review. *Journal of Alzheimer's Disease, 43*(2), 397–413.

Sawatzky, R., Porterfield, P., Lee, J., Dixon, D., Lounsbury, K., Pesut, B., Roberts, D., Tayler, C., Voth, J. & Stajduhar, K. (2016). Conceptual foundations of a palliative approach: A knowledge synthesis. *BMC Palliative Care, 15*(1), 5.

3. Quoted by Dr Robert Twycross in his tribute at the Service of Thanksgiving for Dame Cicely's life, 8 March 2006. www.stchristophers.org.uk/about/damecicelysaunders/tributes

van der Steen, J. T., Radbruch, L., Hertogh, C. M., de Boer, M. E., Hughes, J. C., Larkin, P., Francke, A.L., Junger, S., Gove, D., Firth, P., Koopmans, R.T.C.M., Volicer, L. & European Association for Palliative Care (EAPC). (2014). White Paper defining optimal palliative care in older people with dementia: A Delphi study and recommendations from the European Association for Palliative Care. *Palliative Medicine, 28*(3), 197–209.

World Health Organization. (2020). *Global atlas of palliative care* (2nd ed.). World Health Organization. www.thewhpca.org/resources/global-atlas-on-end-of-life-care

Part three

Supporting people living
with dementia

15 Nutrition in dementia

Nina Herrington and Deborah Thompson

Good nutrition contributes to positive health and wellbeing and reduces the risk of chronic disease. It is also crucial in aiding recovery from acute illness and preventing malnutrition. Conversely, poor nutrition increases the risk of disease, can delay recovery from illness and negatively affects body function, wellbeing and quality of life (NICE, 2006; Public Health England, 2019).

Dementia is associated with numerous nutritional challenges (Droogsma et al., 2013; Volkert et al., 2015). Dementia is also most prevalent in older adults, and the ageing process itself is associated with altered food and fluid intake and increased nutritional needs.

Research shows that risk of malnutrition increases as dementia progresses (Martin et al., 2012; Dos Santos et al., 2018) and early intervention to promote good nutrition and hydration is recommended (Tombini et al., 2016; Volkert et al., 2015; Volkert, 2017).

The NICE guidelines for the care of people with dementia (NG97) (NICE, 2018) include the following:

> 1.10.6 Encourage and support people living with dementia to eat and drink, taking into account their nutritional needs.

In this chapter, we describe some practical solutions to help make this possible. People with dementia may be living in a variety of settings, including their own home, supported accommodation or a care home, or be in hospital, and the information in this chapter applies to all these environments.

Factors influencing nutritional intake

The most common factors that affect nutritional intake in people with dementia include cognitive decline and changes to physical function that result from the ageing process. Chronic disease may also affect nutritional intake. In addition, social context and environment are important factors influencing the nutritional support needs of people with dementia (Public Health England, 2019; Alzheimer's Society, 2020).

Low mood, depression and hallucinations may result in changes in the food and fluid intake patterns and preferences of a person living with dementia. The decline in cognitive function may lead to memory loss, and the person may forget to eat or believe that they have already eaten, resulting in weight loss (NICE, 2018). People with dementia may refuse food if it is not familiar to them or is presented on the plate in a different, unfamiliar form (Alzheimer's Society, 2020). In a hospital or care home, people are sometimes encouraged to choose meals from pictorial menus to facilitate their choices, as the pictures may prompt their recognition of foods. Puréed or mashed food may be recommended if the person has swallowing issues, poor dentition or a painful or sore mouth. However, the person may then reject the food because they don't recognise it when presented in this way. To help to prevent this, puréed foods can be puréed separately and arranged on the plate to appear like a non-purée meal that may be more familiar to them.

Older adults can experience changes to all their senses. Altered taste, sight and smell could result in familiar foods tasting unpleasant and lead to the person not wanting to eat. Taste buds change with ageing; with some health conditions, they can change by up to 65%. These changes alter taste perceptions and sensitivity to sweet, salty or bitter foods, which may influence a person's food choices or readiness to accept meals (Public Health England, 2019; Alzheimer's Society, 2020). Impaired sight and changed perceptions of how something smells can also mean the person is unable to recognise a food or meal and this can lead to food refusal.

People who are restless or agitated will have higher energy requirements. Conversely, their energy requirements are likely to decrease if they become less active due to physical disabilities and ageing. If someone has poor concentration or eats slowly, the food may get cold and become unappetising, or carers may remove the plate before the person has eaten enough. Decline in dexterity and co-ordination can also make it difficult for someone to use cutlery or put food in their mouth, or to peel fruit or unwrap packaged items, such as butter or jam (Alzheimer's Society, 2020). Medication and other medical conditions can also affect appetite and what people are eating.

Dehydration is an ongoing concern for older adults and people with dementia. It can lead to infection and to further ill health. Consistent support from caregivers is essential to ensure that people living with dementia drink enough fluids. In line with this, it is important to consider the following factors: physical and social environment; staff communication strategies; access to drinks; drinking vessels, and individual preferences (Lea et al., 2017; Wilson & Dewing, 2020).

Constipation is a common problem, often caused by dehydration, low fibre intake and/or medication. It can also affect appetite if not treated.

The person may need to be referred to a speech and language therapist and/or a dietitian, who can make recommendations to help improve their nutritional intake if they are having difficulties with eating and drinking.

Learning point 1

Consider the factors that can affect an individual's food and fluid intake, as outlined above.

What can be put into place to help overcome these difficulties? We suggest:

- Find out what foods and drinks the person likes and dislikes.
- Provide a suitable eating environment (not too busy and noisy, so they aren't distracted or distressed), and provide appropriate plates, cutlery and drinking vessels.
- Provide company and support while they are eating.
- Provide appropriate, acceptable meals, snacks and drinks of good quality and nutritional content.
- Help them with cutting up food or with feeding, if needed.
- Use pictorial menus to help people choose their meals and ensure that the actual meals resemble the pictures.

Nutritional requirements in older adults and people with dementia

Eating a healthy, balanced diet means eating a wide variety of foods in the right proportions and consuming the right amount of food and drink to achieve and maintain a healthy body weight.

The Eatwell Guide (Public Health England et al., 2016) sets out government recommendations on eating healthily and achieving a balanced diet. The guide shows how much of what we eat overall should come from each food group. In general, a regular meal pattern of three meals a day and appropriate snacks can help to achieve this balance. However, meeting nutritional requirements can be a challenge for older adults and those with dementia. Eating little and often, meals and snacks, may be particularly preferable if the person has a reduced appetite and is unable to eat full meals.

Energy – Adults should aim to consume enough energy (calories) to maintain their body weight within a healthy range. The body mass index (BMI) is a measure that uses height and weight to work out if a person's weight is healthy. The BMI calculation divides an adult's weight in kilograms by their height in metres squared. A healthy weight for older people may be higher than a healthy weight for younger adults. A BMI of 24–31 kg/m^2 can be considered healthy in people aged 70 years and over (Winter et al., 2014). For adults under 70 years, a BMI of 18.5–25kg/m^2 is considered healthy (NHS, n.d.). Unintentional weight loss should not be considered normal in people with dementia. If this occurs, it is recommended that advice is sought from a healthcare professional. If it is not possible to weigh the person, other signs of weight loss can include changes in physical appearance and clothes becoming looser. To help achieve energy requirements, *The Eatwell Guide* suggests basing meals on starchy carbohydrates. Examples include cereal or toast for breakfast, and pasta, rice, potatoes, yam or bread at lunch and dinner time. Energy-dense snacks, food fortification and nourishing drinks can also help to increase energy intake and can be useful for people who have a reduced appetite and/or are losing weight.

Protein – Protein is required for maintaining and growing new cells. It is recommended that older adults in particular consume enough protein to prevent muscle wasting. Protein foods include meat, fish, eggs, beans and pulses. Having protein as part of the meal at lunch and dinner can help to achieve requirements.

Fibre – Fibre can help to prevent constipation, and the recommendation for adults is 30g per day (Scientific Advisory Committee on Nutrition, 2015). Good sources of fibre for older adults include oats, wholegrain breakfast cereals, sandwiches made with wholemeal bread, fruit and vegetables, and vegetable- and pulse-based soups. In addition to fibre, fruit and vegetables also provide a range of vitamins and minerals. *The Eatwell Guide* recommends five portions of fruit/vegetables per day. However, this may not always be practical in people with dementia, especially as the condition progresses. Including fruit and vegetables at mealtimes and as snacks can help to achieve this.

Fluid – Ensuring the person with dementia is drinking enough can help to prevent dehydration, urinary tract infections, constipation and pressure sores. Adults should aim for six to eight 250ml cups of fluid per day. In addition to drinks, food items such as ice lollies, jelly and soup are good sources of fluid and can help individuals with dementia to meet their requirements.

Vitamin D – Reduced exposure to sunlight and decreased skin synthesis of vitamin D can increase risk of bone fractures and osteoporosis. All adults should consider taking 10ug vitamin D supplement during the autumn and winter months. If access to safe sunlight exposure is limited, a 10ug vitamin D daily supplement is recommended throughout the year (British Dietetic Association, 2019).

The Eatwell Guide also recommends including some dairy or dairy alternatives to help achieve calcium requirements. If using a plant-based milk, a variety fortified with calcium is preferable.

NICE guidelines (2006, 2012) advise a 'Food First' approach to prevent malnutrition. That is to say, nutritional requirements should ideally be met from food and drinks, rather than oral nutritional supplements. Practical ways to achieve this in people with dementia include:

- small, frequent meals
- snacks (e.g. full-fat yogurt, custard, rice pudding)
- finger foods (e.g. small sandwiches, pieces of cheese, small pieces of fruit)
- nourishing drinks (e.g. milk, milkshakes, hot chocolate, malted drinks)
- food fortification (e.g. adding milk, full-fat yogurt, cream, butter or cheese to meals)
- ready meals – easy preparation for individuals living independently
- encouragement to be active.

Oral nutritional supplements

If Food First approaches do not meet an individual's nutritional needs, oral nutritional supplements may be considered. These are available on prescription, and a dietitian can advise about these.

Learning point 2

Consider how people with dementia can be supported to meet their nutritional requirements.
   Examples include:

- nourishing drinks
- fortifying meals
- snacks between meals
- fluid in the form or drinks, ice lollies, jellies and soups
- including fruit, vegetables, protein, wholegrain cereals and dairy (or dairy alternatives) in their diet
- vitamin D supplements as appropriate.

Comorbidities

People with dementia may also have other health conditions that affect their nutritional requirements and intake, such as cancer, gastrointestinal issues and chronic obstructive pulmonary disease. Advice should be sought from a dietitian if someone with these conditions is finding eating and drinking difficult or is unintentionally losing weight.

There is substantial evidence linking dementia with increased risk of obesity, diabetes and heart disease. Dementia can impact on individuals' ability to follow a balanced diet. A diet high in total energy can lead to weight gain and obesity, increasing the risk of heart disease and diabetes (Public Health England, 2019).

People with dementia and diabetes can be at increased risk of hypoglycaemia (low blood sugar levels) if their meal pattern is irregular, meals are not evenly spaced, or they are not eating adequate amounts of carbohydrate foods. Conversely, there is risk of hyperglycaemia (high blood sugar levels) if they consume excessive foods and drinks containing added sugars and large portions of carbohydrate-rich foods. For some people with diabetes, dementia will mean they are less able to manage their diet themselves. Carers need to ensure that nutritional intake is appropriate to meet the individual's needs.

Learning point 3

Consider how the nutritional intake of a person with dementia may be affected by comorbidities. Does the nutritional intake need to be modified or adapted to meet nutritional needs?

Examples include:

- monitor signs of weight changes – are clothes fitting more tightly or loosely?
- encourage individuals to be active
- aim for a balanced diet as per *The Eatwell Guide*
- seek help from a dietitian if an individual is losing weight or finding it difficult to eat or drink
- support individuals with attending appointments regarding management of diabetes or other comorbidities.

Food planning, shopping and mealtimes

Dementia reduces the person's ability to undertake daily activities independently, such as shopping, cooking or food planning. As the disease progresses from mild to severe, daily tasks become increasingly challenging (NICE, 2018).

Shopping

Memory loss can affect routine tasks, particularly for those living independently. The person with dementia may no longer recognise local supermarkets or shops. They may forget preferred brands and usual foods. Carers can provide support by accompanying them to the supermarket or writing a shopping list with them and shopping for them. People can also be encouraged to shop in small stores and avoid large supermarkets. Some people with dementia may be able to manage online shopping, with assistance, if they tend to become distressed or confused at the supermarket.

Meal preparation

The ability to plan and prepare meals is likely to decline as dementia progresses. Meals that were once liked may no longer be enjoyed. Some people with dementia may revert to foods they preferred as a child. Caregivers could talk to family members to find out the person's food preferences. Regular chats with the person about preferred meals and favourite snacks will promote choice and independence. For those living independently, a pictorial chart can aid menu planning. Use of snacks and finger foods can help reduce safety issues with cooking and so promote independence.

Feeding

To help with eating, a regular meal pattern and routine to maintain continuity and ensure adequate time for feeding is recommended; a person's anxiety levels may increase if mealtimes are rushed. Where possible, self-feeding should also be encouraged to promote independence, and use of adapted cutlery can help with this. Use of plain plates can also be helpful as patterned crockery may increase confusion and anxiety. Drinks can be served in a clear drinking vessel to help monitor how much the person has drunk.

Learning point 4

Think about creative and practical ways to support people with dementia when going shopping. How might you encourage a calm and relaxed environment during mealtimes?

Examples include:

- go shopping with the person with dementia, or consider online shopping, with them if possible
- discuss food preferences with the individual and their family
- encourage a regular meal pattern and allow time for meals to be completed
- use clear drinking vessels and plain plates.

The role of the dietitian

Dietitians are qualified and registered health professionals who assess and treat dietary and nutritional problems. If a person living with dementia is losing or gaining weight, having difficulties with eating and drinking or requires dietary support due to other medical conditions, they can be referred to a dietitian. In the community, this may be someone who visits them at home or sees them as an outpatient at their GP practice or local hospital. The GP can make a referral. If the person is in hospital, they can usually be referred by a doctor or nurse on their ward to the hospital dietitian. Dietitians working in palliative and hospice care can also be involved with patients with dementia. The dietitian will carry out an assessment and provide a plan to optimise nutritional intake.

Speech and language therapists can also be involved with an individual's food and fluid intake. See Chapter 16 for further information.

Conclusion

Dementia is a progressive condition that, when coupled with the ageing process, can impact negatively on what a person eats and drinks and their general physical health. This chapter has discussed a range of nutritional issues that can occur in people who have dementia. These issues include, but are not limited to, poor or excessive food and fluid intake, inability to meet nutritional requirements, gastrointestinal issues, the management of comorbidities, and practical issues with regards to food preparation, food choice, food consumption, presentation of food and mealtimes.

Numerous factors can influence nutritional intake for people living with dementia, often in combination. This chapter also highlights the importance of staying alert to and addressing these issues and provides practical suggestions for supporting and encouraging people with dementia and their carers to maintain a healthy and, above all, enjoyable diet for as long as possible.

References

Alzheimer's Society. (2020). *Changes in eating habits and food preference.* www.alzheimers.org.uk/get-support/daily-living/changes-eating-habits-food-preference

British Dietetic Association. (2019). *Vitamin D: Food fact sheet.* www.bda.uk.com/resource/vitamin-d.html

Dos Santos, T.B.N., Fonseca, L.C., Tedrus, G.M.A.S. & Delbue, J.L. (2018). Alzheimer's disease: Nutritional status and cognitive aspects associated with disease severity. *Nutricion Hospitalaria, 35*(6), 1298–1304

Droogsma, E., van Asselt, D.Z.B., Schölzel-Dorenbos, C.J.M., van Steijn, J.H.M., van Walderveen, P.E. & van der Hooft, C.S. (2013). Nutritional status of community-dwelling elderly with newly diagnosed Alzheimer's disease: Prevalence of malnutrition and the relation of various factors to nutritional status. *The Journal of Nutrition, Health & Aging, 17*(7), 606–610.

Lea, E.J., Goldberg, L.R., Price, A.D., Tierney, L.T. & McInerney, F. (2017). Staff awareness of food and fluid care needs for older people with dementia in residential care: A qualitative study. *Journal of Clinical Nursing, 26*(23–24), 5169–5178.

Martin, M.A., Barrera Ortega, S., Dominguez Rodriguez, L., Couceiro Muiño, C., de Mateo, S.B. & del Rio, M.P.R. (2012). Presence of malnutrition and risk of malnutrition in institutionalized elderly with dementia according to the type and deterioration stage. *Nutricion Hospitalaria, 27*(2), 434–440.

NHS. (n.d.). What is the body mass index? www.nhs.uk/common-health-questions/lifestyle/what-is-the-body-mass-index-bmi/#:~:text=For%20most%20adults%2C%20an%20ideal,the%20 18.5%20to%2024.9%20range.

NICE. (2006). *Nutrition support for adults: Oral nutrition support, enteral tube feeding and parenteral nutrition.* Clinical guideline 32. NICE. www.nice.org.uk/guidance/cg32

NICE. (2012). *Quality standard for nutrition support in adults.* Quality standard 24. NICE. www.nice.org.uk/guidance/qs24

NICE. (2018). *Dementia: Assessment, management and support for people living with dementia and their carers*. NICE.

Public Health England (PHE). (2019). *Dementia: Comorbidities in patients: Data briefing*. Public Health England.

Public Health England, in association with the Welsh government, Food Standards Scotland and the Food Standards Agency in Northern Ireland. (2016). *The eatwell guide*. www.gov.uk/government/publications/the-eatwell-guide

Scientific Advisory Committee on Nutrition. (2015). *Carbohydrates and health*. The Stationery Office.

Tombini, M., Sicari, M., Pellegrino, G., Ursini, F., Insardá, P.P. & Di Lazzaro, V. (2016). Nutritional status of patients with Alzheimer's disease and their caregivers. *Journal of Alzheimer's Disease, 54*(4), 1619–1627.

Volkert, D. (2017). Nutrition in dementia. *Der Internist, 58*(2), 141–148.

Volkert, D., Chourdakis, M., Faxen-Irving, G., Frühwald, T., Landi, F., Suominen, M.H., Vandewoude, M., Wirth, R. & Schneider, S.M. (2015). ESPEN guidelines on dementia. *Clinical Nutrition, 34*(6), 1052–1073.

Wilson, K. & Dewing, J. (2020). Strategies to prevent dehydration in older people with dementia: A literature review. *Nursing Older People, 32*(1), 27–33.

Winter, J.E., MacInnis, R.J., Wattanapenpaiboon, N. & Nowson, C.A. (2014). BMI and all-cause mortality in older adults: A meta-analysis. *American Journal of Clinical Nutrition, 99*(4), 875–890.

16   I was finding it hard to eat and drink and got referred to speech and language therapy! What's that all about?

Dara Brown

Speech and language therapists (SLTs) work with people who have communication and swallowing difficulties. Our title is often a point of confusion, especially when people are referred for swallowing issues. In this chapter, we will discuss some of the main communication and swallowing difficulties that arise for people living with dementia, practical strategies for people with communication or swallowing difficulties and their carers, and when you might need to see an SLT for specialist assessment and advice.

When might I see a speech and language therapist?

SLTs work with people living with dementia in a range of different settings, from your own home to acute hospital wards. The sort of input you have from an SLT is likely to vary, depending on where you are seen. This is because the needs of a person living with dementia will change over time and may fluctuate, particularly when they are unwell.

In hospital, you are likely to be unwell, and eating, drinking and communicating may be more difficult than usual. With you, your family and your medical team, the SLT will plan how to best manage any swallowing difficulties. This will include thinking about the risks of eating and drinking; if and how quickly the medical team expect you to recover; and if you have currently, or previously, expressed views about what you would want if your swallow became unsafe. If you still need speech and language therapy when you are medically ready to leave hospital, you will be referred to a community SLT.

In the community, your SLT may see you at home, in a care home or in an outpatient clinic. Unlike in hospital, it is more likely that swallowing or communication difficulties will be linked to progression of the dementia rather than another illness. Changes may be long term, and this might affect your views on how you would like any swallowing difficulties to be managed.

Your SLT will talk to you, your family and your medical team (such as your GP or nurses in your care home) about what is normal for you and any recent changes. They may also help you with advance care planning – we will talk about this in more detail further on in the chapter.

For people experiencing communication difficulties early in dementia, there may be the opportunity to attend a communication support group or one-to-one session with a close family member or friend. This *conversation partner* training often focuses on understanding the communication strengths and difficulties in your pair and giving you both the skills to try to repair communication breakdowns when they happen.

How might dementia impact my swallowing?

All forms of dementia can impact on the ability to safely and effectively eat and drink, particularly in the advanced stages.

The medical term for difficulty swallowing is *dysphagia*. It has been estimated that 45% of people with dementia living in care homes will have some degree of dysphagia. One of the main reasons for this is probably the complexity of the swallowing mechanism itself.

The act of swallowing (moving food from the mouth to the stomach) involves 26 pairs of muscles moving in co-ordination. It can take as little as one second or more than a minute to complete. Different types of dementia impact swallowing differently, and this can change over time. Table 16.1 lists some of the more common difficulties associated with eating, drinking and swallowing that someone with dementia might experience.

Table 16.1: Difficulties with eating, drinking and swallowing in dementia

Sensory changes	• Changes in perception of taste, temperature and texture • Reduced sensation of food or drink in the mouth • Vision or hearing impairments make engaging in mealtimes more difficult
Motor changes	• Difficulty using utensils • Difficulty sitting upright during meals • Reduced strength or difficulty co-ordinating and sequencing the muscles used for chewing and swallowing
Cognitive changes	• Difficulty recognising foods or utensils • Not recognising thirst or hunger • Forgetting to eat, or that you have already eaten • Difficulty paying attention during meals
Oral hygiene changes	• Missing teeth or ill-fitting dentures make it difficult to chew and control food • Poor oral hygiene can cause infections or sores in the mouth. Pain may reduce inclination to eat • Excess bacteria in the mouth can result in chest infections for people with dysphagia

Neuro-psychiatric changes	• Low mood can reduce appetite and motivation to eat or drink • Rarely, some people with dementia may experience untrue beliefs – for example, that their food has been poisoned

The consequences of swallowing difficulties can be severe, particularly if not identified early. This includes malnutrition, dehydration, weight loss, and food or drink 'going down the wrong way' – called aspiration. Aspiration is the medical term for food, drink, saliva or medication dropping down into the lungs, rather than the stomach, and it can lead to a chest infection called aspiration pneumonia.

It is important that anybody supporting somebody with dementia to eat and drink can identify signs of aspiration (Table 16.2) and that they contact the GP if they are concerned.

Table 16.2: Signs of aspiration you might see

Immediate signs of aspiration	Long-term signs of aspiration
Coughing during or after swallowing Regular throat clearing when eating or drinking Gurgly voice when eating or drinking Pain or discomfort when swallowing Breathlessness during or after eating or drinking	Unexplained weight loss Regular chest infections Avoidance of food or drink

What might the options be if I have difficulty swallowing?

Food is not just vital for physical health; it is important to recognise the social and emotional value of eating. It is central to how many of us engage with others, from chatting over a cup of tea to sharing a celebratory meal.

When swallowing difficulties arise for a person living with dementia, an SLT will create a person-centred care plan, taking into account not just which foods they can manage safely but also the support and environmental changes that will help them to eat and drink as independently as possible (Table 16.3).

Often, simple adjustments such as reducing distractions during mealtimes can be enough to support somebody with dementia to concentrate, as it reduces the amount of information they have to process at once.

For people experiencing dysphagia, SLTs may recommend modifications to the texture of food or drink, such as softer or puréed foods to reduce the need for biting and chewing, or thickened drinks. This can reduce the risk of aspiration or choking.

However, modification of food and drinks does have possible limitations and downfalls, including reducing the enjoyment of meals, which may cause the person to eat or drink less overall. It is important that anybody experiencing dysphagia is assessed by an SLT and monitored by a dietitian.

For some people, even with strategies and modifications, there may still be a risk of aspiration. In these circumstances, the aim will be to make eating and drinking as comfortable, pleasurable and safe as possible.

Some people ask about tube feeding when swallowing difficulties occur. The current evidence shows that tube feeding does not improve (and may even worsen) outcomes for people living with dementia, including length and quality of life, developing aspiration pneumonia, and weight gain.

Therefore, careful handfeeding is usually the recommended option in the UK for people in the advanced stages of dementia.

Table 16.3: Strategies to support a person with eating, drinking or swallowing difficulties

Support strategies	• Reduce distractions during mealtimes – e.g. turn off the television/remove clutter from the table. Quiet music may be helpful • Eating meals together can support attention and prompt eating and drinking • If a person is having difficulty feeding themselves, try holding the cutlery with them, talk about which food they would like next, and go at their pace by checking when they have swallowed • Taste preferences may change; sweeter or stronger flavour foods may be enjoyed more
Equipment	• Adaptive cutlery, crockery and cups may be recommended by the SLT or occupational therapist • Plain coloured plates can help the person to identify foods (e.g. it may be difficult to see white fish on a white plate on a white tablecloth). Avoid patterns
Oral hygiene	• Daily mouth care is very important. Maintain usual routines, such as brushing teeth in the bathroom at a regular time
Positioning	• It is important that the person sits as upright as possible when eating, drinking or taking medications. Adapted seating may be required to support them to remain upright
Diet and fluid modification	• Foods that are easy to chew or moistened with sauce may help people with mild dysphagia • Some people may need to avoid higher-risk foods – e.g. tough meats, raw vegetables, nuts and sweets, or 'stringy' foods such as celery • Foods can be mashed or puréed to further reduce the need for chewing. Presentation should always be considered (avoid blending everything together into a mush) • SLTs may recommend drinks are thickened to make them easier to feel and control • Some medications can be given as liquids instead of tablets; talk to the GP or pharmacist about this

Learning point 1

Careful handfeeding is often recommended for people in the advanced stages of dementia. However, it is not something that many of us have experienced in adulthood. To help you understand what it feels like to be fed, you may want to try the following task with somebody you trust:

• Have somebody else feed you a meal.

- Think about the positioning and pace (e.g. Are you facing each other at eye level? Can you see what you are being fed? Do you feel in control of how much and how quickly you are being fed?).
- Is there anything that makes being fed more comfortable?

How might dementia impact my communication and how can people support me?

Communication refers to the exchange of information between people, through speech, writing, gesture and body language. Communication difficulties are a feature in all types of dementia.

Some types of dementia have a greater impact on communication early in the disease: these are the language-variant frontotemporal dementias, also called primary progressive aphasia (PPA). People with PPA are likely to require earlier SLT support.

Below are some of the most common communication changes associated with dementia.

Cognitive communication changes

Cognition, or thinking skills, such as attention, memory and understanding of social rules, are vital to help us engage effectively in social interactions. Difficulty with communication due to cognitive changes is called cognitive communication difficulties. Top tips to support somebody with cognitive communication difficulties include:

- Get the person's attention before talking to them.
- Reduce background distractions.
- Don't rush. Give one piece of information at a time. Break down instructions into small, manageable chunks.

Language changes

Dementia can disrupt the way we understand, process or use language. In the early stages of dementia, some people forget the names of items or people, or find it difficult to understand complex sentence structures. In the later stages, most people experience language difficulties and will rely on non-verbal communication. Emphasising touch, tone of voice and facial expressions can be particularly important to facilitate meaningful interactions without relying on words. Top tips to support somebody with language difficulties include:

- Avoid asking questions you know the answer to. Instead, make comments to stimulate conversation (e.g. rather than 'Who came to visit you today?' you could say, 'Jacquie came to visit you today, how was that?').

- If somebody is struggling to find a name for something, ask if they can describe it or show it to you (with words, gestures or objects).
- Check that you have both understood each other correctly.

Sensory changes

Many people with dementia also have sensory impairments, such as hearing or sight loss, and some may experience perceptual changes in the way their brain processes what they see, feel, or hear. Tips to support somebody with sensory changes include:

- Ensure glasses, hearing aids and dentures are well-fitting. Keep prescriptions up to date where possible and ensure batteries in hearing aids are changed regularly.
- Avoid excessive background noise and highly patterned surfaces, such as elaborate tablecloths.
- Face each other when talking.

As language skills decline, a person may express their needs through behaviour rather than words. Considering the meaning behind a person's actions may help to de-escalate any challenges and improve relationships and quality of life for the person and their carers. For example, becoming upset or angry when getting dressed may suggest the person is feeling scared, embarrassed or out of control. Support understanding and independence by keeping calm and giving simple instructions or asking them to complete small steps themselves.

Non-verbal communication, such as body language and facial expression, is a core part of communication and is especially important for somebody with language difficulties. Carers may need to anticipate a person's needs, as well as find ways of engaging that do not rely on language, such as touch, smell, pictures, objects and music.

Learning point 2

For a person experiencing difficulties with language or cognition, it may be difficult to process all the environmental, non-verbal and verbal information needed to communicate effectively. Next time you have a conversation think about:

- The environment – what are the background noises? Can you easily see the person you are talking to? Are there distractions?
- The non-verbal communication – what facial expressions, body language, gestures and objects are you using to help communicate?
- The verbal communication – who is doing most of the talking? Are you giving each other enough time to think and respond? If giving instructions, are these broken down into manageable chunks?

What decisions might I need to make and how can SLT help me?

We all make choices every day – from what to wear or eat to larger decisions about medical treatment, finances or where to live. The law protects an individual's right to make decisions for themselves. This is called 'mental capacity'.

The principles of mental capacity are set out in UK law in England and Wales under the Mental Capacity Act 2005 (different Acts apply in Scotland and Northern Ireland). This defines mental capacity as the ability to do four things:

- understand the information relevant to a particular decision
- retain that information for long enough to make the decision
- weigh up the information
- communicate their decision.

People living with dementia are likely to experience times where they have difficulty making an informed decision. SLTs play an important role in helping people with communication difficulties understand information and communicate their choices. This might include providing information in an accessible format – for example, writing down key points or using pictures to help them understand and remember the important parts of discussions.

In the advanced stages of dementia, most people will experience communication difficulties. It can therefore be helpful for carers and healthcare professionals to know a person's wishes regarding routines, preferences, living situation and medical treatments. Having these discussions early will allow you to express what is important to you. This can be done informally (through discussion with somebody you trust, such as a relative or healthcare professional) or formally (including in an advance care plan or appointing a Lasting Power of Attorney (see Chapters 4, 12 and 13).

Learning point 3

To help with advance care planning, you may want to help the person with dementia consider what their preferences would be if they experience dysphagia. Below are some key questions that you might discuss with them:

- Are there any foods, drinks, or routines that are particularly important to you?
- Would you want to try modified foods or thickened drinks if they were more comfortable or safer for you?
- How would you feel about short-term tube feeding if your swallowing deteriorated when unwell with a reversible condition (such as an infection)?

Conclusion

For most people living with dementia, communication and swallowing difficulties are likely to be a part of their journey. SLTs advocate for those with dementia, ensuring that communication skills are optimised, and that eating and drinking remains dignified, pleasurable, and as safe as possible.

Further reading

The following publications explore the above issues in more detail:

Kindell, J. (2002). *Feeding and swallowing disorders in dementia.* Speechmark Publishing Ltd.

National Institute for Health and Care Excellence (NICE). (2018). *Dementia: Assessment, management and support for people living with dementia and their carers* (NG97). NICE. www.nice.org.uk/guidance/ng97

Rahman, S. & Howard, R. (2018). *Essentials of dementia: Everything you really need to know for working in dementia care.* Jessica Kingsley Publishers.

Royal College of Physicians and British Society of Gastroenterology. (2010). *Oral feeding difficulties and dilemmas: A guide to practical care, particularly towards the end of life.* Royal College of Physicians.

Royal College of Speech and Language Therapists. (2014). *Speech and language therapy provision for people with dementia: RCSLT Position Paper.* RCSLT.

Sura, L., Madhavan, A., Carnaby, G. & Crary, M. (2012). Dysphagia in the elderly: Management and nutritional considerations. *Clinical Interventions in Aging, 7,* 287–298.

Teno, J., Gozalo, P., Mitchell, S., Kuo, S., Rhodes, R., Bynum, J. & Mor, V. (2012). Does feeding tube insertion and its timing improve survival? *Journal of the American Geriatrics Society, 60*(10), 1918–1921.

Ticinesi, A., Nouvenne, A., Lauretani, F., Prati, B., Cerundolo, N., Maggio, M. & Meschi, T. (2016). Survival in older adults with dementia and eating problems: To PEG or not to PEG? *Clinical Nutrition, 35*(6), 1512–1516.

Volkmer. A. (2013). *Assessment and therapy for language and cognitive communication difficulties in dementia and other progressive diseases.* J&R Press.

Volkmer, A., Spector, A., Meitanis, V., Warren, J.D. & Beeke, S. (2019). Effects of functional communication interventions for people with primary progressive aphasia and their caregivers: a systematic review. *Aging & Mental Health, 24*(9), 1381–1393.

17 Alternative treatments for insomnia for people with dementia and mild cognitive impairment

Lisa Austin

Dementia leads to a number of challenges, including behaviour and mood changes. Although most people connect dementia with memory problems, it can also lead to significant sleep problems, with up to half of those with dementia being affected (Zeitzer et al., 2010). Typically, this involves wandering at night, and this is a leading reason for people with dementia being admitted into care homes. Some 70% of people with dementia in care homes have sleep problems (Webster et al., 2020).

How does dementia affect sleep?

As we get older, our ability to sleep well declines. However, the changes to sleep with dementia go far beyond what we expect with age and can actually be one of the first clinical signs of the disease. Sleep disturbance can lead to accidents around the home, including falls. These falls can be very serious, especially at night when the lights are off. Many people with dementia are admitted to A&E departments with a broken or dislocated hip, having fallen at night. A significant number are never able to return home.

People with mild to moderate cognitive impairment (MCI) also suffer from poor sleep. In fact, this is more significant in people with MCI than those with dementia – up to 60% of those with MCI are affected (Guarnieri et al., 2012). This has a negative impact – waking at night leads to poorer functioning the next day, and poorer learning, and this actually worsens the memory problems that go with people's cognitive impairment.

In general, a lack of sleep has been found to impact on the immune system, and this is linked to depression and anxiety. Lack of sleep is also associated with weight gain, which can lead to obesity and diabetes. This is particularly problematic in stroke-related (vascular) dementia, as those with this condition are already at risk of developing the condition.

Caring for people with dementia, especially with the added factor of insomnia, can be very wearing, as the carers' disrupted sleep and constant vigilance leads them to be too tired to function.

Learning point 1

- If an elderly person in your family is waking up a lot, getting out of bed in the night and is confused, this could be one of the first signs of dementia. Make an appointment with your doctor if you are concerned.

- Encourage the person with dementia to adopt a regular routine of going to bed at the same time and getting up at the same time.

- If a loved one is waking at night, you could try using a clock by the bed with an LED display, so that they can see the time when they wake up. Try to persuade the person to go back to bed.

- To make the home safe, you could leave a light on in the hallway and toilet and use a nightlight in the bedroom. Make sure that you remove any potential trip hazards, such as a table that might get in their way.

- If light is getting into the room, use black-out curtains to keep it dark and suitable for sleeping. Make sure the temperature is comfortable for sleeping and the person is not too cold or too hot.

- Try things that soothe, such as a warm bath before bed or a soft toy to cuddle.

Sleep disturbance and dementia

One of the most common complaints among older adults and those with dementia is maintaining sleep. Other sleep problems in dementia include 'sundowning' – increased confusion, anxiety, agitation, pacing and disorientation that starts at sunset and continues throughout the night. It is thought that the organic process of dementia may damage the part of the brain that controls circadian rhythms and lead to the release of melatonin, which in turn leads to increased disruption of sleep at night and napping in the day.

It is important to rule out other medical causes of insomnia, such as pain. The issue of pain in dementia is difficult to resolve if the person with dementia cannot communicate it (see Chapter 13). Restless leg syndrome, sleep apnoea and respiratory problems, which often occur with vascular dementia and Alzheimer's disease, can all lead to sleep disturbance too.

Various methods are used for measuring sleep. Polysomnography was first developed in the 1960s. This technique is still used today to monitor sleep cycles, and is generally considered to be the gold standard for confirming sleep disorders, such as sleep apnoea. This method studies the stages of sleep through physiological signals. Typically, wires are attached to the head via a skull cap, which is worn overnight. However, polysomnography can be uncomfortable for some people and therefore is not always suitable for people living with cognitive impairment and dementia. In addition, it requires the person to have the test at a laboratory, where participants may not feel at home or behave naturally. For this reason, actigraphy is preferred as a measure for those with dementia.

Actigraphy involves the use of wrist-worn activity monitors, which look like watches. They record activity over long periods. This method has been shown to work as well as polysomnography, and has been used successfully in dementia research studies, as it is flexible, comfortable and works well in a home setting.

Sleep diaries have also been used successfully with people with dementia, but they may need carer input to ensure they are completed reliably. Diaries are advantageous as they allow researchers an insight into subjective factors, as well as objective data, and also allow the participant to state any problems and issues that might not emerge otherwise.

Learning point 2

A sleep diary can be used to monitor sleep and can be a useful way of seeing which treatments work best for the person concerned. Below is an example of a sleep diary that can be used – just copy your own version on a piece of paper. The diaries include a question about common illnesses or other disruptions that could affect sleep.

If a person's sleep is affected by external factors, the treatment should be tried again when they are better, as it is not a fair test. It is best to try each treatment over two to three days to see if it seems to be working.

Sleep diary

Date:
Treatment tried [e.g. aromatherapy]:
What time did you go to bed?
What time did you go to sleep?
What time did you wake up?
What time did you get up?
Comments: Please write down below if you got up in the night, what time this occurred and how long it was before you went back to bed. Also, please record any events that may affect your sleep, such as illness, surprising news and so forth.
N.B. All information will be kept strictly confidential.

Treatments for insomnia

The most common treatments for insomnia in the UK, including for people with dementia, are drugs – typically benzodiazepines. However, the British National Formulary guidelines state that: 'Patients should be offered non-drug treatment approaches to manage sleep problems and insomnia, including sleep hygiene education, exposure to daylight, and increasing exercise and activity.'[1]

The NICE guidelines on dementia (2018) similarly advise:

> For people living with dementia who have sleep problems, consider a personalised multicomponent sleep management approach that includes sleep hygiene education, exposure to daylight, exercise and personalised activities.

Likewise, the Alzheimer's Society recommends on its website:

> Most experts and the National Institutes of Health (NIH) strongly encourage use of non-drug measures rather than medication.
> Studies have found that sleep medications generally do not improve overall sleep quality for older adults. Use of sleep medications is associated with a greater chance of falls and other risks that may outweigh the benefits of treatment.[2]

Previous benzodiazepine use is of itself thought to be connected with onset of dementia, although the literature is contested: there are studies evidencing either way (see, for example, Gray et al., 2016). However, sedatives such as benzodiazepines carry the risk of 'hangover effects', such as day-time sleepiness and a consequent increase in confusion, risk of falls and injury, cognitive decline and an overall detrimental impact on quality of life, wellbeing and social interaction (Ballard & Fossey, 2008). In addition, their chemical properties make the accumulation of the drug more likely in older people, especially when combined with other medications and if the person has multiple illnesses.

More attention is now being paid to non-medical ways of aiding sleep in people with dementia. Research with people at risk of dementia shows that those who already undertake regular physical activity report better sleep (Saks et al., 2018). Those who do less physical activity have poorer sleep, are more likely to be depressed and overweight, and have more medical conditions. This study suggests the importance of physical activity due to its benefits for health. To tackle sleep disturbance, some researchers have aimed to increase the daily activity of those with dementia, to improve both efficiency and length of sleep during the night. Other care homes try to tackle the sedentary nature of care-home life by avoiding day-time naps and arranging activities and trips out (please see Part 4 of this book). Structure is thought to be helpful in maintaining healthy sleep patterns.

---

1. https://bnf.nice.org.uk/treatment-summaries/dementia
2. www.alz.org/alzheimers-dementia/treatments/for-sleep-changes

Other researchers have tried to change people's sleep habits. Sleep hygiene is an important element of treatment in a sleep clinic. Patients are encouraged to adopt helpful behaviours, such as winding down before bed and having a pre-bedtime routine that is conducive to rest.

Medical engineering charities, such as Designability in Bath,[3] have worked on the development of technology to provide practical measures to assist those with dementia to improve their sleep regimes. For instance, the 'wanderer sensor' detects if an external door is opened during the night and prompts a voice message to urge the person with dementia to go back to bed, reminding them that it is night-time.

Cognitive behaviour therapy for insomnia, known as CBT-I (Kyle et al., 2015), has also been found to be helpful for some people living with mild cognitive impairment and early dementia. In practice, the focus should be on behavioural aspects, such as maintaining a regular time to get up and go to bed, rather than avoiding negative thought traps.

Light therapy, or phototherapy, consists of exposure to bright light, which stimulates the brain and releases melatonin, thereby influencing the sleep cycles. Bright light therapy has been shown to improve sleep for people living with dementia in a care home; controls who did not have the therapy did not show this improvement (Lyketsos et al., 1999). However, all light therapy research to date has involved small numbers and it is therefore not possible to draw firm conclusions from the findings.

It is accepted that the hormone melatonin, produced by the pineal gland in the brain, plays a significant part in the sleep/wake cycle (Sack et al., 2000). Research has shown that melatonin is helpful in aiding sleep in healthy adults. Studies testing melatonin on people with dementia have had mixed results. One research study with people with dementia (Asayama et al., 2003) found that melatonin improved the ability to fall asleep, prolonged sleep and reduced waking at night. However, the NICE guidelines (2018) advise against the use of melatonin with people with Alzheimer's disease, and this is supported in a Cochrane review of a range of medicines for sleep problems in this group (McCleery & Sharpley, 2020).

It is possible that alternative therapies may offer effective and well-tolerated ways to address insomnia for those living with dementia. Aromatherapy is an ancient therapy dating back to 3000 bce and involves the distillation of essential oils believed to have medicinal benefits for the brain, mind and body. The oils can be introduced in a number of ways, including in baths, massages and vaporisation.

Controlled aromatherapy research has found mild benefits for insomnia from lavender oil (Lewis et al., 2005). In the four-week study, insomnia reports were moderately reduced as measured by the Pittsburgh Sleep Quality Index. No side effects were observed. Other studies with stronger scientific rigour confirm the modest benefits of lavender treatment. For example, Goel et al. (2005) found that lavender increased deep sleep in 31 healthy adults. All reported more energy the next day.

---

3. https://designability.org.uk

Aromatherapy treatment has also been shown to be effective in reducing agitation in those living with dementia in care homes. Oils used include lavender, sweet marjoram, patchouli and vetiver. A Japanese study (Takeda, 2017) successfully treated elderly people with dementia in a care home with essential oils – lavender, Japanese cypress and cedar wood. The researchers found that those on the treatment slept longer and woke early less often than they did when they were not using the oils.

In another study, conducted by a team at the University of Bath (Austin, 2015), Melissa essential oil increased sleep time with people with dementia and mild cognitive impairment. Treatment was one drop of Melissa oil administered to the bedclothes at night over two nights, by the person's partner or carer. The comparison was two nights using a base massage oil, which was assumed to have no effect on sleep, and two nights of no treatment. With Melissa oil, the sleep time was on average 45 minutes longer than with no treatment.

Learning point 3

- Some people may respond better to certain treatments than others. It is worth trying several treatments and even combining them.
- Make sure that the person has plenty of daylight and things to do during the day so they do not nap, as this will disturb their night-time sleep.
- Try gentle exercise – it seems to help.
- If you can, take the person outside. The extra sunlight will help keep sleep regulated. If you cannot do this, consider investing in a light box that you can put on from time to time when the person is close by.

Conclusion

Sleep disorders are a significant problem for people with dementia and mild cognitive impairment but are poorly understood and often go unrecognised. This leads to a huge burden, both on those that suffer disrupted sleep and on their carers. While drug treatments are often favoured, they are not recommended in national guidelines. Given the complexity of dementia, single-component interventions are often considered to be too simplistic. Instead, combined approaches are recommended. Research indicates that light therapy, activity, technology, aromatherapy and sleep hygiene practice deliver improvements in sleep for people living with dementia. Complementary non-medical approaches that take into account other factors and address quality of life are increasingly being explored and found helpful.

There is an urgent need for suitable therapies, particularly for those with long-term insomnia and those who are vulnerable to any drug-related impairment or affected by co-morbidities and for whom medication is not advised due to potential interactions. The therapeutic need is growing, given the increased number of people in the community with dementia. People with dementia and cognitive impairment have a right to choices that will enable them to live well.

References

Asayama, K., Yamadera, H., Ito, T., Suzuki, H., Kudo, Y. & Endo, S. (2003). Double blind study of melatonin effects on the sleep-wake rhythm, cognitive and non-cognitive functions in Alzheimer type dementia. *Journal of Nippon Medical School, 70*(4), 334–341.

Austin, L. (2015). *Balanced, cross over, single blind designed trial to assess whether Melissa essential oil is an effective treatment for insomnia for people with dementia and mild cognitive impairment.* Unpublished thesis. University of Bath. https://researchportal.bath.ac.uk/en/studentTheses/balanced-cross-over-single-blind-designed-trial-to-assess-whether

Ballard, C. & Fossey, J. (2008). Clinical management of dementia. *Psychiatry, 7*(2), 88–93.

Goel, N., Hyungsoo, K. & Lao, R. (2005). An olfactory stimulus modifies nighttime sleep in young men and women. *Chronobiology International, 22*(5), 889–904.

Gray, S.L., Dublin, S., Yu, O., Walker, R., Anderson, M., Hubbard, R.A., Crane, P.K. & Larson, E.B. (2016). Benzodiazepine use and risk of incident dementia or cognitive decline: Prospective population-based study. *British Medical Journal, 352*, i90. doi: 10.1136/bmj.i90.

Guarnieri, B., Adorni, F., Musicco, M., Appollonio, I., Bonanni, E., Caffarra, P., Caltagirone, C., Cerroni, G., Concari, L., Cosentino, F. I.I., Ferrara, S., Fermi, S., Ferri, R., Gelosa, G., Lombardi, G., Mazzei, D., Mearelli, S., Morrone, E., Murri, L., Nobili, F. M., Passero, S., Perri, R., Rocchi, R., Sucapane, P., Tognoni, G., Zabberoni, S. & Sorbi, S. (2012). Prevalence of sleep disturbance in mild cognitive impairment and dementia disorders: A multi-centred Italian cross-sectional study on 431 patients. *Dementia and Geriatric Cognitive Disorders, 33*(1), 50–58.

Kyle, S.D., Aquino, M.R.J., Miller, C.B., Henry, A.L., Crawford, M.R., Espie, C.A. & Spielman, A. J. (2015). Towards standardisation and improved understanding of sleep restriction therapy for insomnia disorder: A systematic examination of CBT-I trial content. *Sleep Medicine Reviews, 23*, 83–88.

Lewis, G.T., Godfrey, A.D. & Prescott, P. (2005). A single-blinded, randomized pilot study evaluating the aroma of lavender augustifolia as a treatment for mild insomnia. *Journal of Alternative and Complementary Medicine, 11*(4), 631–637.

Lyketsos, C.S., Lindell Veiel, L., Baker, A. & Steele, C. (1999). A randomised controlled trial of bright light therapy for agitated behaviours in dementia patients residing in long-term care. *International Journal of Geriatric Psychiatry, 14*(7), 520–525.

McCleery, J. & Sharpley, A.L. (2020, November 15). Pharmacotherapies for sleep disturbances in dementia. *Cochrane Database of Systematic Reviews.* https://doi.org/10.1002/14651858.CD009178.pub4

NICE. (2018). *Dementia: Assessment, management and support for people living with dementia and their carers.* NG97. NICE.

Sack R.L., Brandes, R.W., Kendall, A.R. & Lewy, A J. (2000). Entrainment of free-running circadian rhythms by melatonin in blind people. *New England Journal of Medicine, 343*(15), 1070–1077.

Saks, D., Naismith, S.L., Lamonica, H., Mowszowski, L., Pye, J., Lewis, S.J.G., Hickie, I., Grunstein, R. & Duffy, S.L. (2018). Understanding the relationship between physical activity, depressive symptoms and sleep quality in older adults at-risk for dementia. *Alzheimer's & Dementia, 14*(7S), 592. DOI:10.1016/j.jalz.2018.06.665

Takeda, A., Watanuki, E. & Koyama, S. (2017). Effects of inhalation aromatherapy on symptoms of sleep disturbance in the elderly with dementia. *Evidence-based Complementary and Alternative Medicine, 2017*, ID: 1902807. https://doi.org/10.1155/2017/1902807

Webster, L., Costafreda Gonzalez, S., Stringer, A., Lineham, A., Budgett, J., Kyle, S., Barber, J. & Livingston, G. (2020). Measuring the prevalence of sleep disturbances in people with dementia living in care homes: A systematic review and meta-analysis. *Sleep, 43*(4). doi: 10.1093/sleep/zsz251

Zeitzer, D.J., Friedman, L., Noda, A., O'Hara, R., Robert, P. & Yesavage, J.A. (2010). Non-pharmacologic management of sleep disturbance in Alzheimer's disease. *Journal of Nutrition, Health and Aging, 14*(3), 203–206.

18   Being in hospital when you have dementia

Rachael Kelley

This chapter outlines the difficulties people living with dementia can experience if they are admitted to hospital and practical ways in which the person, families and hospital staff can counteract them. Strategies for improving care are discussed at three key stages: when the person is first admitted; during the hospital stay, and around discharge.

Experiences of hospital care for people living with dementia

Many people living with dementia will spend time in a general hospital during their dementia journey. Around a quarter of people in general hospitals have dementia (Sampson et al., 2009), making the care of people with dementia very much part of the work of hospital wards. Although most people will be admitted for a condition other than their dementia (Glover at al., 2014), having dementia is likely to have important impacts on their care needs.

Research exploring hospital care from the viewpoint of people living with dementia highlights how difficult hospital admissions can be (Dewing & Dijk, 2016). Unfamiliar environments, routines and people can be challenging to adapt to and, alongside physical illness, can make people feel more confused or upset than usual. People with dementia may also experience difficulties communicating with staff, maintaining self-care abilities, getting enough to eat and drink and decision-making. Families can also find the experience difficult and stressful (Beardon et al., 2018).

To counteract these difficulties, research has explored how hospital care for people with dementia and their families can be improved. Drawing on this, the following sections focus on what people living with dementia, families and staff can do to make hospital stays more positive.

While this includes a focus on what others can do, the person and their wishes should remain at the heart of any actions undertaken.

When someone living with dementia is first admitted to hospital

What can people living with dementia and families do?

- **Share the person's dementia diagnosis and care needs**

A crucial first step when someone living with dementia is admitted to hospital is ensuring staff know the person has dementia, so that their needs can be met accordingly. Do not assume that a dementia diagnosis will be shared with the hospital or between wards; this is not always the case and symptoms of dementia may not always be recognised by staff (Jackson et al., 2017).

As dementia affects people differently, it is also important that staff understand how the person is impacted and their needs. Many hospitals have a form you can use to share information about someone with dementia to help staff provide better care, including information about likes and dislikes, communication preferences, usual care routines, signs of pain or distress, and what helps them relax. If you are not offered one of these forms, you could ask for one or download one called 'This is me' from the Alzheimer's Society website.[1]

- **Involve families and people living with dementia**

People with dementia and their families report more positive experiences of hospital care when they feel more involved (Bridges et al., 2010). There is growing recognition of the importance of continuing supportive relationships between people with dementia and their families during hospital stays (Beardon et al., 2018; Kelley et al., 2019). If both the person and their family want this, family members should ask how they can be involved, or look for posters/leaflets explaining the options.

Ways to get involved include information-sharing, shared decision-making and, for families, providing social or practical support (e.g. during mealtimes or assessments) (Kelley et al., 2019; Morrow & Nicholson, 2016). Support for families can include open visiting (sometimes via a 'carers passport'), free/concessionary parking, refreshment, overnight facilities and support services (NHS Improvement, 2017). Experiences can vary (Kelley et al., 2019) – in some hospitals you may need to proactively pursue your involvement. It is also important that the level of family involvement does not unintentionally override the needs or wishes of the person (Kelley et al., 2019; NHS Improvement, 2017).

What can staff and hospitals do?

- **Recognise dementia and the person's care needs**

As highlighted above, identifying when someone has dementia is a crucial step in determining their care needs (Dewing & Dijk, 2016). Routine cognitive assessments are recommended to reduce the under-detection of dementia in general hospitals (Jackson et al., 2017) and should form a standard part of initial conversations and assessments with the person and their family. If these reveal diagnosed or suspected dementia, a conversation should take place with the person and their family about

---

1. www.alzheimers.org.uk/get-support/publications-factsheets/this-is-me

their needs and how they can be met. This could include asking them to complete a form providing personal information to inform the person's care (e.g. the 'This is me' form mentioned above). Diagnosed or suspected dementia, and any resulting care needs, should be clearly documented in hospital records and care plans.

- *Seek early engagement with the person and their family*

Early engagement with the person, their family, and other regular supporters (e.g. community/care home services) is a vital part of identifying the person's needs and wishes and incorporating them into their care (Dementia Action Alliance, 2018; Kelley et al., 2019; Morrow & Nicholson, 2016; Moyle et al., 2008; NHS Improvement, 2017). Conversations should take place with the person and their family about how they could be involved to ensure involvement opportunities are clear and mutually agreed (Kelley et al., 2019). Families can be involved in a variety of invaluable ways (described earlier) and some hospitals in the UK have committed to involving families via John's Campaign.[2] Staff should ensure that they are familiar with the arrangements and resources their hospital has in place to support family involvement and convey this information to people with dementia and their families.

Learning point 1

Before reading further, you may like to consider the following questions, or ask them of the person with dementia you are supporting:

- How do you feel about being in hospital? Do you have any worries or concerns?
- What could be difficult about being in hospital for you?
- What might help?

During the hospital stay

What can people living with dementia and families do?

- *Keep conversations flowing*

Staff should continue to involve the person and their family as much as possible throughout the hospital stay. It is important to keep sharing information between you all, so that everyone is kept up to date. Conversations about how things are going can also help to spot and address any difficulties or misunderstandings early on. If at any point you feel less involved than you would like to be, or are unsure of what is happening, you should speak to a member of staff.

A hospital stay is a big disruption to familiar routines, activities and people. Keeping those connections going through visits and by continuing activities or

---

2. https://johnscampaign.org.uk/#/

routines that are feasible in hospital is important (Kelley et al., 2019). Having personal items (e.g. family photographs, a favourite blanket, familiar clothes, books, newspapers, music or hobbies) may provide comfort and activity and stimulate conversation with visitors and staff (Moyle et al., 2008). Ensuring the person has any glasses and hearing aids that they use with them, and that staff are aware of this and know where they are stored, will also help the person to communicate and feel more comfortable (Moyle et al., 2008).

If the person seems more confused than usual at any point during their stay, it is important to let staff know. This could be a sign that the person has delirium (short-term confusion on top of their dementia), which can be treated. Similarly, if the person appears to be in pain or more unwell in any other way, it is important to make the staff aware.

What can staff and hospitals do?

- *Provide person-centred and relationship-centred care*

Guidance is available on how to provide high quality hospital care for people living with dementia and their families (e.g. Dementia Action Alliance, 2018). The cornerstone of this is person-centred care. This includes ensuring care needs (such as personal care, mobility, eating, drinking, sleeping, continence, pain control, social interaction, activity and emotional wellbeing) are met, with close attention to the person's preferences, usual routines and independence levels wherever possible (Dementia Action Alliance, 2018; Dewing & Dijk, 2016).

Relationship-focused care is highly valued by people living with dementia and their families and seen as fundamental to good quality hospital care (Bridges et al., 2010). This highlights the importance of good communication and relationship-building with the person and their family (Dewing & Dijk, 2016; Turner et al., 2017). Finding and using opportunities to interact during busy shifts (e.g. during tasks or when passing the person's bed) is important (Kelley et al., 2019). This is where knowing something about the person (from previous conversations or a 'This is me'-type document) creates valuable shortcuts to meaningful conversations. Knowing what helps someone relax, or their favourite hobbies or conversation topics is also invaluable when someone is anxious or distressed (Dewing & Dijk, 2016). Group activities (such as eating together or reminiscence groups) can maximise opportunities to support several people.

Regular communication with the person and their family will ensure everyone is kept up to date. Continuing to involve families as partners in care and support for their needs remains crucial, particularly as hospital admissions can increase families' physical and emotional difficulties (Beardon et al., 2018). Continuity of staff and wards is also important, for all the reasons above.

- *Provide dementia training for staff and volunteers*

Sufficient staffing levels and skill mix are required to delivery high quality dementia care (Dementia Action Alliance, 2018; Jackson et al., 2017). Hospitals should ensure all staff have good quality dementia training (Dementia Action Alliance, 2018;

NHS Improvement, 2017). Training should equip all staff to understand dementia and its symptoms, to communicate with people with dementia and their families, to recognise and respond to distressed behaviour as expressions of unmet need and to understand issues such as capacity, informed consent and best-interests decision-making (Dementia Action Alliance, 2018; Handley et al., 2017; Moyle et al., 2008; NHS Improvement, 2017).

- *Promote delirium awareness*

Training should include delirium (acute confusion) awareness and staff should monitor for signs of delirium, which is common in people with dementia and has multiple negative outcomes (Jackson et al., 2017). Recognising delirium alongside dementia can be difficult; delirium-specific assessments (e.g. the CAM or 4AT (Jackson et al., 2017)) or asking families about the person's normal cognitive state may help. Delirium prevention and treatment includes encouraging hydration, nutrition, mobilisation, social interaction and orientation, which family members or volunteers could support.

- *Provide specialist staff, services and leadership*

Leadership around dementia care is also key to improving care. 'Dementia champions' can model high quality care, advocate good practice and provide advice and support (Dementia Action Alliance, 2018; Handley et al., 2017; NHS Improvement, 2017). Specialist services, such as dementia or liaison psychiatry teams, can also be beneficial. These teams provide training, assessment and support on hospital wards, resulting in increased cognitive assessment and diagnosis rates and greater staff confidence in caring for people with dementia (Dewing & Dijk, 2016; Handley et al., 2017). Specialist wards offering medical and psychosocial care (via specialist staff, environments and a focus on person-centred care and activities) also provide benefits, including reduced falls and agitation and improved staff–patient interactions and carer satisfaction (Dewing & Dijk, 2016). Trained volunteers can offer valuable input (e.g. social interaction or mealtime assistance) (Dewing & Dijk, 2016). All these roles can be challenging and must be well supported (Dewing & Dijk, 2016).

- *Provide dementia-friendly environments*

Busy, confusing environments can compound the difficulties people with dementia experience in hospital. Hospitals should use dementia-friendly design features, such as good lighting, clearly written and pictorial signage, easy sight of clocks and calendars, colour and distinguishing features to promote wayfinding, removal of unnecessary clutter, and spaces that promote activity and interaction (Jackson et al., 2017; Moyle et al., 2008; NHS Improvement, 2017). Dementia-friendly hospital environment guides (e.g. The King's Fund, 2020; Dementia Services Development Centre, 2013) can inform environmental improvements, many of which will benefit all hospital users. Environmental adaptations that support families (e.g. refreshment and social or overnight areas) are also important (Dewing & Dijk, 2016).

> **Learning point 2**
>
> Before reading further, you may like to consider the following questions or ask them of the person living with dementia you are supporting:
>
> - How is the admission going so far?
> - Are you happy with the care being provided?
> - Do you feel involved enough in what is happening?
>
> If the answers to any of these questions is negative, you should discuss your concerns with the ward staff.

Towards the end of a hospital stay

What can people living with dementia and families do?

- *Ensure you are involved in decision-making*

Hopefully you will have been involved throughout the hospital stay in discussions and decisions about discharge and what will happen afterwards. If you do not feel well informed or involved, then let someone know. It is very important that people with dementia as well as their families are involved in decision-making wherever possible (Kelley et al., 2021). Many people living with dementia can make or contribute to decisions about their care and should be encouraged and supported to do so. Others may require someone, often family members, to do this on their behalf. Families can either be appointed informally or formally (via a Lasting Power of Attorney) to make decisions on behalf of someone lacking capacity to make a particular decision – their role being to understand the person's preferences and determine which decision is in their best interests. Advance directives setting out someone's wishes should they lose capacity can also be helpful (see Chapter 12).

What can staff and hospitals do?

- *Ensure you involve the person with dementia and their family in decision-making*

As described above, it is important to actively involve people living with dementia and their families in decision-making. Early discussions are vital to ensuring discharge planning considers the needs and priorities of all involved (Dementia Action Alliance, 2018; Jackson et al., 2017; Kelley et al., 2021). Particular attention should be given to involving people with dementia wherever possible (Kelley et al., 2021). This includes holding discussions and presenting information in ways that meet the person's communication needs (Bridges et al., 2010). Time and care can be required to make more complex decisions, to ensure risks are balanced against quality of life and assimilate any differing opinions between families, the person and/or staff (Kelley et al., 2021, Jackson et al., 2017). If someone's ability to make an informed decision appears reduced, a decision-specific capacity assessment may be required. Finally, before discharge, it is important that everyone involved (including community services and families providing post-discharge care) is informed and understands the discharge and post-discharge arrangements.

Learning point 3

Finally, you may like to consider the following questions or ask them of the person living with dementia you are supporting:

- Have you been involved in decision-making and discharge planning?
- Do you understand the discharge plans?
- Do you feel happy with the decisions being made?

If any of the answers are 'no', you should discuss your concerns with the ward staff.

Conclusion

Admission to hospital can be confusing for anyone. For people with dementia, the disruption, confusion and potential for distress may be much greater. Hospital care can be improved for people living with dementia in a range of ways. A combination of approaches is likely to produce the best results. People with dementia and their families should be involved as much as possible, and in accordance with their preferences, throughout the hospital stay.

References

Beardon, S., Patel, K., Davies, B. & Ward, H. (2018). Informal carers' perspectives on the delivery of acute hospital care for patients with dementia: A systematic review. *BMC Geriatrics, 18,* 23.

Bridges, J. Flatley, M. & Meyer, J. (2010). Older people's and relatives' experiences in acute care settings: Systematic review and synthesis of qualitative studies. *International Journal of Nursing Studies, 47,* 89–107.

Dementia Action Alliance. (2018). *Dementia-friendly hospital charter.* Dementia Action Alliance.

Dementia Services Development Centre. (2013). *Virtual hospital.* Dementia Services Development Centre.

Dewing, J. & Dijk, S. (2016). What is the current state of care for older people with dementia in general hospitals? A literature review. *Dementia, 15*(1), 106–124.

Glover, A., Bradshaw, L.E., Watson, N., Laithwaite, E., Goldberg, S.E., Whittamore, K.H. & Harwood, R.H. (2014). Diagnoses, problems and healthcare interventions amongst older people with an unscheduled hospital admission who have concurrent mental health problems: A prevalence study. *BMC Geriatrics, 14,* 43. doi: 10.1186/1471-2318-14-43

Handley, M., Bunn, F. & Goodman, C. (2017). Dementia-friendly interventions to improve the care of people living with dementia admitted to hospitals: A realist review. *BMJ Open.* doi:10.1136/bmjopen-2016-015257

Jackson, T.A., Gladman, J.R.F., Harwood, R.H., MacLullich, A.M.J., Sampson, E.L., Sheehan, B. & Davis D.H.J. (2017). Challenges and opportunities in understanding dementia and delirium in the acute hospital. *PLoS Medicine, 14*(3), e1002247. doi:10.1371/journal.pmed.1002247

Kelley, R., Godfrey, M. & Young, J. (2019). The impacts of family involvement on general hospital care experiences for people living with dementia: An ethnographic study. *International Journal of Nursing Studies, 96*, 72–81.

Kelley, R., Godfrey, M. & Young, J. (2021). Knowledge exchanges and decision-making within hospital dementia care triads: An ethnographic study. *The Gerontologist, 61*(6), 954–964.

King's Fund. (2020). *Developing supportive design for people with dementia: Enhancing the healing environment.* King's Fund. www.kingsfund.org.uk/projects/enhancing-healing-environment/ehe-design-dementia

Morrow, E. & Nicholson, C. (2016). Carer engagement in the hospital care of older people: An integrative literature review. *International Journal of Older People Nursing, 11*(4), 298–314.

Moyle, W., Olorenshaw, R., Wallis, M. & Borbasi, S. (2008). Best practice for the management of older people with dementia in the acute care setting: A review of the literature. *International Journal of Older People Nursing, 3*(2), 121–130.

NHS Improvement. (2017). *Dementia assessment and improvement framework.* NHS Improvement. www.housinglin.org.uk/_assets/Resources/Housing/OtherOrganisation/Dementia_Assessment_Framework.pdf

Sampson, E.L., Blanchard, M.R., Jones, L., Tookman, A. & King, M. (2009). Dementia in the acute hospital: Prospective cohort study of prevalence and mortality. *British Journal of Psychiatry, 195*, 61–66.

Turner, A., Eccles, F., Elvish, R., Simpson, J. & Keady, J. (2017). The experience of caring for patients with dementia within a general hospital setting: A meta-analysis of the qualitative literature. *Aging & Mental Health, 21*(1), 66–76.

19 Validation builds relationships and communication

Vicki de Klerk-Rubin

My mother, Naomi Feil, escaped Nazi Germany with her mother and sister and joined my grandfather, who had found a job as a nursing home administrator in Cleveland, Ohio. The family moved into the nursing home, living on the same floor as the old people. As my mother says it, 'They became my friends'. I believe this unique childhood gave her special insight into the world of older people, especially those who are now diagnosed with different forms of dementia.

She began her development of what would later become the Validation Method in the 1960s. She experimented with many techniques and listened carefully to the older adults who guided her process. Her first published work (Feil, 1972) was presented at the 25th annual meeting of the Gerontological Society in that year. In 1982, she published her first book, *Validation: The Feil Method*, now in its third edition (Feil & de Klerk-Rubin, 2015). She spread her then radical ideas by giving workshops all over North America. These ideas included:

- Older people must be accepted as they are; we can't try to change them.
- We caregivers must enter into the older person's world, using empathy, while also understanding that the symbols that they use are tickets to the past. (In Validation, symbols are objects or people who represent things or people from the past that are laden with emotion and personal meaning.)
- These older adults are expressing unresolved issues and unfulfilled needs. There is always a reason behind their behaviour.
- Every person is unique and worthwhile, even when they are disorientated.

I think it is not overstated to say that Naomi Feil was the godmother of 'person-centred' care.

What is Validation?

The Validation Method (Feil & de Klerk-Rubin, 2015) is simply a humanistic way of connecting with older adults who have cognitive decline. It encourages them to communicate and to express their feelings and needs.

Validation has three interdependent elements, which are: the basic attitude; theory, and techniques. The basic attitude is who I am and the skills that I bring to an interaction. The Validation principles, which were developed by Naomi Feil, are based on humanistic and developmental psychology. These principles give an understanding of ageing and disorientation, and guide our actions. They also suggest the goals of the interactions. The verbal and non-verbal techniques are the 'tools' I use to reach those goals.

In this chapter, I will concentrate on the basic attitude, because without integrating these qualities, the techniques are useless. Given that this is a practical book, I will focus on specific things that you can do to learn and practise elements of the validating attitude.

Learning point 1

Develop an open, respectful, non-judgemental and empathetic approach:

- Reflect on how you address older adults.
- Practise being non-judgemental.
- Practise recognising an empathetic response when interacting with older adults.

The basic attitude requires the carer to be respectful, show honour and not judge anyone. It also encourages them to use emotive empathy when interacting with older adults. To be respectful means many things, including addressing the older adult in a way that he or she feels respected. When younger people call me, 'Vicki' instead of 'Mrs de Klerk', I feel disrespected. I come from a generation that has always used a formal address to show respect.

Consider the following questions:

- How do you address older adults usually? Is it by their first names or by their last names?
- When you use the older adult's first name, what are your intentions?
- What was normal when they were young for the older adult you are addressing?

Showing honour to an older adult is not just about giving compliments; it is about acknowledging the history of the individual. In front of you is a person who has lived a lifetime and built up a wealth of experience. This person is worthy of being looked in the eye when spoken to and of being asked instead of being told to do something. Their limits should be respected above the needs of the carer.

A Validation practitioner does not judge the other person. She respects the other as he or she is, in the moment. Judgement is reflected in the words 'should', 'shouldn't', 'good', 'bad', and so on.

An old, disoriented woman says: 'I had a wonderful talk with my mother.' Which of the following possible responses is NOT judgemental?

a.   Isn't that wonderful!

b.   You know Mrs B., your mother passed away many years ago.

c.   Tell me what was wonderful about it?

d.   That was your daughter, Mrs. B. You should recognise your daughter.[1]

In Validation, having empathy with a person who is expressing emotion is a way to connect quickly and to explore what is going on. It is a gateway to communication. In Validation, empathy is putting your own feelings and thoughts aside so that you can observe the other person, calibrating yourself to match what you see and hear as you take in the emotions of the other person. This is emotive empathy. You feel what the other person is feeling, without acting or pretending.

Case study: Mrs Whelan

Mrs Whelan is an 82-year-old woman, who has been living in a memory care unit for the past six months. She is not happy about the move. Even though she has had trouble getting washed and dressed in the morning, as she has very little short-term memory and was disorientated at times, she did not feel that she should mix with all of the 'crazy people.' Mrs Whelan is in the hall shouting, 'Someone stole all my jewellery!'

Which is the most empathetic response?

a.   Mrs Whelan, let me go look in your room. I'll help you.

b.   All your jewellery is gone! (Same voice tone as Mrs Whelan).

c.   Do I understand that you can't find your jewellery?

d.   What is missing this time?[2]

In this case, it is important for the carer to recognise that Mrs. Whelan is not accepting her cognitive decline and is fearfully clinging to what she has not yet lost. She projects her loss of memory onto her jewellery, using her jewellery as a symbol of valued things. She feels deep loss and expresses this by blaming others for stealing from her.

---

1. The correct answer is C. A is pretending or lying; B is reality orientation; D is reality orientation.

2. The correct answer is B. A is taking her seriously and factually, trying to fix the situation. C is using understanding, not emotions; D is not taking her seriously.

> ### Learning point 2
>
> There is a reason behind the behaviour of older adults:
>
> - Recognise that the past often has greater meaning than the present.
> - Recognise that older adults express need and feelings.

Like Mrs. Whelan in the example above, many older adults have not developed enough coping skills to handle the enormity of the aging process. The physical losses are often overwhelming. Someone who used to love walking, hiking and jogging now has to cope with hips and knees that are painful every day. Someone who loved to read can now no longer see well enough to do so. Socially active people who have lost hearing no longer feel that they are part of a conversation because they can't follow it. There are ways of coping with all of these challenges, but you need to have the inner flexibility to find alternatives.

As we age, we lose people we love – friends, family and lifelong partners. Our world grows smaller. If your identify is tied to your work, retirement becomes a difficult life transition. Accepting normal memory loss and being unable to do what you used to do can feel overwhelming. Society doesn't respect older adults with cognitive decline. There are very few advertisements that show older adults in a positive light. Often they are seen as a burden on society. This influences how people think about themselves. Unless we have coping skills that allow us to accept these psychosocial losses, there is an inner struggle.

When these losses become overwhelming, many older people withdraw to an inner reality. Their need to express their needs and feelings, to re-live and resolve old unresolved issues from the past, is stronger than the need to hang onto reality. They let go and move into a final stage of life that Naomi Feil calls 'Resolution'. These people express basic human needs. The need for identity, to feel useful, to express emotions and be heard, to love and be loved – these don't go away when one reaches 80 years of age. They are expressed in creative ways.

Exercise

Identify the needs being expressed in the following case studies.

1. Mr. Brown is 87 years old. He worked in a Ford factory from the age of 19 until his forced retirement at the age of 62. A few years ago, Mr. Brown started getting dressed in the middle of the night and leaving home. This behaviour forced his children to move him to a memory care unit. In this new home, Mr. Brown stands by the locked door trying to get out. When you ask him, 'Where are you going?' he answers, 'To the plant.'

    What need is Mr. Brown expressing?

    a. identity
    b. to feel useful

      c. to express emotions and be heard

      d. to love and be loved.[3]

2. Mrs. Clark mothered five children. She lost one child in a miscarriage, but because she was so busy with the other children, she never had time to grieve. When the children were grown and left home, Mrs. Clark started looking after other people's children in her own home. When she got too old to handle the children, she started to withdraw inward. Now, at the age of 82, she doesn't speak any more and sits all day in her chair with a little blanket that she folds over and over.

    What need is Mrs. Clark expressing?

      a. identity

      b. to feel useful

      c. to express emotions and be heard

      d. to love and be loved.[4]

3. Mr. Dowd was an executive in a big company. He had money, the corner office, a staff and all the things that come with a high-powered job. As he got older and retired, he became sour and mean to everyone. By the time he reached 90 years old, he had lost most of his short-term memory and could no longer care for himself. His move to an assisted living facility was a loss that he could not process, and he moved into his own personal reality. Every morning he got dressed, ate breakfast, and then sat at a table by a window and spent time writing. When he was approached by a staff member, he said, 'I don't have time for you now. Make an appointment with my secretary.'

    What need could Mr. Dowd be expressing?

      a. identity

      b. to feel useful

      c. to express emotions and be heard

      d. to love and be loved.[5]

Learning point 3

Use the techniques below to develop an approach that stimulates communication and builds a positive relationship:

- Learn how to centre yourself – approach the other person openly.
- Find eye contact that is comfortable for the other person.

---

3. The correct answer is B, the need to be useful. He is going to work.

4. The correct answer is D, the need to love and be loved. She misses her lost child perhaps, and is finally grieving over its loss.

5. The correct answer is A, identity. Mr. Dowd identifies with his position and hangs on even when reality has changed.

- Find a respectful distance that encourages communication.
- Use a respectful adult-to-adult tone of voice.

Centring

The first prerequisite technique to learn is how to centre yourself and put your own thoughts and feelings aside for the 10 minutes that you choose to validate. There are many methods to choose from and each person must find out what works best. You can find several exercises on the Validation Training Institute YouTube channel.[6]

By learning how to centre, you make it easier to tune into the emotional world of the other person, and this means that you are less likely to project your own thoughts and feelings onto them. A question that is useful to ask yourself is, 'Whose need am I expressing with my words?' For example:

> Mr Henry is sitting in his wheelchair and is totally absorbed in his inner thoughts. His face is contracted, muscles tense around the mouth, and his eyes are turned down at the corners and closed. You enter his room at around 11.30am to take him to lunch in the dining hall. You've had a rushed morning and have had to deal with a lot of problems at home before work. Then there was too much to do when you arrived.
>
> Mr Henry has immediate needs. He seems to have something emotional going on and does not look like he is in our reality. He may be experiencing physical pain.
>
> You also have needs. You may feel upset and want to get this done as quickly as possible, so that you can get a minute to have a break. Plus, there are five more people to get to lunch before noon.
>
> This is a moment to centre and become aware of your own emotions, pressures, thoughts and needs. You tell yourself 'Okay, I'm stressed'. Take a breath and remind yourself that you can deal with all of your needs later, but for these five minutes you are going to focus on Mr Henry and where he is at. Breathe again, down to your toes, then enter into Mr Henry's world.

Find eye contact that is comfortable for the other person

Remember that older adults often lose peripheral vision. If you are not in front of them, they don't know you are there. It is good practice always to wait until you are in front of the older adult before you start to speak. Second, get on their eye level. Don't stand and talk down to the other person – it can feel demeaning or condescending and sometimes people are triggered by this and react in an angry

---

6. www.youtube.com/channel/UCM9PIB1v5YWqlwkraX7rh1Q

way, even when your words are caring. Others may feel small and child-like when they are spoken down to, and this creates a hierarchical relationship. Try to get down or up to the other person's eye level.

When a person is very withdrawn in her own world, you may have to get very, very close in order to make eye contact. Without eye contact, it's difficult to communicate deeply, and often the older adult won't even hear your words.

Find the appropriate distance

From your own experience, you know how it feels when someone gets too close to you. You take a step back and need 'your space'. When you want to communicate something important, you probably lean in when talking to someone you trust. Older adults have varying needs for distance and closeness. When you want to communicate with an older adult, it's important to become sensitive to his or her needs at that moment. Move closer at a pace slow enough for you to see any changes in the other person. What are the clues that tell if you are too close or too far away?

Exercise

Below is a list of characteristics you can see in another person that might give you cues to finding an appropriate distance. Mark a 'C' for too close, or 'F' for too far away.

- The eyes widen.
- The eyes remain closed.
- The person takes a quick sharp breath inward.
- The chin moves backwards.
- The eyes narrow and the mouth turns down at the edges.
- Arms are crossed.
- The whole body turns away.
- The person is non-reactive to your words, looking away or inward.
- The person shouts.
- The person leans toward you.[7]

When a person is very withdrawn and in their own world, you may need to get closer than you feel comfortable with in order to make contact. You have a choice here – put aside your own need for distance and connect with the other person or maintain your need for distance and do not make a connection.

Use a respectful voice tone

Often caregivers are not aware of how they sound to others. Sometimes the voice tone is high and filled with stress; at other times, frustration or anger can come

---

7. The correct answers are: C, F, C, C, C, C, C, F, C, F

through, even when the caregiver uses the kindest of words. Sometimes your view of older people can be expressed through your voice tone. If you think that older adults behave like children, your voice tone can be like that of a kindergarten teacher. If you think that older adults should be controlled and helped, your voice tone can be syrupy-sweet and directive. When validating, you *always* use an adult-to-adult voice tone, as you would when speaking with a good friend. The voice tone should be pitched slightly lower because it's easier for older people with possible hearing loss.

Exercise

Use your mobile phone voice recorder app. Record a short part of an exchange with a good friend. Also record a short section of your exchange with an older adult. Listen to the recordings and write down what you hear. Here are some qualities to listen for:

- loud
- soft
- high-pitched
- low-pitched
- sharp, clipped words
- stressed
- warm
- slow
- fast
- telling the other person what to do
- asking the other person questions
- voice tone going down at the end of a sentence
- voice tone going up at the end of a sentence.

What does your voice tone remind you of?

When the older person is not expressing a particular emotion, the voice tone should be warm. When the older person is expressing a strong emotion, the voice tone should match. This is part of developing empathy with the other person.

Empathy is reflected through the voice tone, facial expression and posture. If you feel what the other person is feeling, the physical changes will happen automatically.

Once you have integrated these prerequisites to communication, you can start adding verbal and non-verbal Validation techniques. You need to use centring to find the appropriate eye contact and distance and a respectful voice tone to build trust with the other person and engage in meaningful communication.

References

Feil, N. (1972). *Summary of 1972 research data*. Presented at the 25th annual meeting of the Gerontological Society, December 1972. https://vfvalidation.org/wp-content/uploads/2019/05/FeilNaomi_GerontologicalSoc1972PuertoRico.pdf

Feil, N. & de Klerk Rubin, V. (1982/2015). V/F *Validation: The Feil Method* (3rd ed.). Edward Feil Productions.

Further reading

de Klerk-Rubin, V. (2008). *Validation techniques for dementia care: The family guide to improving communication*. Health Professions Press.

Feil, N. & de Klerk-Rubin, V. (2012). *The Validation breakthrough* (3rd ed). Health Professions Press.

20 Rapport-based communication: A practical approach to social inclusion and mutual wellbeing

Matt Laurie

Rapport-based communication (RBC) is a person-centred approach to establishing rapport and building relationships with a person with a severe communication difficulty. I have developed the approach over the 20+ years I have been supporting people with a high level of social need in care and education settings.

The purpose of RBC is:

- to help caregivers build a relationship with the person they support
- to help caregivers understand the theory behind why relationships are an essential element of person-centred care
- to help embed person-centred practice at a service-wide level.

This chapter lays out the rationale for this approach and the benefits that RBC can bring to caregivers and to organisations that support people with dementia in particular.

The importance of building relationships in dementia care

The progression of dementia can make communication difficult and this can be upsetting and frustrating for a person with dementia and their caregivers (Alzheimer's Society, 2020). Building authentic relationships is, therefore, an essential element of a person-centred approach (Brooker, 2007), but this is often seen as being difficult, or even impossible, due to a lack of understanding of the process (Allan & Killick, 2008). RBC offers a straightforward model for this process and is rooted in three existing approaches to establishing relationships with people with dementia: positive person work, relational time, and adaptive interaction.

Positive person work

Brooker (2007, p.6) explains that the primary outcome of person-centred care for people with dementia is to maintain their personhood: 'a standing or status that is bestowed upon one human being by another in the context of relationship and social being' (Kitwood,1997, p.8). Brooker (2007, pp.80–83) describes 17 qualities of positive person work (PPW) that caregivers can embody to create a social environment that supports personhood: warmth, holding, relaxation, celebration, respect, acceptance, acknowledgment, genuineness, validation, empowerment, facilitation, enabling, collaboration, recognition, including, belonging and fun.

Relational time

Relational time (RT) is defined as:

> a time of one-to-one interaction with the person with dementia, and a way of activating and stimulating the person with dementia that begins with the person's unique interests, wishes and capacity, and where the focus is on the person. (Ericsson et al., 2011, p.64)

Ericsson and colleagues (2011, pp.63–79) found that caregivers can help a person open up to a relationship by:

- choosing an appropriate time to approach for interaction
- creating an inviting environment
- respecting the person's wishes
- positioning themselves close to the person with dementia, at the same level (or lower), in a place that makes eye contact possible
- helping the person with dementia feeling like a contributor.

Intensive interaction and adaptive interaction

The learning disability practice of intensive interaction, based on the infant–caregiver work of psychologist Geraint Ephraim and later developed by Mel Nind and Dave Hewett (1994), 'uses body language to communicate with children and adults in a way that establishes attention and emotional engagement' (Horwood & Caldwell, 2008). This is achieved by initially imitating the person's behaviour and developing this into a 'shared language' (Horwood & Caldwell, 2008). This approach has been successfully applied with people with advanced dementia by Ellis and Astell (2017), who named the approach 'adaptive interaction'.

Developing an approach informed by the needs of caregivers

From 2008 until 2018, I worked directly with many care staff who were supporting people with complex needs. My role was to support the staff to build relationships with the service users and I delivered many induction training sessions and mentoring sessions. Over this time, I engaged with the care workers to understand the value of the training I was offering through both formal feedback and informal conversations. As I got to know these people and understood more about their context, the need for a simple language to communicate person-centred practice became apparent, for the following reasons.

First, most of the care workforce is unqualified and poorly paid, with low levels of literacy (Surr et al., 2017). Using plain language therefore makes practice as inclusive as possible to this group, in contrast to existing practice that is often communicated through academic language or lacks clarity (the overlapping principles of PPW being an example (De Bellis et al., 2009, p.25)).

Second, during my interviews with them, support workers explained that building relationships is one of their greatest challenges but also their greatest reward. When a relationship is established with a person with dementia, caregivers feel that their work is meaningful, and the person with dementia feels a sense of wellbeing too (Ericsson et al., 2011). Tickle-Degnen and Rosenthal (1990, p.286) call this mutual experience *rapport*, and so, because the RBC approach was developed in dialogue with caregivers, investigating how to create these important experiences became a priority for me.

The nature of rapport

So, what is rapport and how does rapport underpin RBC? Rapport is defined as the emotional experience of high-quality interactions (Baker et al., 2020, p.2). It is an experience that happens only between people. Tickle-Degnen and Rosenthal (1990, p.286) describe three primary components to rapport:

- mutual *social attention* (which creates a cohesiveness to the interaction)
- mutual *positivity* (feelings of friendliness and caring toward each other)
- mutual *co-ordination* (the immediate, spontaneous, sympathetic responses to the sentiments and attitudes of the other).

Learning point 1 – Three components of rapport

Before you read any further you may like to consider the following questions:

- Can you spot the three components of rapport in your everyday interactions?
- With whom do you experience rapport? With whom do you not experience rapport?
- Think of an interaction when you didn't experience rapport. Can you spot which component(s) of rapport were either missing or at a low level?

Rapport meets fundamental needs and increases wellbeing

According to self-determination theory (SDT), the fulfilment of three basic needs (autonomy, competence and relatedness) is highly influenced by the social environment. Close relationships, and rapport in particular, have a deep impact on whether a person's needs are satisfied and wellbeing is experienced (Baker et al., 2020; Ryan & Deci, 2002).

More specifically, research directly examining how the three needs of SDT are related to rapport found that, when one member in an interaction supports the autonomy of the other person, the other person tends to perceive more rapport in the interaction (Gurland & Grolnick, 2003). Furthermore, Zeilig and colleagues (2019, p.17) describe how wellbeing is dependent on having a feeling of agency, which was demonstrated in their study when a person with dementia assumed leadership of a co-creative group session.

The central practice of RBC, therefore, is to adopt an interaction style that is supportive of a person with dementia's autonomy in order to create rapport, meet psychological needs and increase wellbeing. Having an autonomy-supportive interaction approach means encouraging the person's own initiations in a way that allows them opportunities to make choices (Gurland & Grolnick, 2003). As in adaptive interaction, the simplest way to do this is just to follow the lead of the person with dementia, joining in with what they are doing. This is a technique that is also found in other social interventions and therapies, including dance movement psychotherapy (Coaten, 2011), and early years music practice (Pitt & Arculus, 2018).

Offers

In RBC the starting point for interactions are the in-the-moment interests and behaviours of the person with dementia. Each behaviour is called an *offer* – a term borrowed from improvisational theatre and defined as:

> any new idea that is brought to the stage, for example, a line of dialogue, gesture or mime. An *offer* can either be blocked (preventing an action from continuing or denying the reality of an *offer*) or accepted (embracing and celebrating an *offer*). (Salinsky et al., 2017, p.68, original emphases)

An *offer* in RBC can also be blocked and celebrated:

* to block an *offer* is to ignore, dismiss or criticise what a person is doing
* to celebrate an *offer* is to warmly join in with what the person is doing, with 100% attention.

For example, is the person walking, shaking, vocalising, singing? These are the offers.

Learning point 2 – Offers

- Can you see the offers that the person you support is making? Watch what the person does when they are left on their own and make a list of the things they do.

- Make sure to include behaviours that you might initially judge as 'negative' or 'inappropriate'. While you might later choose not to engage with these behaviours, it is important not to dismiss anything that the person is doing, based on your judgments and opinions.

- Are you making any judgements of the person when observing what they are doing?

The three Cs of RBC

The three Cs have been developed to both support caregivers and facilitate the dissemination and application of the practice after a training intervention. They have proved effective in achieving these goals by providing caregivers with a practice that is easy to remember and that helps to solve their daily challenges in building and maintaining relationships.

- The first C is to 'C' (see) the *offers*. In the context of RBC, an *offer* is anything that a person does unprompted that has the potential to be reciprocated by the caregiver through joining in, copying or reflecting. *Offers* are the potential starting points for an interaction, and it is up to the caregiver to be able to recognise and frame these behaviours as such. Looking for *offers* requires mindful social attention, the first component of rapport.

- The second C is to *copy* the *offers*. The caregiver now joins in with the person, reciprocating their actions and behaviour. When copying the person's actions, the caregiver and the person are co-ordinated and in synchrony –the second component of rapport. The caregiver is implicitly following the lead of the person, offering a sense of autonomy.

- The third C is to *celebrate* the *offers*. The caregiver makes sure to join in and reciprocate warmly, responding as though there is nothing that they would rather be doing and this is the best idea ever. This positive feeling is the third component of rapport.

Learning point 3 – Using the three Cs of RBC

The essence of this practice is to create rapport and develop a relationship by warmly joining in with what the person is doing with 100% of your attention. Do you think that you naturally celebrate the offers of the people you engage with day to day? Reflect on some interactions that you have engaged with recently and consider whether you unconditionally celebrated their offers, behaviours and requests or whether you blocked them.

- What was the result of celebrating or blocking offers in these interactions?
- How might these interactions have been different if you had celebrated the offers?
- How would your interactions with the person you support be different if you use the 3Cs of RBC? Try to unconditionally celebrate some of the offers that you previously listed.

Now try doing the three Cs with a person you support:

- 'C' (see) the offer – observe the person that you care for and list the unprompted things that they do.
- Copy the offer – join in with what the person is doing, using 100% of your attention. (Make sure to choose a behaviour that you are comfortable to join in with.)
- Celebrate the offer – use your facial expressions, tone of voice and body language to communicate warmth.

Case study 1

I observed a person with dementia sitting in an armchair appearing to talk to himself. His face was entirely neutral, without any sign of a smile. Only one in 10 words was intelligible. Care workers were not observed to engage the gentleman socially.

The offers are that the person was sitting down and vocalising. Copying the offers, I also sat down and began to repeat some of the sounds and words. Celebrating the offers, I made sure to communicate warmth, using tone of voice, facial expression and body language. The gentleman began to take an interest, offering eye contact and an occasional smile. Even though there was no 'sense' to the words, a kind of verbal turn-taking ensued, which flowed naturally and resulted in the author feeling engaged and feeling a sense of mutual reciprocity. As the interaction continued, the gentleman became more positive, showing signs of happiness and delight. Together, these qualities indicated the presence of the three components of rapport: social attention, positivity and co-ordination.

Case study 2

I observed a man with dementia walking up and down the hospital corridor, holding and talking to a large doll. A care worker ignored the behaviour – they said that the person 'just does that because they have dementia'.

The *offers* are that the person is walking and holding and talking to the doll (the care worker did not see the *offers* because they were judging the behaviour). *Copying the offers* would involve joining in with the walking and either taking an interest in the person's doll or finding a second doll to hold. *Celebrating the offers* would involve communicating warmth using speech and open, welcoming body language. When I tried this, walking up and down the corridor for several minutes, the person with dementia turned to look, smiled and offered me his doll. We then enjoyed taking turns to hand the doll back and forth between us.

Conclusion

RBC is introduced here as an effective, straightforward yet high-quality communication practice in dementia care that is suitable for anybody supporting a person with dementia, regardless of their level of education or experience. RBC has its roots in person-centred care, relational time, intensive interaction, adaptive interaction and improvisational theatre practice. RBC has the potential to make a significant contribution to the dementia care field. It does so by giving a simple, practical framework for building rapport. It can give satisfaction to both the caregiver and the person with dementia when they find that, through it, they are able to connect in new, improvisational and perhaps even playful ways that value personhood. By clearly identifying the purpose (to find rapport), the starting point of the process (behavioural *offers*) and the process itself (warmly joining in with 100% attention), RBC adds to the existing understanding of person-centred dementia practice.

The building of relationships is also an essential element in other care contexts and therapeutic practices, so RBC can be used effectively in autism, learning disability and mental health care. RBC also offers a language to practitioners from other disciplines to describe and understand the common principles of rapport building.

RBC has been embedded in several care settings with very positive feedback from practitioners and managers. The ease with which RBC can be disseminated contributes to this success and can ensure consistency and continuity of practice – a key issue, given the high staff turnover in this area. The next step for my own research is to empirically study the development of these communities of practice.

References

Allan, K. & Killick, J. (2008). Communication and relationships: An inclusive social world. In M. Downs & B. Bowers (Eds.), *Excellence in dementia care: Research into practice* (pp.212–229). Open University Press.

Alzheimer's Society. (2020). *Communicating and language.* [Online.] www.alzheimers.org.uk/about-dementia/symptoms-and-diagnosis/symptoms/dementia-and-language#content-start

Baker, Z.G., Watlington, E.M. & Raymond Knee, C. (2020). The role of rapport in satisfying one's basic psychological needs. *Motivation and Emotion, 44,* 329–343.

Brooker, D. (2007). *Person-centred dementia care.* Jessica Kingsley.

Coaten, R. (2011). Going by way of the body in dementia care. *Animated, the Community Dance Magazine, Spring,* 24–25.

De Bellis, A.M., Wotherspoon, A.J., Walter, B.K., Guerin, P.B., Bradley, S.L., Cecchin, M. & Paterson, J.B. (2009). *Come into my world: How to interact with a person who has dementia.* Flinders University/Hyde Park Press.

Ellis, M. & Astell, A. (2017). *Adaptive interaction and dementia: How to communicate without speech.* Jessica Kingsley Publishers.

Ericsson, I., Kjellström, S. & Hellström, I. (2011). Creating relationships with persons with moderate to severe dementia. *Dementia, 12*(1), 63–79.

Gurland, S.T. & Grolnick, W.S. (2003). Children's expectancies and perceptions of adults: Effects on rapport. *Child Development, 74*(4), 1212–1224.

Horwood, J. & Caldwell, P. (2008). *Using intensive interaction and sensory integration: A handbook for those who support people with severe autistic spectrum disorder.* Jessica Kingsley Publishers.

Kitwood, T. (1997). *Dementia reconsidered: the person comes first.* Open University Press.

Nind, M. & Hewett, D. (1994). *Access to communication: Developing basic communication with people who have severe learning difficulties.* David Fulton Publishers.

Pitt, J. & Arculus, C. (2018). *SALTMusic: Research report.* National Foundation for Youth Music. http://researchonline.rcm.ac.uk/334/1/SaltMusic-Research-Report.pdf

Ryan, R.M. & Deci, E.L. (2002). Overview of self- determination theory: An organismic dialectical perspective. In E.L. Deci & R.M. Ryan (Eds.), *Handbook of self-determination research* (pp.3–33). The University of Rochester Press.

Salinsky, T., Frances-White, D. & McShane, M. (2017). *The improv handbook: The ultimate guide to improvising in comedy, theatre, and beyond.* Bloomsbury Methuen Drama.

Surr, C.A., Gates, C., Irving, D., Oyebode, J., Smith, S.J., Parveen, S, Drury, M. & Dennison, A. (2017). Effective dementia education and training for the health and social care workforce: A systematic review of the literature. *Review of Educational Research, 87*(5), 966–1002.

Tickle-Degnen, L. & Rosenthal, R. (1990). The nature of rapport and its nonverbal correlates. *Psychological Inquiry, 1*(4), 285–293.

Zeilig, H., Tischler, V., van der Byl Williams, M., West, J. & Strohmaier, S. (2019). Co-creativity, well-being and agency: A case study analysis of a co-creative arts group for people with dementia. *Journal of Aging Studies, 49,* 16–24.

21 Dementia in the workplace

Louise Ritchie, Debbie Tolson and Mike Danson

In the UK, changes affecting the age at which people become eligible for a state pension and the abolition of the default retirement age are resulting in an increasing number of people working into later life. While there are economic benefits to this, there are also costs. It is currently estimated than some 40,000 people with dementia are of working age (i.e. under 65) in the UK (Parkin & Baker, 2021). Earlier diagnosis, coupled with policy changes that extend working years, means the number of people with dementia in employment is likely to increase. Our project, 'Dementia in the Workplace: The potential for continued employment post-diagnosis', was funded by the Alzheimer's Society and explored the experiences of 17 people who had been diagnosed with dementia while still in employment, using a case study methodology.

Drawing on the anonymised stories of our participants, this chapter describes the employment-related experiences of people living with dementia in employment. We highlight the employment practices that can support a person with dementia to continue employment, and we expose the complexities of doing so. We also explore the transition to retirement for people with dementia and the importance of post-employment opportunities to maintain wellbeing and quality of life.

National government policy emphasises the importance of remaining in, or re-entering, the labour market. Yet, while legislation requires that people with disabilities are supported in the workplace through reasonable adjustments (Baumberg, 2014), this is often not the case (Ritchie et al., 2015), with negative effects for their financial, social and psychological wellbeing and that of their families.

Working with dementia: employee perspectives

For people with early onset dementia, the first symptoms are often experienced in the workplace. The initial symptoms include, for example, memory problems and problems with planning and lack of concentration, which are often initially mild but gradually begin to impact on their ability to complete their work tasks (Chaplin & Davidson, 2016; Evans, 2019).

For many, the route to diagnosis is complex and lengthy. Alternative reasons for symptoms that are common in mid-life (e.g. menopause, depression, anxiety) have to be excluded before a diagnosis of dementia can be considered. For this reason, many employees with (undiagnosed) dementia leave their employment or go on sick leave before they receive their diagnosis. It is unlikely that they will be facilitated to return to work once they have a diagnosis, even though this should be possible. Therefore, research suggests that a diagnosis is one of the key resources required to enable continued employment (Ritchie et al., 2020).

Once an employee discloses a diagnosis of dementia to their employer, they should be protected under the Equality Act 2010. Reasonable adjustments are usually formal arrangements put in place by the employer to provide supports for the employee to continue their role (Egdell et al., 2018). However, reasonable adjustments are never straightforward; a comprehensive assessment of the abilities of the employee, the workplace environment and the job requirements is needed to inform recommendations for reasonable adjustments within the workplace.

From our case study research (Ritchie et al., 2018), there is evidence that people with dementia can and do continue in employment post-diagnosis. A variety of formal and informal adjustments to work role and/or environment are being introduced to support people with dementia to continue employment, in some cases for years after their diagnosis. Table 21.1 provides examples of these adjustments.

Table 21.1: Examples of workplace adjustments

Formal adjustments	Informal adjustments
Flexible working hours Change of shift pattern Change of job description Working from home Office move (to reduce noise)	Use of technology (phones/calendars/reminders) Support from colleagues Working longer hours (unpaid) to get the work done Family support

One of our interviewees, Jane, was Head of Business Development and Support with a small charity. When she was diagnosed with dementia in her early 50s, she had an open conversation with her line manager, and they worked together to develop a plan that would support her continued employment. Being open about her specific difficulties led to a change in her job description to allow her to focus on the tasks she could do. Although this change was reflected in a drop in salary, she was happy to be able to continue working. She was confident she could continue to do the job well and contribute usefully to the organisation. This formal arrangement also required forward planning and involved Jane working closely with colleagues to pass on the knowledge she had developed over the years and ensure that, when she did decide to leave, the company wouldn't lose her expertise.

This also meant that, in her day-to-day job, she built up trust in her colleagues and she knew she could ask for help if she needed it.

> It was about looking at what she was capable of, rather than looking at what she couldn't do. (Joan's line manager, Head of Business Support)

For others of our interviewees, continued employment was maintained through informal support arrangements. For example, Phil was working as a safety inspector in a factory when he was diagnosed with frontotemporal dementia at the age of 56. Although he was able to continue with his inspections, his condition meant that he did not have the insight to see the mistakes he was making in his report writing. In this safety-critical role, accuracy in reporting was key, and he was reluctant to disclose his diagnosis to his employer because of fear of losing his job. Rather than make formal arrangements, he enlisted the help of his wife to support him with the paperwork and began bringing work home to ask her to check and help him to write the reports. This arrangement was not sustainable for either of them and ultimately led to him leaving his job.

Informal arrangements used in conjunction with formal adjustments may be the most successful way of maintaining employment for a person with dementia. Another interviewee, Paul, was working as an estates officer in a janitorial role in a large office building when he was diagnosed with dementia at the age of 55. A combination of adjustments to his job description along with support from colleagues enabled him to continue working for six years post-diagnosis. The 'reasonable adjustments' that supported Paul were:

- changing the shift pattern to day shift only
- regular review meetings involving Paul, his employer, his family and his healthcare support
- a standardised task list to follow during his shift (what to do at what time).

In addition to this, Paul's healthcare worker arranged a session with his colleagues to help them understand dementia and how they could support Paul. In understanding the support Paul needed, some of his colleagues developed ways to keep him safe. They were mindful of the importance of ensuring that Paul maintained his independence in the workplace and so tried not to do tasks for him, while also making sure that he had everything he needed to do his job safely and well.

The majority of people who are diagnosed with dementia do not continue in employment (Chaplin & Davidson, 2016; Evans, 2019; Öhman et al., 2001). However, as presented here, our research indicates that people with dementia can continue in employment post-diagnosis if they are given appropriate support. This requires employers, colleagues and healthcare professionals to work with the employee with dementia to develop support packages, concentrating on the contribution they can still make, rather than focusing on their diagnosis (Thomson et al., 2019).

Learning point 1

People living with dementia, can and do continue employment post-diagnosis. A multidisciplinary approach is required to support people living with dementia to maintain employment.

- What is the role of the employer in supporting continued employment?
- What legal protections do employees with dementia have?
- How can healthcare professionals support people with dementia to stay in the workplace?
- What other disciplines might have a role in supporting employment for people with dementia?

Understanding dementia in the workplace: employer perspectives

Recent research has highlighted that, while the majority of employers have an awareness of dementia, this is often not applied to the employment context (Egdell et al., 2019). That is to say, although many people have personal experience of dementia, employers often do not apply that knowledge to understanding the situation of an employee with dementia or to making adjustments to support them. There is a need to improve understanding of dementia in the workplace, to ensure that all employees with dementia have access to appropriate and timely supports.

Employers often do not know where to get support in making decisions about how to support their employee. As a result, they often have to take guidance from the employee or healthcare professionals (Ritchie et al., 2018). Although employers involved in our case studies expressed a desire to do the best by their employee, this was often misjudged and resulted in arrangements for the worker to take early retirement, without adequate consideration of the contribution they could still make in the workplace. One example of this was Alison, a maternity care assistant. Alison was on sick leave when she received her diagnosis, and a subsequent occupational health assessment deemed her unable to continue in the role. Both Alison and her husband felt that she could still work in another role, but this wasn't considered, and she had no option but to take ill-health retirement.

> The redeployment: it was just mentioned and moved on. That was how I got the impression right from then that they were just going down the retirement thing, whether Alison wanted to or not. (Alison's husband)

It may be assumed that in Alison's case the employer felt they were making the best decision for her. However, research by Egdell and colleagues (2019) has shown that employers often make knee-jerk assumptions about the abilities of an employee with dementia.

Therefore, it is recommended that employers engage in dementia-awareness sessions that focus on how dementia affects a person in the workplace. From our case study research, there were many examples of how such training was delivered and how this resulted in positive outcomes and support for the specific employee. For example, Rose was employed as a manager in a large organisation. After she disclosed her diagnosis to her employer, she decided that the best approach to discussing her diagnosis with her team was to deliver her own dementia-awareness session, specifically outlining what she could still do, what she had difficulty with, and what her colleagues could do to support her.

This is one unique example of workplace dementia awareness, and it may not be suitable for all employees who develop dementia. Other examples include awareness sessions delivered by healthcare professionals and sessions delivered by external organisations. There is a growing number of organisations providing resources and training around dementia in the workplace.[1]

Learning point 2

With better dementia awareness, workplaces can ensure that they can support employees living with dementia:

- What is the impact of dementia awareness sessions in the workplace?
- Who benefits from an improved understanding of dementia?
- What are your attitudes towards supporting people with dementia in employment?

Leaving employment

Retirement is commonly thought of as an 'end of an era' and a celebration of the achievements made throughout an individual's working life. For many people who receive a diagnosis of dementia while still in employment, the opportunities to plan for and look forward to retirement can change overnight. For example, one of our case studies featured Edward, who was a judge. He began experiencing symptoms of dementia in his early 60s and started making mistakes in his work. He relied heavily on the support of his team in the absence of formal discussions with his employers. His symptoms and the decline in his performance led to him taking sick leave, during which he received his diagnosis of dementia. At this point, he was told that his employment would be terminated and was given an ill-health retirement package. As with Alison in the previous section, the decision-making about Edward's employment was out of his control.

1. See for example, Alzheimer's Society (www.alzheimers.org.uk/research/our-research/research-projects/guides-support-dementia-workplace) and Age Scotland (https://issuu.com/agescotland/docs/dementia_and_the_workplace).

This affected not only Edward's financial situation but also his self-esteem and emotional wellbeing. An unnecessarily insensitive and undignified exit from a high-status role was demeaning and an unexpected, abrupt end to an otherwise very successful career.

For many people, retirement is a period in life that they look forward to, as they will be making plans to spend more time with loved ones and try new things. However, a diagnosis of dementia challenges the meaning of retirement, particularly where people have been deemed unable to continue to work. People with dementia who have had an unplanned and/or chaotic ending to their working life may require help and support to normalise the transition from work to retirement. Many participants in our case studies were not afforded this opportunity, and many of those who experienced an unplanned workplace exit were left without a reason to get out of bed in the morning, which impacted on their mental health.

Volunteering activities may be one way that people with early-onset dementia can continue to make a meaningful contribution to society if they have to leave employment. Research has shown that workplace-based volunteering schemes can be successful in supporting people with early-onset dementia (Kinney et al., 2011; Robertson & Evans, 2015). Although there are no volunteering schemes like this in the UK, there is potential for finding volunteering roles that allow people to apply the skills they have developed throughout their careers. In our case studies, there were three examples of people who found volunteering opportunities after they left work. Rose, who was mentioned above, began writing a blog post-diagnosis, which led to opportunities to raise awareness of dementia in a wider setting through public speaking. Anna could no longer work as a children's nurse after she was diagnosed with dementia aged 62. However, having always been engaged with her community, she sought other ways to use her skills and found a volunteering role with a local charity supporting refugee families with their basic health needs. Ken was an electrician and found a volunteering role with a local furniture charity where he would test the donated electrical equipment before it was given to people in need. All three said these volunteering opportunities gave them a sense of normality and improved their wellbeing by providing meaningful occupation. Many of the other participants in our case studies said they felt that they still had something to contribute to society but did not know how to access opportunities. There is a need to consider how support around employment for people with dementia addresses the difficulties people experience both in employment and post-employment in order to maintain their wellbeing.

Learning point 3

Employment support for people with dementia should support decision-making around leaving employment and post-employment:

- When do you plan to retire?
- What are your hopes for your retirement?

- What services are available to support your transition from work to retirement?

Conclusion

This chapter has explored the experiences of people who are diagnosed with dementia while still employed. It is clear that people with dementia can and do continue in employment post-diagnosis. However, many do not as they cannot access support and employers do not understand dementia. There is a lack of readily available practical guidance on supporting people with dementia in employment, and this is an area where more research is needed to identify the adjustments that can help people to continue to work in different settings. While there are specialist services that focus on supporting people with employment (such as vocational rehabilitation, employability services and careers guidance), they have not traditionally been focused on issues related to dementia. As our population demographics change and the workforce ages, there will be an increased need for practical support services to address issues around dementia in the workplace.

References

Baumberg, B. (2014). Fit-for-work – or work fit for disabled people? The role of changing job demands and control in incapacity claims. *Journal of Social Policy, 43*(2), 289–310.

Chaplin, R. & Davidson, I. (2016). What are the experiences of people with dementia in employment? *Dementia, 15*(2), 147–161.

Egdell, V., Cook, M., Stavert, J., Ritchie, L., Tolson, D. & Danson, M. (2019). Dementia in the workplace: Are employers supporting employees living with dementia? *Aging and Mental Health,* doi: 10.1080/13607863.2019.1667299

Egdell, V., Stavert, J. & McGregor, R. (2018). The legal implications of dementia in the workplace: establishing a cross-disciplinary research agenda. *Ageing and Society, 38*(11), 2181–2196.

Evans, D. (2019). An exploration of the impact of younger-onset dementia on employment. *Dementia, 18*(1), 262–281.

Kinney, J.M., Kart, C.S. & Reddecliff, L. (2011). 'That's me, the Goother': Evaluation of a program for individuals with early-onset dementia. *Dementia, 10*(3), 361–377.

Öhman, A., Nygård, L. & Borell, L. (2001). The vocational situation in cases of memory deficits or younger onset dementia. *Scandinavian Journal of Caring Science, 15,* 34–43.

Parkin, E. & Baker, C. (2021). *Dementia: Policy, services and statistics.* Briefing paper 07007. House of Commons Library. https://researchbriefings.files.parliament.uk/documents/SN07007/SN07007.pdf

Ritchie, L., Banks, P., Danson, M., Tolson, D. & Borrowman, F. (2015). Dementia in the workplace: A review. *Journal of Public Mental Health, 14*(1), 24–34.

Ritchie, L., Egdell, V., Cook, M., Stavert, J., Tolson, D. & Danson, M. (2020). Dementia, work and employability: Using the capability approach to understand the employability potential for people living with dementia. [Online first]. *Work, Employment and Society.* https://doi. org/10.1177/0950017020961929

Ritchie, L., Tolson, D. & Danson, M. (2018). Dementia in the workplace case study research: Understanding the experiences of individuals, colleagues and managers. *Ageing and Society, 38*(10), 2146–2175.

Robertson, J. & Evans, D. (2015). Evaluation of a workplace engagement project for people with younger onset dementia. *Journal of Clinical Nursing, 24*(15/16), 2331–2339.

Thomson, L., Stanyon, M., Dening, T., Heron, R. & Griffiths, A. (2019). Managing employees with dementia: A systematic review. *Occupational Medicine, 69*(2), 89–98.

22 Does technology have a role in meeting the care and support needs of people living with dementia and their families?

John Woolham

People's lives are increasingly shaped by technology. It makes working lives more productive; it makes it easier to communicate and keep in touch, and it entertains us. It is omnipresent in most societies, and everyday technology already plays a big part in the lives of people living with memory loss and dementia, and their families.

However, over the past two decades, increasing attention is being paid to technology specifically designed to help people with dementia. This chapter will explore what it is, why and how it is used, how effective it is in the UK at the moment and what's needed to make it more effective.

Defining 'technology'

The rapid pace of technological development means that there isn't wide agreement about terminology. *Assistive technology*, an umbrella term, has been defined as:

> any item, piece of equipment, product or system, whether acquired
> commercially, off the shelf, modified or customised, that is used to increase,
> maintain, or improve functional capabilities of individuals with cognitive,
> physical or communication difficulties. (Marshall, 2000, p.9)

This can include things like walking sticks, but also *electronic assistive technologies*, such as medication dispensers that can help people remember to take their medicines, or calendar clocks that can help people keep track of time. *Telecare* is one type of electronic assistive technology. It has been defined as a service that uses:

> … a combination of alarms, sensors and other equipment to help people live independently. This is done by monitoring activity changes over time and will raise a call for help in emergency situations, such as a fall, fire or a flood. (Department of Health, 2009)

Telecare devices collect and send data from a user's home to somewhere else – typically, a call centre. This can be an 'active' process, such as a pendant alarm that a wearer can press to summon help in an emergency. Or it can be 'passive', which means the devices work without the need for user activation. These include environmental sensors of various kinds, such as those to detect carbon monoxide, smoke or flooding. They send information automatically to a call centre. (*Telehealth* refers to the use of similar kinds of technologies to collect and send information about a patient's vital signs – pulse, blood pressure, oxygen saturation levels and so forth – to a clinician.)

A fairly wide range of telecare devices is available. In addition to those referred to above, devices can also detect, for example:

- gas – and temporarily disconnect an unlit appliance (this kind of technology is widely used on most gas appliances in the UK now)
- falls – a wearable device can detect if someone falls and then send an alert
- low environmental temperatures – the device will then automatically switch on the heating, overriding the home thermostat
- nighttime activity – motion lights will automatically switch on if someone gets up at night, or alert a family member that someone has got out of bed
- doors opening – sensors detect if a person enters or leaves the house, sending information so a response can be made if necessary
- activity within the home – sensors can track movement within the home (useful, for example, to establish if someone does not get up, or does not go to bed).

Over time, it may be that further technological progress will make current definitions obsolete. Some already eschew the terms 'telecare' and 'telehealth' in favour of '*technology enabled care*', and '*enabling technology*'. These terms also encompass the use of mobile phone technology and apps, and, over time, the use of the '*internet of things*' (IoT) (the interconnection, via the internet, of computing devices embedded in everyday objects such as freezers, cookers and household goods, enabling them to send and receive data). This technology is already being used in health settings – for example, ingestible sensors (pills) to establish if a patient is really taking their prescribed medication. However, this chapter will focus mostly on electronic and telecare technologies, which we will now refer to as 'telecare', since these are much more widely used at the present time.

> **Learning point 1**
>
> Thinking about how we use telecare today:
>
> - How easy is it for people living with dementia to use?
> - If it's difficult for people with dementia to use it, is this just because of the person's dementia, or because of how technology is designed?
> - Could technology be redesigned to make it easier for everyone to use?

What factors are 'driving' the use of technology and telecare?

Several factors have led telecare to become widely used by local authority adult social care (ASC) departments in the UK. Among these, four stand out. The first is technological progress, which makes possible the manufacture of increasingly sophisticated devices. The second is demography. The UK has an ageing population; the prevalence of dementia increases with age, and the number of people living with this disease is predicted to rise sharply. These demographic changes place increasing pressure on both NHS and ASC services. Third, Department of Health policy (2005) encouraged ASC departments to establish telecare services and get technology into the homes of as many people as they could as quickly as possible, and provided a 'preventive technology grant' (Department of Health, 2006). Fourth, public sector austerity policies have led to cuts in ASC budgets over the past decade, forcing ASC departments to think about different ways to provide care that are more cost effective. Telecare is widely seen as an important way to do this. All ASC departments in the UK are now likely to have telecare services.

Does telecare make a difference to people with dementia and their families?

Although telecare is believed to simultaneously achieve cost savings while improving outcomes and maintaining independence of older people and people with dementia, current research evidence does not support this belief.

Practice guidance (Bjørneby, et al., 1999; Marshall, 2000) first explored the feasibility of introducing technology to supplement the care of people with dementia. This guidance contributed to the creation of a number of small-scale telecare projects in different parts of the UK.

Some of these early studies were evaluations of local projects designed to support people with dementia, and their findings were generally extremely positive. For example, Woolham (2005) found that, compared with a matched comparison group, people given telecare were much more likely to remain living independently and to require fewer hospital stays. These early studies, alongside a series of reports from influential bodies such as the Audit Commission and government select committees, contributed to government policy guidance and the financial support for telecare referred to above.

However, these studies suffered from various methodological shortcomings, and were insufficiently robust to provide evidential support for Department of Health policy. To address this, it commissioned a major evaluation of telecare and telehealth, but only after policy guidance was published. This became known as the Whole System Demonstrator (WSD) project. The WSD was a very large randomised controlled trial (RCT). RCTs are often regarded as the 'gold standard' in research, capable of producing more reliable and trustworthy findings than research using other methods. Participants included people with dementia (most of the participants were older people), but they were not a specific focus of the research.

There was a clear assumption from the outset that this trial would validate policy and funding decisions that had already been made:

> The Whole System Demonstrator programme was set up by the Department
> of Health… To provide a clear evidence base to support important
> investment decisions and show how the technology supports people to live
> independently… (Department of Health, 2011, p.2)

Unfortunately, the findings did not fulfil these expectations. The results produced no evidence that outcomes for telecare users were any better than for those receiving traditional care (Steventon et al., 2013).

Nevertheless, these findings did not lead to any change in policy direction. The Department of Health had previously released findings from an interim report (these were not intended for publication), cautiously suggesting that telecare might produce more positive outcomes. The full report, and subsequent publications, told a different story – but were not publicised. The final results were generally overlooked in policy and practice settings. For example, the Association of Directors of Adult Social Services (ADASS) in England made no mention of them on its website, instead promoting evidence from its own review of local authority practice. Guidance from the National Institute for Health and Care Excellence (NICE) and the Social Care Institute for Excellence (SCIE) similarly overlooked the WSD findings. Perhaps because of this, telecare managers working in ASC departments in England often seemed poorly informed by the final results of this trial (Woolham et al., 2019).

Another RCT (which began shortly after the WSD had ended) focused specifically on people living with dementia. The Assistive Technology and Telecare to maintain Independent Living At home for people with dementia (ATTILA) trial was designed to see if telecare might prolong the ability of people with dementia to live independently, and whether this was cost effective. This trial concluded that it offered no significant increase in the length of time someone with dementia was able to remain living independently; did not decrease carer burden, depression or anxiety, and provided no reduction in health, social care or societal costs (Howard et al., 2021).

Learning point 2

When organisations and professionals say that their policies or practices are evidence based, what does this mean?

- What factors shape what becomes evidence, in policy and practice?
- If there are gaps in evidence, what should policy makers and practitioners do?

Does technology have a role in supporting people with dementia?

Both trials concluded that technology was not effective in improving outcomes, supporting independence or supporting carers, and that it was not cost-effective. However, neither was able to *explain* its findings, leaving open the possibility that telecare's impact and effectiveness might depend on *how* it is used.

The Using Telecare for Older People In Adult social care (UTOPIA) project (Woolham et al., 2018, 2021) conducted a survey of how ASC departments were using telecare. This found that telecare was most frequently used to manage risk and promote safety, and much less to achieve other objectives – for example, to enable or support social contact, or support hobbies or valued activities. This was particularly important for people with dementia. It also found various shortcomings in the way telecare assessments were conducted, and in the nature of the training offered to telecare assessors. Additionally, the survey suggested that only a limited range of devices was used – most commonly, pendant alarms, smoke and fall detectors and bed or chair occupancy sensors. Other research has also highlighted shortcomings in the assessment and provision supply chains (Gibson et al., 2016; Forsyth et al., 2019), consequent disappointment with technology and high rates of discontinuation (Gramstad et al., 2014; Federici et al., 2016). Finally, the survey found that not all ASC departments were able to offer a response service, relying instead on family carers. These findings suggest that changes to the way technologies are provided may optimise their effectiveness in supporting people with dementia and their families.

Learning point 3

Based on the findings from the research, how would you answer these questions?

- Why should technology be used for people living with dementia?
- When should it be used, and when should it not be used?
- What needs to happen so that there is a good match between a person's needs and goals and any telecare or technology that's provided?

- What ethical issues need to be considered when using technology for people living with dementia?

Optimising the benefits of telecare technology

More research is urgently needed into how to optimise the benefits of telecare technology for people with dementia and their families. But existing studies suggest various ways forward in the way technology is currently used.

First, research points to the need to make changes in the way assessments for technology are carried out. Careful matching of need with technology has been identified as a pre-requisite to its effective use (Wey, 2004). Other studies have suggested that technology is often seen as a 'plug and play' solution by ASC departments, rather than as a complex intervention (Greenhalgh et al. 2015, Ganyo et al., 2011). Understanding how people use −or do not use − even simple technologies may require a deep level of understanding on the part of the assessing practitioner. An understanding of how the technology recipient interacts with their social and physical environment is also vital. Without this, a proper understanding of what may be needed will not be possible (Wey, 2006). It has also been argued that the limited range of technologies available in ASC telecare services can encourage assessors to fit the person to the technology, rather than design the technology around the person (Gibson et al. 2016). It has also been suggested that assessments for technology should be seen as a *process*, rather than as a single event.

Second, the kinds of technology prescribed should fully take into account the capacity and capability of the recipient to use it. A pendant alarm is useless, for example, if the wearer is unable to remember to press it in an emergency.

Third, technology should not be used to replace hands-on social care, but to augment it. Reducing social contact for people with dementia will lead to even greater isolation and loneliness.

Fourth, for technology to be valued, it should be used to support a wider range of activities than simply keeping people safe. Using technology to support social contact, hobbies and preferred lifestyles can be especially important for people with dementia.

Fifth, it has been suggested that enabling technology should be designed to be adaptable to meet changing needs (as dementia progresses) and there should be a recognition that people will want to interact with the technology and customise it in different ways to its original intended use (Greenhalgh et al., 2013).

Sixth, telecare services should be better at exploiting new technological possibilities. Social media apps such as WhatsApp and Zoom may be very useful in enabling some people with dementia to keep in touch with relatives living elsewhere. Virtual assistants (for example, 'Alexa') might also have a role in supporting meaningful occupation. Apps have also been developed for mobile phones to promote 'safer walking' and prevent people with dementia from becoming lost (Wood et al., 2015). These technologies were not generally used in ASC telecare services.

Finally, it is important to remember that everyone's journey through dementia is different, and it is very unwise to assume that technology that 'works' for one person will work for all. Technology should never be imposed: co-production of solutions – which may or may not involve the use of technology – is more likely to result in a good match between need and technology, and that the technology is useful and valued.

References

Bjørneby, S., Topo, P. & Holthe, T. (1999). *Technology, ethics and dementia: A guidebook on how to apply technology in dementia care.* Norwegian Centre for Dementia Research/INFO-banken.

Department of Health. (2005). *Building telecare in England.* Department of Health. http://webarchive.nationalarchives.gov.uk/20130107105354/http:/www.dh.gov.uk/prod_consum_dh/groups/dh_digitalassets/@dh/@en/documents/digitalasset/dh_4115644.pdf

Department of Health. (2006). *Local authority circular LAC (2006)5: Preventative technology grant 2006/07–2007/08.* Department of Health. http://data.parliament.uk/DepositedPapers/Files/DEP2009-0073/DEP2009-0073.pdf

Department of Health. (2009). *Whole system demonstrators: An overview of telecare and telehealth.* Department of Health. https://webarchive.nationalarchives.gov.uk/ukgwa/20130107105354/http://www.dh.gov.uk/prod_consum_dh/groups/dh_digitalassets/documents/digitalasset/dh_100947.pdf

Department of Health. (2011). *Whole system demonstrator programme headline findings.* Department of Health. https://assets.publishing.service.gov.uk/government/uploads/system/uploads/attachment_data/file/215264/dh_131689.pdf

Federici, S., Meloni, F. & Borsci, S. (2016). The abandonment of assistive technology in Italy: A survey of National Health Service users. *European Journal of Physical and Rehabilitation Medicine, 52(4),* 516–526.

Forsyth, K., Henderson, C., Davis, L., Singh Roy, A., Dunk, B., Curnow, E., Gathercole, R., Lam, N., Harper, E., Leroi, I., Woolham, J., Fox, C., O'Brien, J., Bateman, A., Poland, F., Bentham, P., Burns, A., Davies, A., Gray, R., Bradley, R., ... & Howard, R. (2019). Assessment of need and practice for assistive technology and telecare for people with dementia: The ATTILA (Assistive Technology and Telecare to maintain Independent Living At home for people with dementia) trial. *Alzheimer's & Dementia: Translational Research and Clinical Interventions, 5(1), 420–430.*

Ganyo, M., Dunn, M. & Hope, T. (2011). Ethical issues in the use of fall detectors. *Ageing and Society, 31(8),* 1350–1367.

Gibson, G., Newton, L., Pritchard, G., Finch, T., Brittain, K. & Robinson, L. (2016). The provision of assistive technology products and services for people with dementia in the United Kingdom. *Dementia, 15(4),* 681–701.

Gramstad, A., Storli, S. L. & Hamran, T. (2014). Older individuals' experiences during the assistive technology device service delivery process. *Scandinavian Journal of Occupational Therapy, 21(4),* 305–312.

Greenhalgh, T., Procter, R., Wherton, J., Sugarhood, P., Hinder, S. & Rouncefield, M. (2015). What is quality in assisted living technology? The ARCHIE framework for effective telehealth and telecare services. *BMC Medicine, 13*(1), 1–15.

Greenhalgh, T., Wherton, J., Sugarhood, P., Hinder, S., Procter, R. & Stones, R. (2013). What matters to older people with assisted living needs? A phenomenological analysis of the use and non-use of telehealth and telecare. *Social Science & Medicine, 93*, 86–94.

Howard, R., Gathercole, R., Bradley, R., Harper, E., Davis, L., Pank, L., Lam, N., Talbot. E., Hooper, E., Winson, R., Scutt, B., Ordonez, V., Nunn, S., Lavelle, G., Bateman, A., Bentham, P., Burns, A., Dunk, B., Forsyth, K., Fox, C., Poland, F., Leroi, I., Newman, S., O'Brien, J., Henderson, C., Knapp, M., Woolham, J. & Gray, R. (2021). The effectiveness and cost-effectiveness of assistive technology and telecare for independent living in dementia: A randomised controlled trial. *Age and Ageing, 50*, 882–890.

Marshall, M. (Ed.). (2000). *ASTRID: A social & technological response to meeting the needs of individuals with dementia & their carers. A guide to using technology within dementia care.* Hawker Publications.

Steventon, A., Bardsley, M., Billings, J., Dixon, J., Doll, H., Beynon, M., Hirani, S., Cartwright, M., Rixon, L., Knapp, M., Henderson, C., Rogers, A., Hendy, J., Fitzpatrick, R. & Newman, S. (2013). Effect of telecare on use of health and social care services: Findings from the Whole Systems Demonstrator cluster randomised trial. *Age and Ageing, 42*(4), 501–508.

Wey, S. (2004). One size does not fit all: Person-centred approaches to the use of assistive technology. In Marshall, M., (Ed.), *Perspectives on rehabilitation and dementia* (pp.202–210). Jessica Kingsley.

Wey, S. (2006). 'Working in The Zone': A social-ecological framework for dementia rehabilitation. In Woolham, J. (Ed.), *Assistive technology in dementia care: Developing the role of technology in the care and rehabilitation of people with dementia: current trends and perspectives* (pp.85–103). Hawker Publications.

Wood, E., Ward, G. & Woolham, J. (2015). The development of safer walking technology: A review. *Journal of Assistive Technologies, 9*(2), 100–115.

Woolham, J. (2005). *The effectiveness of assistive technology in supporting the independence of people with dementia: The Safe at Home project.* Hawker Publications.

Woolham, J., Steils, N., Fisk, M., Porteus, J. & Forsyth, K. (2018). *The UTOPIA project: Using telecare for older people in adult social care: The findings of a 2016-17 national survey of local authority telecare provision for older people in England.* King's College London.

Woolham, J., Steils, N., Fisk, M., Porteus, J., & Forsyth (2021). Outcomes for older telecare recipients: The importance of assessments. *Journal of Social Work, 21*(2), 162–187.

Woolham, J., Steils, N., Forsyth, K., Fisk, M., & Porteus, J. (2019). Making use of evidence in commissioning practice: Insights into the understanding of a telecare study's findings. *Evidence and Policy, 17*(1), 59–74.

23 Improving independence, self-esteem and safety with better design for people with dementia

Mary Marshall

Mrs Rossi reported that her husband was very frustrated and bad tempered in the morning because he could no longer lay out the breakfast, something he had done every day of their married life. He could not find things any longer. Mrs Rossi was advised to take the doors off the cupboards or buy glass-fronted doors. She did this and reported that her husband was now able to continue this routine and had returned to his normal cheerful self.

Mrs Gruber was not eating well in the dining room of her care home. She sat with her fists clenched and her whole body tense. One of the staff had a decibel counter on her phone and, to her astonishment, the noise levels were dangerously high for everyone. A large sound-absorbent picture panel was mounted on the dining room wall, soft table mats were used on the tables and staff training on noise awareness was undertaken. Mrs Gruber visibly relaxed as the noise levels were reduced and she began to eat better.

Mr Mackie was not sleeping during the night, having previously been a good sleeper. This was affecting his mood and competence. After much careful investigation, it was realised that an office across the street had changed to 24-hour working and had its lights on all night. This meant that his bedroom was bright all night. Blackout curtains were installed. Mr Mackie was also encouraged to sit in a lounge with lots of bright light in the mornings, to reset his body clock. After a couple of weeks, his sleep/awake cycle was restored, and he was more relaxed and competent.

Design is an important non-pharmaceutical intervention that can make a huge difference to the wellbeing of people with dementia. Most younger people just make the best of the design of a house, day centre or care home, without understanding the impact of some features on vulnerable people, who are usually unable to explain or deal with their problem. If we understand the main impairments of older people and people with dementia, we can easily see why some aspects of buildings are problematic.

It is not difficult to design for people with a single impairment, such as using a wheelchair; it is more difficult to design for people experiencing the complex combination of old age and dementia. However, it is possible to improve their independence, self-esteem and safety. This chapter is a very basic introduction to the issues involved. For more detail, see the *World Alzheimer Report 2020* on dementia and design (Fleming et al., 2020) and the specific books referred to in the text. Bowes and Dawson (2019) provide a literature review of design and dementia.

Impairments of old age

Generally speaking, many impairments are inevitable as you age. Muscles and bones deteriorate, affecting mobility, reach, grip and so forth. Often neglected are shoulder and neck muscles, which mean that most older people stoop to some degree. They therefore need signs, important information and pictures lower down. Toilet signs, for example, are best at 1.2 metres from the floor.

The muscles of the hands can become weaker, which means, for example, that the large press-button flush systems in public toilets can be very difficult. Lung muscles are crucial to breathing well, yet they often deteriorate, meaning that people get less oxygen. This is crucial to the functioning of the brain. Stuffy lounges will mean that people are less alert. Annie Pollock (2021) has written a useful guide to all aspects of air quality and people with dementia.

Eyesight deteriorates for most older people – the world looks hazier. This means that colours will seem less bright. Indeed, many people will struggle to differentiate between colours at the blue and violet end of the spectrum unless there is a lot of light or they are outside. Thus, for example, pale blue and pale purple may look the same. It is important not to rely on colour to assist older people to find their way.

It is crucial to understand the significance of contrast in designing for older people and people with dementia. Objects may be invisible unless there is a good contrast. A chair the same colour as the carpet, for example, may mean that people fall over it because they cannot see it. Wording on signs needs to be larger and contrasting. Contrast is a function of 'tone'. It is the extent to which light is reflected by a surface and is measured in LRV (Light Reflectance Value) – zero LRV is black (no light reflectance) and 100 LRV is pure white. To ensure good contrast, the LRV between two colours/tones has to be 30 or more.

Learning point 1

Being aware of the importance of good contrast (and conversely no contrast where necessary) is perhaps the most important and least recognised design feature:

- Using the camera app on your mobile phone, switch it to 'greyscale'. If you now look at an object, you will be able to see clearly if there is adequate contrast. Try it on floor coverings. If the contrast is strong between two areas of different flooring, someone with dementia might see a step and fall over.
- Next time you are in a hardware shop, look at a Dulux paint chart and you will see that the LRV is given beside each colour square. If you then pick out another very different colour set, you will see that some have the same LRV. This demonstrates that different colours side by side may not contrast.

Light is important for the ageing eye (McNair et al., 2017). Many people at home could cope better and be less likely to fall if the lighting was improved. Indeed, some people with dementia will tell you that they can no longer knit or read the newspaper, when the reality is that they can see if there is enough light. Aim for double the levels of lighting that a 45-year-old with normal sight would want. Natural light is a great deal brighter than most artificial light, so ensure this is maximised – for example, by avoiding curtains and pelmets that reduce the light through windows. However, the ageing eye is very sensitive to glare, so blinds or voile curtains will be required where there is direct sunlight shining in.

Hearing gets less acute, especially at the higher frequencies (R. Pollock, 2021). This can mean that lots of low sounds become indistinguishable: for example, conversation in a busy café. The care assistant in Mrs Gruber's care home did well to realise that noise might be a problem. Dining rooms can be particularly noisy places – the clatter of knives and forks on the table, the dishwasher in the background, hard surfaces that reverberate and so on. Soft table mats and other sound-absorbing changes can make a big difference, but the main change needs to be in staff – noise awareness is crucial.

Learning point 2

Noise is an invisible problem that causes much of the distressed behaviour of people with dementia. Becoming noise aware is not difficult if you stop and listen. You might like to download a decibel app onto your phone.

- Try counting the number of sources of noise next time you are in a café.
- Next time you are startled by a noise, imagine what it might be like to be an anxious person with dementia who cannot understand where the sound is coming from.
- Watch older people in busy cafés and notice how many of them are tense and often leaning forward in their attempts to hear conversation.

Impairments of dementia

As far as design is concerned, there are four key impairments that can result from dementia to consider. The first is impaired memory. Mr Rossi could not remember where the cereal, tea and coffee were kept. Things need to be more visible so people can rely less on memory. Open-plan kitchens with glass cupboard doors and shelves can all help.

People with dementia can slip back in time in their efforts to make sense of their world – sometimes to their childhoods. In terms of environments, our most vivid memories of rooms and places are when we were adolescents and young adults. This means, for people who are now in their 80s, we should try to design places that make sense for those seeing them through 1950s and 1960s eyes. It does not mean trying to make rooms look like they were in the 1950s – people have very different tastes so it would be impossible to get it right for everyone. It does mean that rooms have to give a lot of clues about their purpose. Lounges need to look like lounges, dining rooms like dining rooms and so on. Multi-purpose rooms can be very confusing.

Along with being age appropriate, it is important to be culturally appropriate, which can be a challenge in communal places. Increasing numbers of older people resident in the UK were born elsewhere. They may be making sense of the world through very different eyes as they forget the adjustments they made when they moved to the UK.

Making spaces age- and culturally appropriate is not straightforward. In very general terms, it is sensible to aim for 'traditional' and then add specific things to meet the needs of the actual people living there. Liz Fuggle's book (2013) on interiors is very helpful. Personal spaces, such as bedrooms, can be made fully appropriate for the individual.

The second key impairment in dementia is learning. People may, for example, not be able to learn where the toilet is, so good signage is crucial. They may not know where they are living, even though they have been told many times. Making a place feel welcoming and genuinely homely will be reassuring, even if someone does not know that they are in a care home, for example. Ensuring a care home bedroom is full of familiar objects can be reassuring. Photographs are not enough unless they are old ones, as people with dementia can forget who is in them. One recurring problem is carers' frequent unwillingness to bring in 'Mum's old rubbish'. This is a mistake – objects trigger memories, even if they are old and worn. Julie Christie, in her book on resilience and people with dementia (2020), specifically mentions objects as being helpful in reinforcing identity.

The third impairment is problem-solving. Mrs Gruber, above, was unable to understand or explain why she found the dining room so stressful. Impaired problem solving is often underestimated. It can make independent living really difficult. People may lose the ability to switch on the radio or light the cooker. This impairment is not helped by the fact that both kitchen and bathroom equipment is endlessly modernised in design. Working out how to use a hands-free tap or a modern kettle that looks like a jug may be beyond many people with dementia. The design solution is to make things intuitive/obvious.

A related issue is murals (Marshall, 2019), which are increasingly common in care homes and hospitals. These are photographs printed onto wallpaper and stuck on walls. They should be used with caution. People with dementia may be unable to work out that these are not real. Sometimes the murals are windows onto a garden or nature, which is potentially very confusing because the seasons do not change and the view may be quite different from the view from the actual windows. Sometimes, there are doors that are not doors to anywhere. Many people with dementia may like them, but others will be frightened or confused.

The fourth important impairment is sensory challenge. Sensory challenges are faced by many people with dementia as the brain no longer interprets the information it is receiving effectively. We really should describe dementia as leading to 'cognitive and sensory impairments', since the latter are so common.

Among the most common are what are called 'perceptual problems': something goes wrong between the eye and the back of the brain that interprets the information coming through the eye. If you combine this with the normal visual impairments of old age, it is highly problematic. As in Learning point 1, people may see a step when there is a lot of contrast of tone (more than 5 LRV) between one area of flooring and another. People with dementia may also struggle with shiny floors, perceiving pools of water. Complicated patterns can look like insects, wavy lines can seem to be moving and stripes can look like bars. Avoid highly patterned carpets, vinyl, wallpapers and fabrics.

Other senses can be affected too. Agnes Houston and Julie Christie (2018) have written a very useful book on all the senses.

The dementia design challenge

The challenge in design is understanding the possible impact of the impairments common in older people and those that can occur for people with dementia, and the additional problems when they go together. Mr Mackie above could probably neither remember nor understand that the bedroom was too light for him.

Learning point 3

Consider the vulnerability of older people with dementia in their environment. They can often neither understand it nor change it if it is causing them problems. The more impaired they are, the more they are victims of it. We have a responsibility to ensure that environments are as enabling and not damaging as possible. If you are in contact with people with dementia, try to experience the environment as they might:

- Try switching off the TV and see if they look more relaxed.
- Try providing more light and see if they look around with interest.
- Try opening the window and see if they perk up.
- Try a new, clear sign on the toilet and see if it is easier for people to find their way.

There is a great deal we can do to help if we have empathy and knowledge, and much of what is needed is not expensive or difficult to achieve. Designing a building from scratch means a lot of good design can be built in from the start – such as making it easy for people to understand and navigate, even with a poor memory. However, most staff and relatives will be making small adaptations to an existing house, day centre or care home to enable people with dementia be more independent and less stressed. The test of an enabling environment is usually in the detail. Are the floors all the same tone? Is there enough light? Is it easy to understand how to work the taps? And so on.

We must not forget outside spaces

All the design considerations above apply equally to outside spaces. Going outside is essential for several reasons:

- to get fresh air and exercise
- to synthesise vitamin D (between April and October in the UK). Vitamin D is essential for muscles and bones
- to ensure the body clock is working effectively (the photo-sensitive ganglions in the eye absorb bright light, which is needed to set the body clock)
- because outside is usually quieter than indoors
- because nature is really important for our mental health. Even looking out onto nature is beneficial. However, it is better to get outside (see Gilliard & Marshall, 2012)
- because a lot of people have spent a great deal of their lives outside, and they will get very restless if they are confined indoors.

There are often barriers to going outside. Not being able to find or open the door can make it impossible; a change in the tone of flooring/paving slabs can be alarming; being unable to see a seat can be off-putting if you are a bit lacking in confidence, and so on.

We have to remember that really familiar outside spaces vary hugely from one person to another. Jane Gilliard and I collected descriptions of many different kinds of outside spaces in Marshall and Gilliard (2014). For a full guide to designing outside spaces, see Annie Pollock's book (2018).

Learning point 4

Getting it right for outside spaces is as important as getting it right indoors. When you are next in a park or garden:
- Look at a bench: does it look like a bench? Does it contrast with the paving? Would you be able to see it clearly enough to trust to sit on it?
- Imagine you grew up in a farming community. Would the outside space you are in now make sense?

- Consider the paving and paths. Do they have strong contrasts? Might a person with dementia see a step that isn't there, and then hesitate and fall?

References

Bowes, A. & Dawson, A. (2019). *Designing environments for people with dementia: A systematic literature review.* Emerald Publishers.

Christie, J. (2020). *Promoting resilience in dementia care.* Jessica Kingsley Publishers.

Fleming, R., Zeisel, J. & Bennett K. (2020). *Design, dignity and dementia: Dementia-related design and the built environment. World Alzheimer Report 2020.* Alzheimer's Disease International (ADI).

Fuggle, L. (2013). *Designing interiors for people with dementia.* Dementia Services Development Centre.

Gilliard, J. & Marshall, M. (Eds.). (2012). *Transforming the quality of life for people with dementia through contact with the natural world: Fresh air on my face.* Jessica Kingsley Publishers.

Houston, A. with Christie, J. (2018). *Talking sense: Living with sensory changes and dementia.* The Dementia Centre/HammondCare.*

Marshall, M. (2019). *Talking murals: The use of murals in places where people with dementia live.* The Dementia Centre/HammondCare.*

Marshall, M. & Gilliard, J. (Eds.). (2014). *Creating culturally appropriate outside spaces and experiences for people with dementia.* Jessica Kingsley Publishers.

McNair, D. & Pollock, R., with Cunningham, C. (2017). *Enlighten: Lighting for older people and people with dementia.* Dementia Centre/HammondCare.*

Pollock, A. (2018). *The room outside: Designing outdoor living for older people and people with dementia.* Dementia Centre/HammondCare.*

Pollock, A. (2021). *A breath of fresh air. The importance of air quality in aged care design.* Dementia Centre/HammondCare.*

Pollock, R. (2021). *Acoustics in aged care. Optimising environments for older people with dementia.* Dementia Centre/HammondCare.*

* These resources are free to download from the resources/design area of the Dementia Centre/ HammondCare website: www.dementiacentre.com.au

24 How can gardening enrich the lives of people with dementia?

Sarah Swift and Margaret Brown

Gardening, whether at home, in community spaces or in residential care, has the potential to enrich the lived experience of dementia, reducing social isolation, positively affecting mood and engagement, and improving wellbeing. Moreover, gardening can enable people with dementia to develop a more positive sense of self, cultivate a sense of place, and demonstrate resistance against the stigma associated with their condition.

Despite increasing acknowledgement of the potential of gardening for promoting a more positive experience of dementia, and the development of innovative gardening and forestry projects, opportunities for people living with the condition to enjoy garden spaces remain few. Resources intended to guide carers in supporting people with dementia to spend time outside remain largely focused on risk avoidance, rather than facilitating meaningful, enjoyable outdoor engagement.

In this chapter, we will explore the meaning and value of gardens for people living with dementia and offer practical suggestions for empowering them to enjoy garden spaces. We will also explore the ways in which technology can be used to enable people living with dementia to engage with gardens when physical ability presents a barrier to accessing outdoor environments.

Learning point 1

Learning from the lived experiences of those living with the condition can help us to gain a deeper insight into the meaning and value of gardening for people with dementia:

- Keep your gardening group small to help to ensure that everyone feels included and able to contribute. Jarrott and Gigliotti (2010) recommend including no more than eight people in each group.

- Involve your gardening group members in planning gardening activities. Ask your participants what they would like to do, and incorporate their ideas into your sessions. Following through with your group members' suggestions can help them feel meaningfully involved in the process.

- Invite your group members to share their gardening stories. By learning more about their experiences, you will be able to tailor sessions to their interests and abilities, and they may even be able to lend their expertise to the gardening sessions.

The importance of gardening for people with dementia

Gardening holds a variety of benefits for people with dementia, contributing to increased wellbeing (Hewitt et al., 2013), improving mood and engagement (Jarrott & Gigliotti, 2010) and relieving stress and anxiety (Robertson, 2012). Beyond the reduction of clinical symptoms associated with the condition, gardening possesses the potential to enrich the lived experiences of people with dementia, enabling individuals to express their identity, assert a sense of agency and demonstrate resistance against the stigma associated with dementia (Noone & Jenkins, 2018).

The garden carries a variety of meanings throughout the life course, from a site of play and creativity in childhood to an opportunity to express one's identity and continuing ability to make worthwhile contributions in later life. Gardening becomes an increasingly appealing pastime in later life, with 62% of UK adults over the age of 65 expressing an enjoyment of gardening in their spare time (Milligan & Bingley, 2015).

For older people, the meaning of the garden may be connected to its role as a site of embodied practice, enabling those in later life to express a sense of self and status through their physical actions and navigate the changing relationship between an individual and their home, garden and body in retirement. Engaging with the garden can support an older person in maintaining a sense of identity and independence, becoming a symbol of their resistance against the perceived loss of control and identity experienced as they transition into the third and fourth ages (Milligan & Bingley, 2015).

It may be assumed that the experience of gardening of a person with dementia is informed in part by the factors affecting the wider older population, as most people living with dementia are aged 65 or older (Prince et al., 2014). However, the meaning of the garden may be more complex and profound for people living with dementia, as they face a dual loss of identity – not just due to getting older but also due to the impact of dementia on sense of self. Furthermore, the additional barriers faced by people with dementia when seeking to access activities such as gardening may heighten the value of the experience for them.

A significant proportion of people with dementia are deprived of regular contact with nature; Gilliard and Marshall (2012) report that 50% of care home residents with dementia never go outside, with a further 25% going outdoors only rarely. In other research, 74% of people with dementia living in the community said they lacked the confidence to spend time outdoors, citing a variety of factors, including transportation and physical access to outdoor spaces, lack of self-confidence and fear of stigma, and insufficient availability of dementia-friendly information and activities at nature sites (Mapes et al., 2016).

Concerns regarding the perceived risks associated with outdoor environments such as gardens further limit the ability of people with dementia to enjoy gardening, particularly when those reservations are held by care providers. Almost three-quarters of carers who responded to a recent Natural England survey (Mapes et al., 2016) expressed a reluctance to encourage people with dementia to spend time outdoors, due to worries over safety. Such concerns are well intentioned, but by restricting the ability of people with dementia to access natural environments, they may contribute to the social exclusion and isolation that many experience (Kane & Cook, 2013). They also deprive people living with dementia of the opportunity to enjoy the plethora of benefits associated with being outdoors.

Creating an empowering, enjoyable garden space for people with dementia

Risk enablement in the garden

Gardening and other outdoor activities are commonly considered to be inherently high risk for people with dementia (Cook, 2016). Many of the existing guidelines concerning gardening and dementia (e.g. Alzheimer's Society, 2013) focus on minimising risks and avoiding injury. Although decisions rooted in risk aversion are well intentioned, family and professional care providers may unwittingly negatively affect the emotional and mental wellbeing of a person with dementia in the quest to avoid physical harm. Taking a risk aversive approach to planning gardening activities with people with dementia can negatively impact on their experiences in the garden, removing their freedom of choice (Clarke et al., 2011) and discouraging them from undertaking an active role in gardening tasks.

Conversely, adopting a risk-enablement approach to working with people with dementia can elevate their experiences in the garden by empowering them to participate in decision-making and exercise their autonomy. Working *with* people with dementia to determine their level of risk tolerance, rather than deciding *for* them, can encourage meaningful participation in gardening activities and offer individuals with dementia an opportunity to assert their agency and independence.

Learning point 2

Information on dementia-friendly garden design focuses largely on the design of the physical space, including safety considerations, adaptations and sensory elements. However, we argue that the way people with dementia are involved in gardening activities – guided by a risk-enablement philosophy, with opportunities for meaningful participation in decision-making – is equally essential to engaging people with dementia in gardens.

- Ask your group participants about the activities they would like to undertake in the garden – this can give helpful insight into their level of risk tolerance.
- Ensure you obtain verbal consent from your gardening group members before each task and ask whether they have any worries about taking part in a particular activity.

Meaningful involvement in decision-making

The dementia activism movement is underpinned by the notion that there should be 'nothing about us without us' (Bryden, 2015). However, in the garden, whether at home or in the community, decisions are often made *for*, rather than *with*, people with dementia, perpetuating the disempowerment and loss of agency experienced by many people living with the condition. When people with dementia are meaningfully involved in decision-making concerning gardening activities and the overall development of the space, the garden becomes the embodied articulation of agency and a space for the expression of identity and selfhood and the development of lasting social connections as a result of sharing experiences and working together to achieve goals (Noone & Jenkins, 2018). Furthermore, involving people with dementia as decision-makers can increase engagement with gardening activities and promote more positive outcomes for participants, as activities can be tailored to their abilities and interests, and may even contribute to the development of new skills and knowledge.

How does your garden grow?

In the summer of 2016, I (Sarah) collaboratively created a community garden with a group of people with dementia as part of my doctoral research. I sought to challenge the limitation I had noticed in previous studies in this field, in which people with dementia had been positioned in a passive role, rather than invited to play an active part in the development of the garden.

Following each gardening session, I discussed with the gardeners the activities they would like to try the following week, and I planned the next session based on the group's ideas. Some of the group members were experienced gardeners, whose knowledge and skills far outweighed mine. Others were curious novices, who wanted to try activities such as growing vegetables and planting hanging baskets but were unsure where to start. All of the gardeners shared suggestions over the course of the project, and every activity undertaken in the garden was chosen by the group.

By meaningfully involving the gardeners in the decision-making process, the project benefitted from the extensive knowledge of the group's more experienced members and offered the gardeners an opportunity to indulge their curiosity and learn new skills. In doing so, we demonstrated that people with dementia can contribute a wealth of knowledge and experience to communal activities and embrace the opportunity to develop new abilities, challenging some of the negative stereotypes encountered by many people living with dementia.

Using technology to help people with dementia enjoy gardens

The digital world has opened a range of possibilities for gardens and gardening for people with dementia. New technology, such as tablets, wearable devices, smart home systems, gaming systems involving body motion, and augmented and virtual reality (Astell et al., 2019), is greatly expanding the potential to support people living with dementia in a range of settings. The following project is one way of using everyday digital technology to meet the needs of a person living at home with a recent diagnosis of dementia.

Our virtual garden

This local project for people with dementia was set in a church garden. The group was supported by the local NHS community mental health team for older people. The team explored the use of a digital solution for people who had been diagnosed with dementia and were unable to visit the real garden site, whether due to a physical condition affecting mobility, depression or a reluctance to engage with strangers. The aim was to support the person to become part of the garden group. A practitioner would visit the person and, using their tablet, link with the established garden group to make a digital bridge for the person with dementia. The person could chat, choose plants or give advice to other people with dementia and practitioners during the gardening experience. This broke down barriers and could provide a pathway to them attending the group in person. A short film outlining the project is available at www.youtube.com/watch?v=-xiR6XxxWLU

The current digital apex of augmented and virtual reality systems would seem to offer the richest experience of gardens and open spaces. This would seem ideal for the garden environment, with its rich, multi-sensory encounters. These bespoke environments are intended to surround the person with images and sound, immersing them in the experience. Research on this approach to gardens is sparse but the use by care homes of virtual headsets to immerse the person with dementia in range of different spaces is being explored (see, for example, BBC News, 2019). A pilot study in an Australian care home created a virtual forest on a large, interactive digital screen, using gaming technology, including motion sensors, vivid images and a soundtrack (Moyle et al., 2018). The residents involved were rated to have greater pleasure and alertness during the experience, but they also had higher levels of fear and anxiety. The use of such a digital experience with people with sensory and neurological changes due to age and dementia needs more study. Being transported to a new and unfamiliar environment successfully would depend on the person's understanding and previous experience.

Less dynamic digital opportunities may be offered by lower-level technology, such as digital sound applications that play birdsong or replicate the weather and movement in the garden. Visual stimulation can be achieved by films of gardens, whether standard professional films or television programmes. Families may be willing to film their own or the person's garden through the year, supporting the person to reconnect with the changing of the seasons. Digital photograph frames with images of the garden and planting may be a slower form of technology where people with impaired cognitive function can maintain interest.

Alongside these virtual options, a table with gardening equipment, plant pots, compost and plants can augment the experience by involving the key senses of smell and touch.

Learning point 3

When actual gardening is not possible, either temporarily or permanently, technology offers a way into the experience. If this can also be augmented by planting and plant care indoors, having a view of the garden outside and creating the sounds and smells of the garden can enhance the experience.

- Ask family members to share their gardening experiences by using their tablet or phone to video what they are doing.
- Work with the person and family to take photographs of their garden through the seasons and upload them to a digital photo frame. This can be used for cognitive stimulation activities.

Conclusion

Gardens and gardening at home in the community or with digital support has the potential to inspire and enrich the daily lives of people living with dementia. This is an opportunity to reduce loneliness, improve mental wellbeing and challenge the stigma associated with the condition. There is a range of very positive initiatives developing across community and care home settings but a lack of robust research to inform guidance and resources. In this chapter, the significance of gardens for people living with dementia is identified and emphasis is placed on a risk-enablement approach. This has potential to empower them and reduce barriers to their accessing the pleasures of the garden.

References

Alzheimer's Society. (2013). *Taking part: Activities for people with dementia* (3rd ed.). Alzheimer's Society Publications.

Astell, A.J., Bouranis, N., Hoey, J., Lindauer, A., Mihailidis, A., Nugent, C. & Robillard, J.M. (2019). Technology and dementia: The future is now. *Dementia and Geriatric Cognitive Disorders, 47*(3), 131–139.

BBC News. (2019, September 13). *How virtual reality is helping people with dementia.* www.bbc.co.uk/news/av/business-49654052/how-virtual-reality-is-helping-people-with-dementia

Bryden, C. (2015). *Nothing about us, without us: 20 years of dementia advocacy.* Jessica Kingsley.

Clarke, C.L., Wilcockson, J., Gibb, C.E., Keady, J., Wilkinson, H. & Luce, A. (2011). Reframing risk management in dementia care through collaborative learning. *Health and Social Care in the Community, 19*(1), 23–32.

Cook, M. (2016). How woodlands and forests enhance mental well-being. *Journal of Dementia Care, 24*(3), 20–23.

Gilliard, J. & Marshall, M. (2012). Introduction. In J. Gilliard & M. Marshall (Eds.), *Transforming the quality of life for people with dementia through contact with the natural world: Fresh air on my face* (pp.11–16). Jessica Kingsley.

Hewitt, P., Watts, C., Hussey, J., Power, K. & Williams, T. (2013). Does a structured gardening programme improve well-being in young-onset dementia? A preliminary study. *British Journal of Occupational Therapy, 76*(8), 355–361.

Jarrott, S.E. & Gigliotti, C.M. (2010). Comparing responses to horticultural-based and traditional activities in dementia care programs. *American Journal of Alzheimer's Disease & Other Dementias, 25*(8), 657–665.

Kane, M. & Cook, L. (2013). *Dementia 2013: The hidden voice of loneliness.* Alzheimer's Society.

Mapes, N., Milton, S., Nicholls, V. & Williamson, T. (2016). *'Is it nice outside?' Consulting people living with dementia and carers about engaging with the natural environment.* NECR 211. Natural England.

Milligan, C. & Bingley, A. (2015). Gardens and gardening in later life. In J. Twigg & W. Martin (Eds.), *Routledge handbook of cultural gerontology* (pp.321–328). Routledge.

Moyle, W., Jones, C., Dwan, T. & Petrovitch, T. (2018). Effectiveness of a virtual reality forest on people with dementia: A mixed methods pilot study. *The Gerontologist, 58*(3), 478–487.

Noone, S. & Jenkins, N. (2018). Digging for dementia: Exploring the experience of community gardening from the perspectives of people with dementia. *Aging & Mental Health, 22*(7), 881–888.

Prince, M., Knapp, M., Guerchet, M., McCrone, P., Prina, M., Comas-Herrera, A., Wittenberg, R., Adelaja, B., Hu, B., King, D., Rehill, A. & Salimkumar, D. (2014). *Dementia UK: Update.* Alzheimer's Society.

Robertson, L. (2012). Allotments. In J. Gilliard & M. Marshall (Eds.), *Transforming the quality of life for people with dementia through contact with the natural world: Fresh air on my face* (pp.106–113). Jessica Kingsley.

25 Nature's role as a coping mechanism for people living with dementia

Wendy Brewin

Access to nature is increasing, with the number of weekly visits per person in England to urban green spaces increasing from 1.3 to 1.7 since 2009 (Natural England, 2019). However, many of us don't yet fully understand the pivotal role nature can play in our healthcare, despite emerging NHS models demonstrating the importance of contact with it. GPs now prescribe contact with nature as part of patients' treatment (RSPB, 2018), and there is even an NHS Forest project,[1] where health sites are working together to realise the healthcare and wellbeing benefits of their green spaces – both examples of how nature is recognised as having significant health benefits. Yet people living with health challenges are more likely to face barriers that limit access to outdoor benefits. Our work with people living with dementia demonstrates the significant physical, emotional and social wellbeing that can be gained from nature-based activities, when barriers to access are overcome (Brewin & Stoneham, 2018).

Barriers for people living with dementia

People living with dementia often experience barriers to accessing nature. Increased anxiety, depression and social stigma can transform the outside world into a place of inaccessible environments and uncomfortable situations. Research into social isolation and loneliness has discovered that the same brain pathways that are triggered by physical pain are also triggered by loneliness (Harrington & Swilinski, 2020), which indicates that isolation and loneliness are the social equivalent of physical pain. So, staying at home may feel the safer option, but unfortunately it brings its own issues, which can intensify negative emotions for all those involved.

---

1. www.nhsforest.org

Learning point 1

- Identify the barriers affecting someone's access to the outdoors. First, make a list of their nature interests (this can be simply watching wildlife from the window) and their level of ability.
- Some barriers may be outside your influence. Look at tackling small barriers to trigger big impacts. For example, short indoor activities can lift confidence levels and, by encouraging a move to spending short periods outside, lead to increased social interaction.

The benefits of connecting with nature

Introducing nature-based approaches into someone's daily life early after a dementia diagnosis can bring benefits throughout their ongoing care. Increased access to nature can have a positive impact on reducing the need for medication and help people with dementia and their carers cope better with dementia-related challenges (Brewin & Stoneham, 2018). This supports a constructive mental health outlook and encourages self-esteem.

Physical and physiological benefits

Many people with dementia have comorbidity or multimorbidity (one or more additional health issues). They are likely to have difficulty undertaking high-impact exercise. However, there is still value in moving at a reduced pace. Any level of physical activity outdoors increases oxygen levels in vital muscles and organs, like the heart and the brain. Walking gently in nature can be enough, as shown in emerging health movements like forest bathing and forest therapy (Farrow & Washburn, 2019). These therapies report benefits such as reduced blood pressure and decreased anxiety by elevating levels of the brain chemicals that make us feel happier.

Natural sunlight is important for maintaining our sleep/wake system, or circadian rhythm. Studies have shown that sunlight can reduce cognitive deterioration and symptoms of depression (Riemersma-van de Lek et al., 2008), both of which can impact negatively on sleep for people living with dementia. Plants also play a vital part in human health, as evidenced in research into chemicals known as phytoncides, produced by plants as part of their own immune systems. Findings suggest that, when we inhale phytoncides, they both stimulate the action of the body's white blood cells, which help fight infections, and increase the number of these cells in our bodies (Li et al., 2009).

Mental health benefits

Emotional wellbeing plays a large part in how we see ourselves and interact with others. Nature provides that 'feel-good' factor – the more the person connects with nature, the better they feel (Richardson & McEwan, 2018).

Spending time outside in natural sunlight helps our bodies produce 'happy' chemicals: dopamine, oxytocin, serotonin and endorphins. These chemicals increase our sense of wellbeing and act as neurotransmitters in the brain. The Attention Restoration theory (Kaplan & Kaplan, 1989) suggests that the 'effortless attention' of being in and observing natural environments allows the cognitive brain to recharge, so that it is later able to focus on tasks that require deeper concentration.

Social health benefits

Immersion in outdoor landscapes inspires our creativity and motivates us to repeat the experience or explore new experiences. It also provides access to social opportunities, which are vital for creating meaningful relationships and developing social skills (ten Brink et al., 2016).

For many people, dementia closes doors to social opportunities. Loud and crowded situations can be difficult because they overstimulate their senses. Low self-confidence can make a once-habitual trip to the pub seem daunting. Public green spaces provide environments that can feel welcoming and safe. If these are quiet places, they provide solitude and peace. Large, open spaces offer opportunities for social interaction without the person with dementia feeling overwhelmed.

Learning point 2

Although discussed separately, the physical and mental health benefits – which include interacting with others – work together to support someone's quality of life. If one of these factors improves, this will have a positive impact on the other factors.

- Spend more time in the garden or the park and try walking further. Do you notice any of the following:
  - benefits from increasing your physical exercise
  - reduction in stress
  - more opportunities to interact with others?

- If there is difficulty in getting outdoors, introduce some indoor plants into the home of the person living with dementia. These plants still provide health benefits, albeit to a lesser degree than plants and trees that are growing outside. The house plants also produce phytoncides, increase oxygen levels indoors, are a focus for conversation and introduce sensory stimulation.

Nature as a coping mechanism

A systematic review by researchers at the European Centre for Environment and Human Health (Orr et al., 2016) shows that older people engage with nature on various levels. Whether sitting indoors looking out of the window or being physically active outdoors, we all engage with nature in our own ways. For people with dementia, however, previous outdoor hobbies may no longer be possible, or even desirable, anymore. The good news is that nature provides so many other activities and resources to help someone cope with life's problems.

At Sensory Trust,[2] we use nature-based approaches and environments as 'tools' to help people enjoy physically active lives that are mentally stimulating and sociable, for as long as possible. We develop new activities and adapt established ones to help people with dementia cope with issues like anxiety and depression. Nature activities can also be used as communication tools to help someone who is living with dementia feel involved in daily life. Just creating a collage using images of gardens, landscapes, outdoor activities and structures cut out of magazines can engage someone in designing or redeveloping an outdoor space.

People can access nature through indoor activities, such as bulb-planting or making Christmas decorations using 'green' materials. Other enjoyable activities include looking at nature websites, online magazines[3] and videos. Our carers' blog provides free resources that support families living with dementia and help them to engage with each other and the outdoors.[4] There is also the bonus of enjoying virtual tours of people's gardens via smart phones and tablets.

In our Creative Spaces project, we demonstrate the importance of devising and using activities that are led by the individual's wishes and capabilities. The type and length of any activity is guided by their level of interest and knowledge. This in itself is a coping mechanism. It helps our beneficiaries to see that they have contributed to and often led the activity. It raises their sense of self-worth and confidence, which are strong foundations in helping them to feel that they are better able to cope with dementia-related issues.

Learning point 3

Nature-based approaches are not 'one-size-fits-all' solutions. People have different levels of confidence, and outlooks on life. Please consider the following:

- Engaging with nature is not always about walking or gardening. Sitting by a window and looking out at the view can calm the mind and reduce tension. It has both mental health and social benefits. It encourages the person with dementia to talk to others and stimulates a desire in them to go outside.

- Include family carers in activities, where possible. Relatives and carers will also benefit from participating in activities (such as planting bulbs in a pot indoors), as these can provide much needed support for their own health.

---

2. www.sensorytrust.org.uk/
3. www.countryfile.com
4. www.sensorytrust.org.uk/blog

Nature activities

Sensory Trust's activities are designed on an asset-based approach that responds to what people can still do, rather than activities that people now find too difficult. These activities build on common interests, such as walking, which are more likely to be included in daily routines.

Physical activities

Low-intensity activities get people moving in a gentle way and are suited to people with limited movement, or who need some persuasion to increase their level of activity. Short activities like seed-sowing, dead-heading flowers or a slow stroll won't overstretch people. For people who are also living with reduced mobility or stamina, these are safe starting points towards making small physiological improvements.

Mid-intensity activities get the heart beating just a little faster and trigger a small amount of additional exertion. These activities are helpful to people who want to be more active but perhaps have reduced stamina. Activities that encourage a little more stretching and bending are appropriate. Participants can engage in most of these activities from a sitting position when they become tired.

Nature Palettes is an activity in which participants create palettes made from natural materials that catch their eye. Participants collect outdoor materials that they are drawn to. This requires bending, stretching and walking. They then use the sticky-coated palettes to display them. They are exercising without realising it. As observers, we can notice the sensory connections that they are making outdoors and can create further activities for them, based on their interests.

High-intensity activities depend on the stamina and mobility of a person with dementia. The person with dementia may enjoy taking a brisk walk of several miles in a hilly landscape or spending the afternoon digging compost. We have worked with people who have mild dementia on a gardening project that involved a couple of afternoons of intensive gardening at an Age UK centre, where they cleared ground cover and branches and planted bulbs to brighten up a dreary garden. This activity was physically exhausting at times, but the sense of achievement that they felt lasted for some time afterwards.

Activities that support mental health

Low-intensity activities for mental health are useful in helping someone with dementia to build up their self-confidence and develop a more positive outlook. Simple, short indoor activities are ideal for this. Our *Memory Postcards* activity uses people's recollections of past events to share their stories with each other. This stimulates conversation and increases people's knowledge of their social network. It is based on writing a postcard, and so is familiar to many adults.

At mid-intensity level, we use a nature activity to encourage people with dementia to exercise their brain without exhausting it. At this level, people are still experiencing the attention restoration of focusing on nature in a 'soft' manner, without thinking too hard about what they are doing. Our *Go Find It* game is an outdoor treasure hunt card game. People are given cards with single words on them, like 'prickly' and 'sticky', and they find items outside that fit these descriptions. It can be used as a team game or as a one-to-one activity.

High-intensity activities give the brain a good 'workout' without creating feelings of inadequacy. The focus on working and enjoying the activity together, rather than on its completion. In this respect, nature's role works in bringing the focus onto the sensory aspects of the materials, working the brain through exploration of touch, smell, sight and so on. *Fibonacci in Nature* is a mentally stimulating activity that we designed for use in a cognitive stimulation therapy session. It involves learning and understanding a short sequence of the Fibonacci numbers that can be found in many aspects of nature,[5] and then applying that sequence to finding spirals in nature, such as sunflowers, snail shells and pinecones.

Social activities

Nature-based activities, indoors or outdoors, stimulate social interaction. The intrinsic connection between humans and nature is the one thing we all have in common, so social activities are important to those living with dementia who have lost many of their previous social connections.

Low-intensity social activities are useful in helping someone reconnect with their community. Public green spaces are ideal environments to enable this to happen. Our *Creative Spaces* outdoor walking and activity groups are often referred to as 'ambles, not rambles'. To foster independence, group members are encouraged to take the lead in decision-making, and we have observed an increase in the confidence of many of our members as a result of this balance of independence and social connections. Walking makes people living with dementia fitter and improves their mental health, while giving them an opportunity to socialise with others. It is also an ideal activity to help begin the process of getting back outdoors.

Mid-intensity social activities are ideal for people who have gained some confidence in being outdoors with others, and who feel comfortable in sharing their skills and knowledge. We have found that working in partnership with creative organisations brings an extra level of support to our beneficiaries. We often discover talent within them that neither we nor they knew they had. Our *Wednesday Wanderers* group is run in partnership with the Bernard Leach Pottery Studio in St. Ives. For four years, the Wanderers have enjoyed three walks a month, followed by a studio session where they have worked with clay and natural materials, producing objects inspired by nature.

---

5. https://en.wikipedia.org/wiki/Fibonacci_number

High-intensity social activities can be tricky as this might mean meeting a group of strangers or being in a busy social situation like an outdoor event. It is best to check with people beforehand as to what they are most comfortable with and only put someone in this situation if they feel happy to be there. In our outdoor activity groups, we invite new people along without any commitment and make it clear that they can leave at any point. Often it is the thought of a situation that is the barrier but knowing that they have control over the situation can help to alleviate anxiety and put people more at ease. A female member of one of our walking groups joined because she found herself physically and socially isolated at home. After enjoying the walking group for several months, she gained confidence in being with others and successfully applied to volunteer in a community café kitchen. She had been a baker for many years, and she enjoyed putting her skills to use once more. It not only increased her social circle but also improved her sense of self-worth. Being outdoors and making friends had encouraged her to strive towards participating in high-intensity social activities.

Learning point 4

- Activities that people are enjoying will engage them for longer. If people enjoy walking, encourage them to walk a little further or enjoy the view a little longer.
- Regardless of the level of intensity, any activity should be guided by the individual. Putting them in the 'driving seat' helps to increase their self-value and confidence.
- There are no right ways or wrong ways to do any activity. When doing a creative, practical activity, it is not about the quality of the object or completing the task. The real benefits come from the time spent in conversation when doing the activity together.

Conclusion

People's relationship with nature is vital to the quality of their lives. The barriers that people with dementia face can drastically reduce their access to the outdoors, and as a result they experience additional burdens on their health. Nature-based approaches can be used to encourage people outdoors again. A simple activity like walking, or more creative approaches like Nature Palettes and Memory Postcards, enable people to regain lost confidence and self-worth. Connecting with nature for just a few minutes each day can make a big difference to their health, improve the quality of life for people with dementia, and foster their feelings of independence for longer.

References

Brewin, W. & Stoneham, J. (2018). *Creative spaces in the community: Evaluation report*. Sensory Trust. www.sensorytrust.org.uk/uploads/documents/Creative-Spaces-Evaluation-2018.pdf

Farrow, M. R. & Washburn, K. (2019). A review of field experiments on the effect of forest bathing on anxiety and heart rate variability. *Global Advances in Health and Medicine, 16*(8), 2164956119848654.

Harrington, K. & Swilinski, M.J. (2020, August 4). The loneliness of social isolation can affect your brain and raise dementia risk in older adults. *The Conversation*. https://theconversation.com/the-loneliness-of-social-isolation-can-affect-your-brain-and-raise-dementia-risk-in-older-adults-141752

Kaplan, R. & Kaplan, S. (1989). Fascination. In R. Kaplan & S. Kaplan, *The experience of nature: A psychological perspective* (pp.192–197). Cambridge University Press.

Li, Q., Kobayashi, M., Wakayama, Y., Inagaki, H., Katsumata, M., Hirata, Y., Hirata, K., Shimizu, T., Kawada, T., Park, B.J., Ohira, T., Kagawa, T. & Miyazaki, Y. (2009). Effect of phytoncide from trees on human natural killer cell function. *International Journal of Immunology and Pharmacology, 22*(4), 951–959.

Natural England. (2019). *Monitor of engagement with the natural environment: The national survey on people and the natural environment. Headline report 2019: Analysis of latest results (March 2018 to February 2019) and ten years of the survey from 2009 to 2019*. Natural England.

Orr, N., Wagstaffe, A., Briscoe, S. & Garside, R. (2016). How do older people describe their sensory experiences of the natural world? A systematic review of the qualitative evidence. BMC Geriatrics 6, 116. https://doi.org/10.1186/s12877-016-0288-0.

Richardson, M. & McEwan, K. (2018). 30 days wild and the relationships between engagement with nature's beauty, nature connectedness and well-being. *Frontiers in Psychology, 9*. https://doi.org/10.3389/fpsyg.2018.01500

Riemersma-van de Lek, R.F., Swaab, D.F., Twisk, J., Hol, E.M., Hoogendijk, W.J. & Van Someren, E.J. (2008). Effect of bright light and melatonin on cognitive and noncognitive function in elderly residents of group care facilities: a randomized controlled trial. *JAMA, 299*(22), 2642–2655.

RSPB. (2018, October 10). *Here is your prescription for nature*. [Blog]. RSPB. https://community.rspb.org.uk/ourwork/b/scotland/posts/here-is-your-prescription-for-nature#:~:text=RSPB%20Scotland%20has%20recently%20launched,health%20as%20well%20as%20physical

ten Brink, P., Mutafoglu, K., Schweitzer, J-P., Kettunen, M., Twigger-Ross, C., Baker, J., Kuipers, Y., Emonts, M., Tyrväinen, L., Hujala, T. & Ojala, A. (2016). *The health and social benefits of nature and biodiversity protection*. A report for the European Commission (ENV.B.3/ETU/2014/0039). Institute for European Environmental Policy.

26   Finding safety: A monthly Rainbow Memory Café meeting for LGBTQ+ people affected by dementia

Sally Knocker and Lucy Whitman

It's a safe place and that's a good thing. It's quite easy to just talk. There's no one asking questions about who you are. (David, caring for husband Elmar, living with dementia)

The Rainbow Memory Café was set up by Opening Doors London in October 2017, following a consultation and publicity event in the summer. It is a monthly two-hour meeting for LGBTQ+ people living with dementia, their partners and friends, and LGBTQ+ people concerned about their memory and wanting to know more about dementia.

The 'Café' title was used as this creates a more informal feel and is a recognised description in the UK for a meeting for people with dementia and their families. The concept of the memory café goes back to the late 1990s and the work of the Dutch psychiatrist Bere Miesen, and has been embraced and adapted by a number of organisations throughout the world, including the Alzheimer's Society in the UK. The word 'café' does imply a drop-in session, whereas the group is actually a set time of two hours. The word 'memory', rather than dementia, means it is more open to those without a formal diagnosis, but there was some debate about whether having 'dementia' in the title was important.

Opening Doors[1] (formerly Opening Doors London) is the biggest UK charity providing information and support services specifically for lesbian, gay, bisexual, trans and queer (LGBTQ+) people over 50. Opening Doors is a membership organisation providing regular social opportunities, a befriending service and a range of consultancy and training services.

---

1. www.openingdoors.lgbt

Why a specialist group for LGBTQ+ people?

Many might argue that all good services and support groups should be welcoming to everyone and that someone's sexual orientation or gender identity should be irrelevant. There is a common response that, 'We don't discriminate. We treat everyone the same.' However, this attitude of treating everyone the same critically fails to capture what person-centred care really is all about. As a guide produced by Age UK and Opening Doors London, *Safe to be Me* (Knocker & Smith, 2017), explains:

> It is through recognising and giving regard to difference in a positive way, that services can distinguish themselves.

Some care professionals, perhaps because they consider themselves not prejudiced, fail to realise the extent to which experiences of hatred and rejection might impact on people's ability to trust health and social care services. For an older generation of LGBTQ+ people, who have lived through a time when they were criminalised or seen as 'sick' or had to hide who they were for fear of losing family, jobs, homes or even their children, trust is a huge issue. Some LGBTQ+ people can feel genuinely fearful about contacting care services when they need support. Richard Ward (2000) first highlighted more than 20 years ago how fearful the 'gay community' is about dementia-related care needs and having to conceal their sexualities in care spaces to avoid prejudice and discrimination. Roger Newman, who founded the original Alzheimer's Society LGBT carers' group, expresses this vividly:

> A new and threatening world suddenly arises for the 60 or 70-year-old gay carer who has to divulge his or her personal circumstances at the hospital, the doctor's surgery, or on the phone to a social worker, and this all happens at a time when the pressure, emotion and isolation of being a carer can be at its greatest. (Newman, 2010, p.150)

'Coming out' is often perceived as a one-off event, but for many trans, gay, lesbian and bisexual people, our invisibility (particularly as we age) means that we face frequent decisions as to if, when and how we feel safe to be open about our life story (Knocker, 2012; Knocker et al., 2012). A pioneering survey by Stonewall found that older LGBT+ people are more likely to be single and less likely to have children, and are therefore potentially more likely to be isolated and in need of support services. Yet, in the same survey, six out of 10 lesbian, gay and bisexual people said they weren't confident that social care and support services would understand or meet their needs (Stonewall, 2015). In a further report, Stonewall found that 72% of patient-facing staff have not received any training on the health needs of LGBT people, the rights of same-sex partners and parents or the use of language and practices that are inclusive of the LGBT+ community (Somerville, 2015). In the same study, there were some shocking attitudes expressed about trans people. A doctor made the following memorable comment:

Somebody's sex is determined by his chromosomes and this cannot be changed. Being transgender is mainly a mental condition. (Somerville, 2015, p.9)

Effective care for LGBTQ+ individuals affected by dementia must include sensitive recognition of the way our lives and experiences have been informed by our sexuality and gender identity – and how our life stories have been different from those of many of our peers in mainstream society. Being gay does not just concern who we are attracted to or who we sleep with; it also shapes many other aspects of our life and our identity in terms of the books we read, the music and films we enjoy, our politics, humour and our friendships. This is well expressed by Caroline, who said:

> If I didn't have sex with another woman for the rest of my life, I would still be a lesbian. It's as integral to my identity as a mother, the job that I do and the beliefs that I hold dear. It's not the whole of me, but it's a big part. (Knocker & Smith, 2017)

Taking time to understand and respect someone's gender identity and sexual orientation is as integral to true person-centredness in dementia care as valuing cultural diversity. All care services rightly focus on safeguarding older adults and vulnerable individuals. The need to include safeguarding people's emotions and recognising psychological safety has increased resonance for minority groups, including black and minority ethnic and LGBTQ+ communities (Westwood & Knocker, 2016).

Making all services welcoming and inclusive to LGBTQ+ people

In many geographical areas, it might not be easy or possible to set up an LGBTQ+-specific group. Even in London, where there is a larger population, it has been hard to expand the group beyond about eight to 10 regular attendees. It might, therefore, be important for other professionals working with people with dementia to look at the ways in which they can make their regular support groups inclusive to people who are transgender, gay, lesbian and bisexual. *Safe to be Me* (Knocker & Smith, 2017) offers a helpful checklist for practical actions to ensure services are being positive and proactive in reaching people who are LGBTQ+, which can be a good starting point. Where specialist groups cannot be offered, additional efforts need to be made to ensure that LGBTQ+ people feel safe to be open within mainstream services.

Learning point 1

Those providing support services for people living with dementia and their families and friends need to recognise the specific experiences of those who are LGBTQ+ that might impact on how safe they feel in mainstream services:

- What could you do to help LGBTQ+ people feel comfortable?

- When organising activities that involve reminiscence and entertainment, how can you ensure they are inclusive of LGBTQ+ memories and lives? (Many traditional reminiscence activities are very heteronormative in relation to marriage, children and so on. One entertainer who came to the Rainbow Café started with a very obviously heterosexual love song and was teased about this!)

- You meet a younger man and a much older man together at a group, or two older women who are living together. What assumptions might be made in these situations and how might you avoid them? How would you enable people to talk about their relationships?

- If you think someone attending a group might be trans, gay, lesbian or bisexual, how would you make it clear that they can talk openly with you? Some organisations use the popular Rainbow flag symbol to indicate that they are LGBTQ+ friendly, for example.

- If you were to make an explicit statement to all members that a) the group is welcoming and inclusive to LGBTQ+ people, and b) prejudice will not be tolerated, how would you word this and when and how often would you say it?

- How will you measure how well you are doing in relation to being inclusive? (For example, Opening Doors runs a 'Pride in Care' process you can work through to achieve their quality standard. They also run a range of training courses for care providers in all settings to help develop understanding and make practical changes towards being more LGBTQ+ friendly.)[2]

Structuring the group

The DEEP (Dementia Engagement and Empowerment Project)[3] offers some helpful guidance on setting up new groups for people living with dementia, emphasising that decisions about the group should be made by the members.

At the Rainbow Memory Café, the first members were asked at the outset what their hopes and expectations of the group were, and this was reviewed on an ongoing basis to check that the group was meeting everyone's needs. A few only came once and didn't return, and it was also useful to check in with them why the group wasn't something they wanted to continue to attend.

The two-hour meeting currently combines the following elements (but not always in this order):

- An opening circle 'check in' – people introduce themselves, if there are any new members. The facilitator may sometimes provide a theme to the 'checking

---

2. https://openingdoorslondon.eu.rit.org.uk/training-for-professionals
3. www.dementiavoices.org.uk/

in': for example, 'something good' or 'something that's been difficult' since the last meeting. This gives an indication for the facilitator of those who might need some more time to talk and get support.

- A topic for the day – this might include an invited speaker giving a presentation or leading a discussion. The presentations that have worked best have included an interactive element: for example, dividing into pairs or small groups to discuss something connected to the topic. This helps hold interest and involves everyone. It is helpful if guest speakers are well informed about experiences and issues that are particularly relevant to LGBTQ+ people.

- A social activity of some kind – for example, inviting everyone in the group to share a piece of music that has some memory or meaning for them. Another group invited members to talk about places in the world they have visited or would like to explore. Occasionally the group has had a visiting entertainer come in to sing or play music.

- Tea and cake – time to chat informally and socialise with other group members. Good-quality refreshments are an important component, and make sure you include vegan options!

- Telling the group news about upcoming events or initiatives that may be of interest to members.

The Rainbow Memory Café co-ordinator has to field requests to attend the group from well-meaning professionals, including researchers who want to consult with the group. While this effort to be inclusive is welcome, it is important to remember that the group is principally there to support its members, not to serve the needs of these external organisations. Generally, the co-ordinator will ask the group members in advance whether they are happy to welcome a visitor to their meeting, and a set time will be allocated to this within the session.

The pandemic lockdowns made it impossible to provide in-person dementia support for more than a year. The Rainbow Memory Café began to meet on Zoom, and members (not all of whom were able to take part digitally) were also supported by emails and a regular newsletter. Although nothing can replace the warmth and directness of face-to-face contact, we found that there were certain advantages to holding groups online: we could now reach LGBTQ+ people affected by dementia who do not live in London and who may be isolated in their local neighbourhood. We were actually able to expand our dementia support, and two additional online-only groups were created, one for LGBTQ+ carers and one for LGBTQ+ people with a dementia diagnosis. The Rainbow Memory Café now has some members outside London, and currently meets alternately in person and online.

Learning point 2

- When setting up a new support group, what kind of group do you want to create (education, peer support, social, online and so on)?

- How will you ensure that the group meets the needs both of people living with dementia and their partners or carers? What are the challenges of doing this in the same group?

- What processes can you develop and put in place to constantly review these needs as the group evolves, especially when new members join?

Building up group membership through outreach and publicity

The Rainbow Memory Café was initially publicised through the existing Opening Doors London membership newsletter, as well as via wider social media and existing organisations throughout London, such as local Age UK groups, carers' organisations and LGBTQ+ voluntary organisations. A consultation event in the summer before the group started was well attended by health and social care professionals, and 'word of mouth' obviously still plays an important part. Channel 4 News also created a short film about the Rainbow Memory Café, featuring two of the couples attending the group (Channel 4 News, 2018). This has been viewed by many thousands of people. Interviews with group members have featured on BBC London News and BBC Radio London, and in the Alzheimer's Society magazine *Dementia Together*. It is important to maximise all opportunities for publicity, and in particular to make sure that local council, NHS and voluntary sector services are aware of the existence of specific support for LGBTQ+ people affected by dementia and can refer people accordingly. There is, therefore, an ongoing need for information to be distributed to GP surgeries, memory clinics, day services, libraries and so forth, to raise the profile of these services.

The pioneering work of the Rainbow Memory Café has inspired similar support groups to spring up round the country, as well as a nationwide network known as the LGBTQ+ Dementia Advisory Group,[4] which was established during the pandemic. The aims of the advisory group are to share knowledge, ideas and resources and to disseminate best practice on how to support LGBTQ+ people affected by dementia. Anyone interested in setting up a dedicated support group or making an existing group more inclusive is encouraged to get in touch.[5]

---

4. https://www.lgbtqdementiaadvisorygroup.net/home
5. Email lgbtq.dementia@gmail.com

Learning point 3

- What would you include in a plan to launch a new group or attract new members to an established group?
- How would you organise this work and who would be involved?
- How might you implement specific initiatives to reach out to people from trans or bisexual communities or those who are from black and minority ethnic groups to make it very clear that the group welcomes them?
- Have you considered confidentiality issues in relation to involving group members in any publicity initiatives? (In the 2018 Channel 4 film, only first names were used, which was a good decision, as there were some very shocking and hateful comments and responses to this film, as well as many positive ones.)

Conclusions

Some of the themes explored in this chapter are not exclusive to the needs of people who are LGBTQ+. Setting up and maintaining any support and social group requires a range of skills, including creative publicity and networking efforts, good group facilitation, ongoing consultation with the group members and efforts to include an interesting range of helpful topics and activities to meet the changing needs of group members. Everyone attending a support group of any kind needs to feel safe and free to be themselves, but this is particularly important for a community of people who have experienced additional layers of prejudice, exclusion and rejection in their lifetime. To end with the words of Elmar, a group member living with dementia:

> It has brought me a lot of security and comfort level coping with it all. It's been wonderful.

References

Channel 4 News. (2018, April 21). *The gay couples living with dementia*. www.channel4.com/news/the-lgbt-dementia-cafe

Knocker, S. (2012). *Perspectives on ageing: Lesbians, gay men and bisexuals*. Joseph Rowntree Foundation.

Knocker, S., Maxwell, N., Phillips, M. & Halls, S. (2012). Opening doors and opening minds: Sharing one project's experience of successful community engagement. In R. Ward, I. Rivers & M. Sutherland (Eds.), *Lesbian, gay, bisexual and transgender ageing: Biographical approaches for inclusive care and support* (pp.150–164). Jessica Kingsley Publishers.

Knocker, S. & Smith, A. (2017). *Safe to be me: Meeting the needs of older lesbian, gay, bisexual and transgender people using health and social care services– a resource pack for professionals.* Age UK/ Opening Doors London. www.ageuk.org.uk/our-impact/programmes/safe-to-be-me/

Newman, R. (2010). Surely the world has changed. In L. Whitman (Ed.). *Telling tales about dementia: Experiences of caring* (pp.145–151). Jessica Kingsley Publishers.

Somerville, C. (2015). *Unhealthy attitudes: The treatment of LGBT people within health and social care services.* Stonewall.

Stonewall. (2015). *Lesbian, gay and bisexual people in later life (2011).* Stonewall.

Ward R. (2000). Waiting to be heard: Dementia and the gay community. *Journal of Dementia Care,* 8(3), 24–25.

Westwood, S. & Knocker, S. (2016). One-day training courses on LGBT* awareness – are they the answer? In S. Westwood S, Price, E. (Eds.), *Lesbian, gay, bisexual and trans* individuals living with dementia: Concepts, practice and rights* (pp.155–167). Routledge.

27 Supporting people living with dementia from Black, Asian and minority ethnic communities

David Truswell

Many people in the UK Black, Asian and minority ethnic communities believe that dementia is less common in these communities than in the White majority population. This is one reason why those from Black, Asian and minority ethnic communities are reluctant to seek diagnosis and care (Berwald et al., 2016). However, research shows that the African-Caribbean, South Asian and Irish communities may be more at risk of dementia than the majority White UK population (Truswell, 2013).

As responses to pharmacological treatments can vary due to ethnicity (Woods et al., 2015), including people from Black, Asian and minority ethnic communities in pharmacological research is important. A literature review by Cantarero Arevalo and colleagues (2016) on Black, Asian and minority ethnic communities and the use of pharmacy in Denmark recommended the involvement of people from these communities in the design of pharmacological research studies for clinical trials, stressing the importance of understanding how people may combine pharmacological treatments with traditional healing methods.

There has been a lack of representation of people from Black, Asian and minority ethnic communities in news accounts of dementia and information material produced by dementia charities. I and others argue (Truswell, 2019) that the poor engagement of Black, Asian and minority ethnic communities with UK dementia services, research and dementia charities is a result of the complex dynamic interaction of a number of factors, including stigma, cultural insensitivity of services, lifetime experience of discrimination and fear of loss of independence.

Currently, there is more discussion in research literature and the mainstream media on understanding and improving the experience of dementia support for

Black, Asian and minority ethnic communities (Kenning et al., 2017; Johl et al., 2016; Juttla, 2015), but significant other communities remain under-researched – for example, the Polish and Jewish communities.

Practice implications

Despite some excellent local initiatives, it is a constant challenge for clinicians, families and those living with dementia to find information and resource materials that:

- provide appropriate and relevant information for Black, Asian and minority ethnic carers and those living with dementia
- can educate frontline social care and clinical staff about cultural issues, and
- identify good practice and resources for support.

This challenge applies throughout the dementia pathway, from timely access to diagnosis to end-of-life care.

When we work with community groups that support Black, Asian and minority ethnic carers and those living with dementia, the following themes regularly emerge:

- anxiety about stigma in the community regarding dementia that lead people living with dementia in these communities to withdraw from the community
- fear of experiencing discrimination or a lack of understanding from dementia services that makes people reluctant to seek help
- lack of information on dementia that feels relevant for people's own personal circumstances
- belief that dementia is a natural part of ageing and nothing can be done
- frustration with services' lack of provision for language issues and cultural practices that have an impact on the day-to-day care and support
- overwhelming anxiety about the loss of independence in those living with dementia after a lifetime of self-reliance and resilience.

Providing dementia care and support is complex and these themes usually interact in individual cases. Not everyone from a given culture will see stigma, for example, as the main issue that concerns them. Even within a single family, there may be widely different viewpoints.

Providing care and support can be further complicated by cultural stereotyping by the professional service or culturally inappropriate approaches used by the service. The limitations found with clinical services include:

- staff uncritically assume that families will 'look after their own'
- diagnostic materials used for assessing cognitive function are not appropriate due to language barriers or the patient's history

- lack of culturally appropriate reminiscence materials and materials for social interventions
- staff are unfamiliar with working with the family group, so carers feel undervalued and not consulted
- staff are unfamiliar with working with an interpreter
- staff lack information on the local Black, Asian and minority ethnic community that could assist with providing resources and support
- pharmacology and ethnicity interactions are unknown
- pharmacology and traditional medicine interactions are unknown
- staff are unfamiliar with the patient and family's cultural expectations about preparing for death and dying.

Learning point 1

Education about dementia is key to supporting those living with dementia in Black, Asian and minority ethnic communities and their carers:

- How can you use visual aids to encourage discussion about living with dementia for people from Black, Asian and minority ethnic communities?
- What basic information on dementia do you have available in community languages?
- How would you explore cultural issues with the person living with dementia and family carers to develop a personal support plan?

Supporting people living with dementia from Black, Asian and minority ethnic communities and their carers

For families and those living with dementia, the illness is commonly the most complicated and emotionally challenging experience of their lives. With the wide ethnic diversity of the UK population, dementia care staff cannot be experts on every culture that they encounter in their clinical work. Improving the support given to carers and people from Black, Asian and minority ethnic communities living with dementia requires supporting their ability to act as partners in the care provision, drawing on their potential and any available local Black, Asian and minority ethnic community resources for resilience, information and support. Understanding and responding to the support needs of carers and those living with dementia must be shaped by understanding the individual and how their history and cultural identity inform their individual support plans.

Managing the reluctance to seek help

Research indicates that people from Black, Asian and minority ethnic communities living with dementia approach GP surgeries at a later stage in the progress of their dementia than the White UK majority. Often they and their family members are reluctant to discuss their concerns or dismiss them as a sign of 'getting old'. Video resources such as Health Education England's *Finding Patience*[1] and the Dementia Alliance for Culture and Ethnicity video resource page[2] have material to inform carers and the general public about dementia in Black, Asian and minority ethnic communities.

Some TV news programmes have explored dementia in Black, Asian and minority ethnic communities, and some local and community radio programmes have featured items on dementia in these communities. Dementia services can work with local community groups by giving talks on dementia at community events, local faith groups or through community radio. This helps to 'normalise' the conversation about dementia in Black, Asian and minority ethnic communities, and reduce stigma.

Learning point 2

Professional staff should never automatically assume Black, Asian and minority ethnic families 'look after their own'. All family carers need help and support with their carer role as it is likely to be one of the most challenging in their lives.

- How can you support Black, Asian and minority ethnic carers?
- How can you work with community groups in the local area that can offer support to Black, Asian and minority ethnic carers?
- How can you help with concerns about stigma creating social barriers for the person living with dementia or family?

Working with cultural difference

Many of those who came to the UK as first-generation migrants may be living alone in later life, and even for those with family, it should not be assumed that the family will be able to undertake a carer role. There may be safeguarding issues for families who struggle to cope with the demands of caring but feel unable to acknowledge this due to fear of being socially shamed. Cultures are not homogenous and dementia support services must work with the individuals living with dementia in their own personal cultural context.

---

1. www.hee.nhs.uk/our-work/dementia
2. www.demace.com/video-resources

Care services need to sensitively explore with family carers their understanding of dementia and their ability to sustain support in the long term. This discussion should include consideration of the use of Lasting Powers of Attorney (LPAs, see Chapter 12) for both financial matters and care needs. Late presentation to diagnostic services can mean that the person living with dementia may lack the capacity to register a Lasting Power of Attorney.

Professional interpreters working with the care team can be a valuable source of information on cultural expectations and norms.

The person living with dementia and family members often welcome the opportunity to talk about their cultural background and how this affects their care and support needs. This conversation is an important part of relationship-building in developing the personal care and support plan. Cultural sensitivity training for staff can be a way of developing this skill, but each person's case must be understood through his or her individual personal circumstances.

Two books that provide comprehensive accounts of the perspectives of the experience of different Black, Asian and minority ethnic communities are Botsford and Harrison Dening's *Dementia, Culture and Ethnicity: Issues for all* (2015) and Truswell's *Supporting People Living with Dementia in Black, Asian and Minority Ethnic Communities: Key issues and strategies for change* (2019). Both include testimonies of individuals living with dementia and carers from Black, Asian and minority ethnic communities.

Learning point 3

Staff do not need to become cultural experts but do need to be open minded and comfortable when discussing cultural values and expectations with those living with dementia from Black, Asian and minority ethnic communities and their family carers.

- Imagine you were in a foreign country with a serious and long-term health problem. What would you want the care service to know about your cultural needs?
- If you were asked to talk about your cultural background to a stranger, what would you talk about?
- Which aspects of the personal care plan of someone living with dementia from a Black, Asian or minority ethnic background might be most affected by their cultural beliefs and values?

Developing appropriate resources

Psychological and social approaches to care and support for those living with dementia have achieved remarkable benefits in engaging those who may display limited capacity in everyday verbal interactions. These approaches include using singing, music and dance. In group-based settings, these can often stimulate shared storytelling by participants.

The Culturally Sensitive Reminiscence Tool is an online resource available from the Pearl Support Network,[3] and is useful for working with a number of Black, Asian and minority ethnic communities, although its African and African-Caribbean resources are the most developed at this point. Every Generation Media has developed a storytelling board game celebrating the contributions of the Windrush generation and other migrants.[4]

The Irish in Britain's webpage on its initiative Cuimhne – Irish Memory Loss Alliance has useful information and a video on supporting those from the Irish community living with dementia and their carers.[5]

Jewish Care are the largest provider of health and social care services for the Jewish community in the UK and their website includes a number of videos of people talking about their personal experience of living with dementia.[6]

From a South Asian perspective, Meri Yaadain have case studies on their website that are helpful in gaining insight.[7]

Local community organisations and community radio have an increasing interest in raising awareness about dementia and promoting more social inclusion for community members living with dementia. Many Black, Asian and minority ethnic community groups support carers of people living with dementia and elders who are living with dementia. These groups can be a rich source of material for supporting reminiscence and encouraging engagement. They will be familiar with community oral traditions, stories and wider cultural touchstones, such as popular songs, dances and films.

Opportunities should be created for people living with dementia to participate in social activities or events that are meaningful, reflecting what feels culturally validating and evocative for them.

National organisations in the UK, such as the Dementia Alliance for Culture and Ethnicity,[8] Culture Dementia UK[9] and Scotland's MECOPP,[10] have a focus on the experience of dementia in Black, Asian and minority ethnic communities, and their websites are useful sources of information.

The Alzheimer's Society also has a comprehensive resource page for professionals working with Black, Asian and minority ethnic communities.[11]

---

3. https://pearlsupportnetwork.org.uk/

4. www.windrushgame.co.uk

5. https://bit.ly/3sJjKMr

6. www.jewishcare.org/about-us/our-stories

7. www.meriyaadain.co.uk/case-studies/

8. www.demace.com/

9. www.culturedementiauk.org/

10. www.mecopp.org.uk/carer-support-services

11. www.alzheimers.org.uk/dementia-professionals/resources-professionals/BAME-communities

Learning point 4

There are some good-quality video-based resources on the internet that can help with informing staff, those living with dementia, their carers and the general public about the experience of dementia in the Black, Asian and minority ethnic communities.

- What information resources on dementia appropriate for the Black, Asian and minority ethnic communities are available in your locality?
- How can you develop more of these resources with the support of local community groups?

Working with interpreters

Truswell and Tavera (2016) developed guidance for memory services working with Black, Asian and minority ethnic communities in the Central and North West London NHS Trust, with detailed recommendations for clinical staff working with interpreters for the patients and their families referred to memory services.

Key points are:

- using professional interpreters to gain insight about cultural norms and/or the significance of non-verbal cues in the treatment setting
- not assuming that younger family members will be fluent in the language of the elders they are supporting
- first-generation migrants who were raised in a rural community may be speaking a version of their language with outdated terms and forms of expression that may challenge even an experienced interpreter's understanding
- translated documents are not always a benefit; the person living with dementia may not be literate or the translated material may be of poor quality
- there may be issues with the choice of interpreters due to stigma and anxiety about confidentiality.

Learning point 5

People living with dementia, their family carers and professional interpreters are the best source of information as to how cultural beliefs and expectations may impact on their day-to-day support needs in individual care planning.

- How can you find out about Black, Asian and minority ethnic community events or faith group meetings in your locality that you could attend to talk about dementia?

- What do you think are the most important issues when working with interpreters in dementia care?
- How would you find out about non-verbal cultural cues from an interpreter?

Summary

People from Black, Asian and minority ethnic communities experiencing early signs and symptoms of dementia are reluctant to discuss this or approach a GP. Clinical teams should engage with local community opportunities to normalise a discussion about dementia and seeking treatment. This could include short presentations to faith groups or participation in local radio and TV features. Community groups should be supported by providing information on the local pathway for access to dementia diagnosis and treatment. Clinicians should be aware of the cultural bias of diagnostic methods and ensure that their clinical practice reflects current recommendations for Black, Asian and minority ethnic patients.

Developing the care plan should involve discussion with the person living with dementia and any family carers about their cultural beliefs and values. This may concern what they eat, how they dress and their personal grooming. Often religious practices have exemptions for those who are ill – for example, doctrines that require fasting periods usually say people who are unwell should not fast.

Opportunities for participation in valued cultural activities should be encouraged. Reminiscence material should be appropriate for those from Black, Asian and minority ethnic communities.

Dementia services should work with qualified interpreters familiar with interpreting in a medical setting to ensure that communication meets an appropriate clinical standard and that the clinical team can be made aware of any relevant non-verbal cues.

Online practical resources from community organisations

These are some useful sources of resources for those working with and/or supporting people with dementia from Black, Asian and minority ethnic communities and their families/carers.

Irish community

Cuimhne – Irish Memory Loss Alliance – Developed by the organisation Irish in Britain that covers all aspects of memory loss in later life, including dementia – https://bit.ly/3sJjKMr

African-Caribbean community

Pearl Support Network – An information resource on services supporting people from Black, Asian and minority ethnic communities living with dementia, with a well-developed section on the African-Caribbean communities – www.pearlsupportnetwork.org.uk

Nubian Life – Offers day support for older Black, Asian and minority ethnic clients with a range of critical health issues, such as dementia, diabetes and physical and visual impairments – www.nubianlife.org.uk

South Asian community

ADAPT – This multi-agency research project, the South Asian Dementia Pathway (ADAPT) study, has developed an online toolkit to support better dementia care and support for the South Asian community, drawing on in-depth research on the experience of South Asian families. This can be found on the Race Equality Foundation's website – https://raceequalityfoundation.org.uk/adapt

All communities

Dementia Alliance for Culture and Ethnicity (DACE) – A hub organisation for groups supporting carers and people living with dementia in Black, Asian and minority ethnic communities. The DACE website has a number of text and video-based resource materials – www.demace.com

Culture Dementia UK – works with many community groups and has successfully developed community conferences in various parts of England. The organisation is primarily focused on carers – www.culturedementiauk.org

Central and North West London NHS Foundation Trust – has developed a handbook for its memory service, available on the website – www.cad-brent.org.uk/wp-content/uploads/2016/01/Memory-Services-Handbook-final.pdf

References

Berwald, S., Roche, M., Ademan, S., Mukadam, N. & Livingston, G. (2016). Black African and Caribbean British communities' perceptions of memory problems: 'We don't do dementia.' *PLoS ONE, 11*(4): e0151878. doi:10.1371/journal.pone.0151878

Botsford, J. & Harrison Dening, K. (Eds.). (2015). *Dementia, culture and ethnicity.* Jessica Kingsley.

Cantarero Arevalo, L., Traulsen, J. & Nørgaard, L. (2016). Addressing ethnic inequalities in medicine use in Denmark: Selected theory-based interventions Public Health Panorama, 2(4), 477–493.

Johl, N., Patterson, T. & Pearson, L. (2016). What do we know about the attitudes, experiences and needs of Black and minority ethnic carers of people with dementia in the United Kingdom? A systematic review of empirical research findings. *Dementia (London), 15*(4), 721–742.

Juttla, K. (2015). The impact of migration experiences and migration identities on the experiences of services and caring for a family member with dementia for Sikhs living in Wolverhampton, UK. *Ageing and Society, 35*(5), 1032–1054.

Kenning, C., Daker-White, G., Blakemore, A., Panagioti, M. & Waheed, W. (2017). Barriers and facilitators in accessing dementia care by ethnic minority groups: A meta-synthesis of qualitative studies. *BMC Psychiatry, 17,* 316.

Truswell, D. (2013, November). Black, Asian and minority ethnic communities and dementia – where are we now? *Better Health Briefing 30.* Race Equality Foundation.

Truswell, D. (Ed.). (2019). *Supporting people living with dementia in Black, Asian and minority ethnic communities: Key issues and strategies for change.* Jessica Kingsley.

Truswell, D. & Tavera, Y. (2016). *An electronic resource handbook for CNWL memory services: Dementia information for Black, Asian and minority ethnic communities.* Central and North West London NHS Foundation Trust. www.cad-brent.org.uk/wp-content/uploads/2016/01/Memory-Services-Handbook-final.pdf

Woods, D.L., Mentes, J.C., Cadogan, M. & Phillips, L.R. (2015). Ageing, genetic variations, and ethnopharmacology. *Journal of Transcultural Nursing, 28*(1), 56–62.

Part four

Creative approaches
to dementia

28   Mindfulness for people living with dementia and their carers

Cath Arakelian and Jonathan Barker

Mindfulness practice is at its core a simple meditation technique to help reduce stress, anxiety and the psychological effects of pain (Williams & Penman, 2011). It allows you to observe your thoughts and feelings without self-criticism and be more compassionate to yourself and others. Over time, mindfulness brings about long-term changes in mood and levels of happiness and wellbeing. Participants are led by a teacher in simple exercises designed to increase their awareness of the present moment. At first the mind wanders constantly, but with practice we learn to sustain our attention and direct it more skilfully. This helps break the grip of unhelpful mental habits, judgements and impulses, making way for greater calm and for more helpful, kinder and more rational thinking about all aspects of life.

Scientific studies have shown that mindfulness practice can relieve day-to-day stress, depression and irritability (Wax, 2016). Mindfulness is being used in a wide variety of therapeutic settings to improve staff and patient wellbeing, and is recommended by the National Institute for Health and Care Excellence in its 2022 *Mental Wellbeing at Work* guideline:

> 1.6.4 Offer all employees (or help them to access) mindfulness, yoga or meditation on an ongoing basis. This can be delivered in a group or online, or using a combination of both. (NICE, 2022)

Mindfulness links our mind, body and heart through the interwoven threads of thoughts, emotions and bodily sensations. The teaching of mindfulness practice is systematic, with a strong emphasis on kindness and compassion to ourselves and others (Kabat-Zinn, 2013). It is not physically taxing and can be practised seated, standing up or lying down. The basic skills are easy to learn and pass on and, with commitment, they are easy to maintain (Puddicombe, 2012). It seemed to both of us that mindfulness might offer a way for carers to enhance their skills and provide an inner peace and renewal that people experiencing dementia may rarely access.

In 2016 the Oxford Centre for Mindfulness[1] offered us an Access Fund to develop our ideas and Shaw Healthcare[2] made available a residential setting so we could deliver mindfulness to staff and residents. The full report of the project is available online.[3] There were many questions to explore. How could we teach mindfulness to busy staff and encourage them to use it with their residents? How would we work collectively with a group of people with differing levels of concentration? What modifications to the established forms of teaching mindfulness would be needed?

What we discovered was that a combination of multi-sensory input and mindfulness exercises, delivered in weekly 40-minute sessions, had a beneficial effect on the wellbeing of people living with dementia in a care home setting. The positive responses to the mindfulness teaching within the staff group itself were as important. This suggested that staff were experiencing less stress and a greater sense of wellbeing at work. Some of the care staff were confident enough to continue the gentle exercises with individual residents, which was very much encouraged. As an activity, a mindfulness session combined with sensory work and touch meditations can be delivered in small groups, but it is our belief that the mindfulness approach is even more widely applicable to many existing care practices, without special time being set aside. So, developing a culture of mindfulness in everyday work and life seems to have a cumulative impact on creating peace and wellbeing.

Learning point 1 – Getting started

Before you read any further, you may like to consider the following questions:

- Have you or any of your care workers attended a mindfulness course?
- Are any of your care workers, volunteers or staff able to teach mindfulness already?
- Could one of your care workers train as a mindfulness teacher and teach other care workers?

Dementia and psychological therapies

In 1997, clinical psychologist Tom Kitwood exploded the myth that a person with organic brain disease no longer has a mind (Kitwood, 1997). Since then, a keen interest has developed in how psychological therapies can be adapted for therapeutic use with people living with dementia (for example, Evans et al., 2019; White et al.,

---

1. www.oxfordmindfulness.org/

2. www.shaw.co.uk/

3. The report on the original project is available from www.oxfordmindfulness.org/

2018). Kitwood described how low expectations and poor relationships could lead to 'malignant social positioning', based on the idea that people with dementia had 'lost their minds' and could no longer be treated as persons. He observed that, under optimal social conditions, a person continues actively to use their mind to make sense of the world, stimulating the healthy parts of the brain. There is now extensive neurological evidence to support this observation (e.g. Schore, 2016; Solms & Turnbull, 2018). The brain has plasticity and flexibility. It is possible to grow new brain cells and to adapt, even when under severe attack from disease. The neurologist Oliver Sacks has shown what extraordinary feats the brain can accomplish if it is surrounded by a beneficial environment (1985).

As Dr David Sheard, among others, has demonstrated, it is possible to alleviate some of the worst symptoms of dementia through changing the environment in which the person is living (Sheard & Alzheimer's Society, 2007). When surrounded by loving people who are in touch with their own emotional lives and know how to communicate with and without words, a person with dementia can lead a more qualitatively satisfying life in the community or in a residential home. Multi-sensory therapy, such as the Sonas Programme[4] used in two out of three care homes in Ireland, has been demonstrated to connect profoundly with people experiencing the dementia symptoms that impede communication (Moniz-Cook & Manthorpe, 2009). The principles of this interventionist programme are incorporated into the structure of the sessions we present in this chapter.

The issue became how to create these optimal conditions for people living with dementia to flourish. One key idea is that a person with dementia is a *feeling* person, rather than a *thinking* person. This means that it is not the cognitive part of the brain that should be appealed to in communication or therapy. Practically, this means not asking direct questions (requiring cognitive responses), but instead presenting options and watching for non-verbal signs of co-operation or agreement. Another central idea is that successful communication is more successful if 'recalling' is used, rather than 'remembering' (e.g. James, 2009). We now know that it is a different brain activity to recall a feeling or information from a sensory prompt (picture, song, spoken poem, scent, taste) than to be asked to remember something from a verbal, and therefore abstract and decontextualised, prompt. Similarly, the deep inner structures of our psyche and our emotions are best stimulated by indirect means that make use of the sensory pathways to the brain rather than the cognitive ones. Contentment is not to be coerced. It must be coaxed.

Learning Point 2 – Communication with people with dementia

- Think about the ways your clients who live with dementia communicate non-verbally with you – for example, making a specific sound for approval or disapproval, or smiling with their eyes.

---

4. https://engagingdementia.ie/sonas-programme/

- How do you already use creative ways to communicate with people with dementia that you could pass on to others?
- Thinking of a particular client, what brings them a sense of peace or wellbeing?

Third, the quality of care we offer ourselves, how we look after our own emotional and psychological health, determines how well we can care for others. Looking after a person experiencing the symptoms of dementia involves hard emotional labour. It is never merely bodily care. Emotional labour is a relatively new concept (Theodosius, 2008). This describes the use of your own emotional capacity to deal with the negative emotions of loss, fear, anger or sadness that lie at the heart of the experience of dementia. However, if we support care staff emotionally, then they will have energy to draw on this capacity, both to avoid excess stress and burnout and to connect with their clients in even more meaningful and enriching ways.

Learning point 3 – Caring for ourselves

- In what ways do you use your emotions in your work?
- In what ways are you already looking after your emotional and psychological health while at work?
- What are your favourite ways to relax away from work – for example, take a walk, have a long bubble bath, watch a cooking programme or a film?

What mindfulness and multi-sensory group sessions feel like

What we offer here is a narrative account of the first and three subsequent sessions and some suggestions as to how you might include the practical elements in your existing activity programme. They can easily be adapted into individual sessions, as might be necessary in (for example) an infection control environment. For individual sessions, we recommend keeping the length to 20 minutes so as not to overtire the person. It is a good idea for all connected with the care delivery, from managers and administrators to care staff, cleaners and volunteers, to receive their own mindfulness training so that they feel confident to act as enablers.

These specimen sessions are intended as inspiration for your own creativity. Please personalise and adapt the exercises to the people you are caring for.

Session 1 – Theme: Taste

The group session lasts around 40 minutes. There is a mixed group of about 15 people with dementia and four carers as enablers, supporting the residents. We begin with music. The method is to use the same opening and closing music each week and to recycle the meditation techniques to help embed the practice. The leader begins by welcoming everyone individually by singing their name in a welcome song: 'Welcome, Doris, we welcome you...' This acknowledges the identity of each person and gathers the group's attention.

Each session is themed on one of the senses and the mindfulness meditations are heralded by a chime to draw people's attention. The group is encouraged to listen to the sound of the bell. This seems to resonate with the memories of this group, perhaps reminding them of a school bell, and many say how they like the actual sound too. For the first meditation on the theme of taste, we hand round sultanas to each resident. Some people eat them straight away, others don't like them and some follow the instructions to eat them slowly and thoughtfully.

The group listens to the leader reading half a proverb. The game is to complete the proverb (for example, a bird in the hand is worth two...). A well-known poem, Wordsworth's 'Daffodils', is read, which some people recognise and join in with.

The second meditation, to draw attention to our body in space, is called 'Feet on floor, bottoms on chairs'. Some residents find it hard to engage with this and instead are encouraged to gently rub their feet on floor, stroke their hands on their thighs and rub their hands together. This seems to focus participants' attention and they enjoy the sensations.

The second mindfulness exercise is a finger breathing meditation.[5] Here we concentrate on the sensation of the index finger of one hand moving up and down the thumb and fingers of the other hand. Some residents can do this exercise on their own. Others prefer a member of staff to enable the exercise by using their finger to trace an outline of the resident's hand. There is a strong sense of people being attentive to the physical sensations. (This was possibly the most successful exercise in the project and was continued by some members of the staff afterwards.)

At the end of the session, everyone is asked to close their eyes as the leader says: 'May you be well, may you be happy, may you be free of pain and worry.' Interestingly, some residents, unbidden, put their hands together in a prayer posture. We play music at the end.

At the end, we write up our journal to record what worked for each person and how we can adapt the exercises and meditations further. We note any requests for poems or songs from residents or staff.

Session 2 – Theme: Touch

The same structure is used, but this time with a theme of 'touch'. The touch meditations worked well in the previous week, and we want to consolidate this feeling of focused wellbeing. This emphasis on repetition and patterned sequencing of the elements is essential to settling the group and re-conditioning the brain.

---

5. This is a technique Jonathan learnt on a course for using mindfulness in schools: https://mindfulnessinschools.org/

Music is very important in reaching parts of the brain that generate good mood. Each person is welcomed by song. In this week we hand round small objects such as soft toys and smooth stones for residents to touch, talk about and enjoy. A resident responds to the title of a well-known poem, Edward Lear's 'The Owl and the Pussy-Cat', and chooses to read it out loud. Again, the group is drawn together by the sound of the bell as a signal for meditation.

Session 3 – Theme: Sounds

This week we explore listening to sounds, as well as repeating the touch meditations. The leader plays six minutes of Beethoven's *Moonlight Sonata* and asks people to bring their attention to listening closely to the sounds, as much as they are able. To begin with, some of the group are quite restless, but as the music continues, everybody falls into a deep silence, as if transfixed by the sound.

A new meditation is introduced in this session. Each resident is asked to hold up the palm of one of their hands against someone else's palm, either their neighbour sitting next to them or one of the care workers. The group very much enjoys this exercise and seems very attentive to the sensations of the other person's palm. The leader then encourages some residents to move their hand slowly for their partner to follow, and then try it the other way round. Some people become very engaged with this too.

Session 4 – Theme: Smell

We focus on the sense of smell. The leader welcomes everyone by song, which people recognise and enjoy. We include the proverbs game again. Later, the leader reads Lewis Carroll's poem 'Jabberwocky'. For the meditation, droplets first of lavender and then of vanilla are spread on tissues and handed around to each participant. The residents seem to enjoy this experience, although some find it hard to identify vanilla and get a sense of its smell. The touch meditations are repeated and the chime that introduces them is now recognised.

Learning point 4

- What aspects of mindfulness might be most helpful to you in your work?
- If there is something sensory that you enjoy (for example, the scent of flowers, the feel of sand on your toes), could you share this?
- What do you think about keeping a journal to record your own mindfulness practice and the work you have done with others, so you can review this?

Ten tips

We have 10 tips for mindfulness teachers or people new to leading these activities with this population:

1. Reduce or omit altogether cognitive explanations of why mindfulness works.

2. Work for up to 40 minutes and close the session if you feel it's getting too long.

3. Use the bell to signal the start of a mindfulness input – to gather a peaceful focus.

4. Focus on sensual activities – such as taste and texture, nice smells on tissues, objects to look at and hold, finger meditation.

5. Don't expect quiet in the room – noise often indicates participation.

6. Repeat and recycle exercises in subsequent sessions to re-activate neural networks.

7. Consider using exact words of instruction with pared-down simplicity. And repeat exactly the same words four times – once to each 'side' of the circle.

8. Vary activities but contain them within a predictable sequence for each session.

9. Create opportunities for group participation, such as singing, reciting, holding hands.

10. Create incentives for the staff group to maintain daily practice for themselves and the people they care for.

Conclusion

The approach we have outlined in this chapter is delivered in a type of activity session that mixes multi-sensory stimulae with mindfulness meditations and body exercises adapted to suit the personal preferences and needs of the group. We omit cognitive explanations of why mindfulness works. It is recommended that the leader is a person who has been able to attend a mindfulness training in order to cascade the knowledge to the enabling staff and volunteer group. The peace and wellbeing generated in the 40-minute group session can extend into the daily activities of the setting. In developing a mindful culture through activities and personal practice, mindfulness could become a simple way of life in the care home, with staff singing instructions, reciting poetry with residents, using touch mindfully, enabling residents to enjoy the sensation of water, or becoming attentive to the taste and texture of food.

References

Evans, S., Garner, J. & Darnley-Smith, R. (2019). *Psychodynamic approaches to the experience of dementia: Perspectives from observation, theory and practice.* Routledge.

James, O. (2009). *Contented dementia.* Vermilion.

Kabat-Zinn, J. (2013). *Full catastrophe living: How to cope with stress, pain and illness using mindfulness meditation.* Piatkus.

Kitwood, T.M. (1997). *Dementia reconsidered: The person comes first.* Open University Press.

Moniz-Cook, E. & Manthorpe, J. (2009). *Early psychosocial interventions in dementia: Evidence-based practice.* Jessica Kingsley.

NICE. (2022). *Mental wellbeing at work.* NG212. NICE. www.nice.org.uk/guidance/ng212

Puddicombe, A. (2012). *Get some headspace.* Hodder & Stoughton.

Sacks, O. (1985). *The man who mistook his wife for a hat.* Duckworth.

Schore, A.N. (2016). *Affect regulation and the origin of the self: The neurobiology of emotional development.* Routledge Classic Edition.

Sheard, D.M. & Alzheimer's Society. (2007). *Being: An approach to life and dementia.* Alzheimer's Society.

Solms, M. & Turnbull, O. (2018). *The brain and the inner world: An introduction to the neuroscience of subjective experience.* Routledge.

Theodosius, C. (2008). *Emotional labour in health care: The unmanaged heart of nursing.* Routledge.

Wax, R. (2016). *A mindfulness guide for the frazzled.* Penguin Life.

White, K., Cotter, A. & Leventhal, H. (2018). *Dementia: An attachment approach.* The Bowlby Centre Monograph Series. Routledge.

Williams, J.M.G. & Penman, D. (2011). *Mindfulness: A practical guide to finding peace in a frantic world.* Piatkus.

29 Trauma-informed yoga for older people living with dementia

Josephine Norrbo and Eleonore Wesén

In December 2019, a project started in Sweden that aimed to develop a yoga method for older people in nursing homes, delivered by the NGO Yoga for All Sweden.

Yoga for all Sweden is a non-profit organisation that strives to make yoga accessible to groups that don't have easy access to yoga. The organisation facilitates yoga that is trauma informed. Trauma-informed yoga considers the impact of trauma on the entire body-mind system and promotes an environment that is empowering and safe. Yoga for All has offered yoga since 2016, mainly to refugees, but also to young people, people with long-term health conditions, unemployed people and older people.

During 2018, Yoga for all Sweden offered a weekly yoga class at a nursing home in Malmö, Sweden. The yoga was appreciated by the participants, but we also encountered challenges when participants experienced restriction in movement, anxiety and/or chronic pain. We became curious about how we could improve the classes and make yoga more accessible for older people.

After dialogue with older people and staff in the nursing home, it was clear that more knowledge was required. Although yoga already exists in care services for older people, no specific yoga method for older people has been developed, and there is limited knowledge as to how older people themselves wish to practise yoga. This is why the Yoga Throughout Life project was set up. In 2019, Yoga Throughout Life was granted three years' funding from Allmänna Arvsfonden (the Swedish General Inheritance Fund) to run from December 2019 until December 2022.

What is yoga?

Yoga has its origins in the Vedas, the oldest recorded Indian culture. The word 'yoga' has many different interpretations, but the most common meaning is 'to unite' or 'to come together' (Desikachar, 1995). This could be interpreted as joining the body and mind, or oneself, with God. There are many views as to how to practise yoga in the 'right way'. At Yoga for All, we promote the view that anybody can practise yoga. Desikachar puts it like this:

> Anybody who wants to can practise yoga. Anybody can breathe; therefore, anybody can practise yoga. But no one can practise any kind of yoga. It has to be the right yoga for that person. (Desikachar, 1995)

Yoga is a system of practice that has developed over time. In the Yoga Sutras, presumed to have been written by the Indian sage Patanjali, eight important aspects of yoga are presented (Stephens, 2010). These include ethics, physical forms, breathing exercises and various ways of turning the awareness inwards to attain enlightenment. Over the years, yoga has developed into different schools and approaches. Even though yoga originated as a Hindu practice, today yoga is largely seen as a secular activity that can be practised in a non-religious context and by people of any faith. At Yoga for All, we promote secular yoga as a way to make yoga accessible for all. One way to do this is to exclude mantras and religious symbols. Yoga can be practised by anyone; there is no right way or wrong way of doing yoga. We aim to let this view of yoga permeate our work.

Contemporary research has been conducted that shows the benefits of yoga specifically for people with dementia. An experimental study undertaken in Taiwan in 2011 examined the effects of yoga on a group of people with mild-to-moderate dementia. It was noticed how participants' physical health improved: for example, they had lower blood pressure, a lower respiration rate, increased muscular flexibility, improved balance and movability, and a significant reduction in depression (Fan & Chen, 2011).

A literature review in 2017 also supports the conclusion that yoga can be an effective intervention for improving older people's physical health and mental wellbeing (Mooventhan & Nivethitha, 2017). Another study from India investigated the impact of yoga on older people's cognitive functions. After six months of daily yoga, the yoga group showed significant improvements in both verbal and visual memory in comparison with the control group (Hariprasad et al., 2013).

Learning point 1

Before you continue reading, please reflect on the following questions:

- What do you imagine yoga to be?
- Do you have any picture of what a person doing yoga looks like? Is it a young or an old person? Are they flexible? How are they dressed?
- Do you agree that anyone can practise yoga?

Eleonore Wesén, a yoga teacher, will now share her personal experiences of teaching yoga to older people living with dementia.

I was asked to guide yoga classes for a group of older people living with different types of dementia. It was a mixed group, where some of the participants were in wheelchairs. Other people in the group had difficulties walking but were still able to do so with the help of a walker. Several of the people were walking without any help. Their cognitive abilities varied as well, and to start with not everyone knew who I was or where they were. After a few weeks spent working together, they were all aware of who I was and what we would do during the time that we spent together.

The project initially continued for 10 weeks, but at the end of those weeks we had seen such wonderful progress that the project was extended, and I ended up working with the group of older people for 18 months.

When I was asked to work with this specific group in a yoga setting, I agreed without hesitation, as I hoped that encouraging the participants to do physical movement would improve their daily lives. I had previous experience of working with people with dementia, and I loved interacting with and supporting this group, who experienced different types of dementia.

I wanted to give the participants the chance to be treated as 'normally' as possible, knowing that sometimes it is easy to underestimate people with dementia.

I decided to keep each yoga class to 90 minutes in length. The time included an introduction to the theme of the day. I chose themes like the turning of the seasons, acceptance, knowledge of the body and self-love. I often had a poem or a short text with me that touched on one of these themes. I invited the participants to share their reflections, and to say whatever popped up for them that could be related to the theme. Then I introduced a physical theme that we were going to explore during the class. I worked with different parts of the body.

First of all, I introduced the theme in words; then, as a part of the practice, I asked the participants to bring their attention to a specific part of their body, and then to a physical sensation, such as through a particular movement. It could be the sensation from letting the fingers touch the surface of the skin on the face, neck, arms and hands; then noticing how the skin was being touched by the fabrics of their clothes, and by the air surrounding them. I asked them to explore what the sensation felt like when they moved their arms or legs. Then, we started a more traditional yoga asana practice. Mostly they did this sitting on a chair or in a wheelchair, and I chose physical exercises that would invite the participants to cross the mid-line of the body – like moving the right arm to the left, for example. We did some twisting and stretching while sitting down, and this was followed by a short sequence where the participants had the choice of standing up. Those who needed support could use the back of a chair or their walker to lean on. The standing sequence was aimed at building and maintaining balance and strength. I noticed that they enjoyed the challenge. When the participants felt supported and safe, they could challenge themselves. This led to an improvement in their strength and balance and the feeling of joy when they actually got to try something new and succeeded at it.

After the standing sequence, we returned to sitting on the chairs and ended the class in a guided meditation, when delegates were asked to stay silent for a few moments and observe their inner landscape. I had some concerns regarding the meditation and stillness, thinking that it might not work with this particular group, but I was wrong. They were very good at finding a sense of peace and presence.

I worked with the breath through breathing exercises. I also asked participants to pay attention to the breath's movement through their bodies, which enabled me to encourage them to work with their bodies as well. I could see how it had a calming effect to trace the breath through the body without doing anything more than just breathing. The breath is always there, and most of us are aware of it.

Before starting to work with this group, I expected that the participants would not remember the exercises between classes. I prepared very simple cues to lead them into the physical body and the movement itself. After a couple of weeks, I noticed that they seemed familiar with the movements, and soon they started to begin the movements and positions ahead of me. They remembered the order – or rather their bodies did.

Before moving on, you are welcome to try a breathing exercise used by Eleonore.

Exercise: Awareness of breath

Find a comfortable seat, either sitting on a chair or on the floor. Maybe you can notice the contact between your body and the floor and the weight of your body towards the ground. If you like, place one or two hands somewhere on your upper body – on your stomach or chest. Without changing your breath, see if you can notice the movement of your breath in your body. Maybe you can notice how your hands are lifted up on your in-breath and sink back on your out-breath? Maybe you are noticing your stomach or chest is expanding on your in-breath and sinks back on your out-breath. Can you feel your breath anywhere else in your body? Can you feel your breath in your upper back, in your hips or maybe somewhere else? Stay like this, following your breath in your body for as long as you like. When you feel ready, let your palms sink back down, and in your own time open your eyes.

Learning point 2
- How did this breathing exercise make you feel?
- Was it easy or difficult for you to follow your breath in your body?

Yoga Throughout Life – project description

The aim of Yoga Throughout Life is to improve the quality of life and health of older people who are living in nursing homes by encouraging them to practise yoga. The project wishes to explore whether yoga can be a way of giving older people the possibility to improve their own wellbeing. To make the results as applicable as possible, we have not developed a yoga method just for the target group; rather, we have worked in partnership with them to create a helpful method for teaching yoga.

The result of this project will be a method for teaching yoga to older people in nursing homes. Some of these people will have dementia; others will not. The method will be developed by combining available research with lived experience. We will teach yoga in three Swedish cities, with nine different yoga groups. The yoga classes will be evaluated in bi-monthly focus groups and by observations during classes.

When we started the classes, the question was where to begin. After researching the topic, we decided to start with classes based on some theories, information from the nursing homes, and our own experiences. Eleonore's experiences of teaching yoga to older people with dementia became a valuable source of information. Another helpful source of information was Lucia McBee's book, *Mindfulness-Based Elder Care* (McBee, 2008). McBee is a US social worker who specialises in working with older people. In her book, McBee presents ways of working with yoga, meditation and relaxation in residential nursing homes. When sharing these exercises with people with dementia, McBee writes that, even though it might seem that you need to have some cognitive functions to follow mindfulness instructions, these practices seem to 'transcend the residents' cognitive conditions'. The key aspect is to follow the group and meet them where they are. As an example, McBee explains how she would use different kinds of music, aromatherapy and movement, depending on whether the group was anxious or tired. Even though there might be periods of agitation during sitting meditation or relaxation, McBee writes that, 'by meeting this with acceptance and redirection, the whole group usually settles down'. Another important factor is how to communicate and the importance of using visceral cues as well as verbal ones (McBee, 2008).

Another source of inspiration is Tania Plahay's book *Yoga for Dementia* (2018). In this, yoga teacher Plahay describes her personal experience of sharing yoga with people with dementia. The book is aimed at those living with dementia and their caregivers. Plahay's method is based on traditional yoga philosophy and a range of yoga techniques, which include more traditional techniques and modern interventions. Plahay says that the techniques have been tested over many years, and that she herself has seen the benefits of the practices in her yoga groups (Plahay, 2018).

Several of the yoga teachers in the project group have trained in Trauma Center Trauma-Sensitive Yoga (TCTSY). TCTSY is a complementary treatment developed at the Center for Trauma and Embodiment at the US-based Justice Resource Institute for people with complex PTSD or complex trauma. One main component in TCTSY is the view that trauma is relational and involves power dynamics (Emerson, 2015). As Judith Herman writes:

> No intervention that takes away power from the survivor can possibly foster recovery, no matter how much it appears to be in her immediate best interest. (Herman, 1992)

We intend to bring this view on power relations into Yoga Throughout Life. Being of old age, with restricted mobility and possibly decreased cognitive functions, makes you dependent on other people, and it can create a sense of disempowerment. Yoga can be a helpful tool for regaining a sense of agency.

The project consists of four phases. In the first phase, we established focus groups and had initial meetings with the project management group. After this, the classes began – one class per week, each of 20–45 minutes in length. The yoga teacher maintains an ongoing dialogue with the residents and staff at the nursing homes. In this phase, the focus groups meet regularly until the end of the project, to make sure that the target group is involved all the way through. The method takes form through the focus group meetings and continuous dialogue with residents and staff. Ultimately, we will present the project in a book.

We are also developing a 20-hour course for staff in nursing homes called 'Yoga Inspirer'. The aim is to train staff to introduce the yoga method in their nursing homes on their own. In this way, the nursing homes are not dependent on the project, and the method can live on beyond this project. In the last phase, we will spread the knowledge gained nationally.

Learning point 3

When developing a yoga teaching method with a target group with special needs, you need to be mindful of relationships. As a yoga teacher, you always hold the most power in the room. Take some time to consider the following questions:

- How can you become aware of power dynamics in a relationship?
- If you are the person with more power in the room (as a yoga teacher you always do have more power), how can you share that power?
- How can you become more aware of your own views and beliefs? Are you ready to let go of your ideas if they are not helping the target group?

References

Desikachar, T.K.V. (1995). *The heart of yoga: Developing a personal practice*. Inner Traditions International.

Emerson, D. (2015). *Trauma-sensitive yoga in therapy: Bringing the body into treatment*. W.W. Norton & Co.

Fan, J. & Chen, K. (2011). Using silver yoga exercises to promote physical and mental health of elders with dementia in long-term care facilities. *International Psychogeriatrics, 23*(8), 1222–1230.

Hariprasad, V.R., Koparde, V., Sivakumar, P.T., Varambally, S., Thirthalli, J., Varghese, M., Basavaraddi I.V. & Gangadhar, B.N. (2013). Randomized clinical trial of yoga-based intervention in residents from elderly homes: Effects on cognitive function. *Indian Journal of Psychiatry, 55*(S3), 357–363.

Herman, J. (1992). *Trauma and recovery: The aftermath of violence – From domestic abuse to political terror*. Basic Books.

McBee, L. (2008). *Mindfulness-based elderly care: A CAM model for frail elders and their caregivers*. Springer Publishing Company.

Mooventhan, A. & Nivethitha, L. (2017). Evidence-based effects of yoga practice on various health related problems of elderly people: A review. *Journal of Bodywork & Movement Therapies, 21*(4),1028–1032.

Plahay, T. (2018). *Yoga for dementia: A guide for people with dementia, their families and caregivers*. Jessica Kingsley Publishers.

Stephens, M. (2010). *Teaching yoga: Essential foundations and techniques*. North Atlantic Books.

30 Improvisatory movement and dance for family carers and others

Richard Coaten

This chapter presents some simple, practical approaches involving improvisatory movement and dance that can be used to help generate spontaneity, creativity and the maintenance of relationship in everyday care. While professional and amateur dancers, including dance movement psychotherapists, community dance workers and others, have been doing this for some years now, the focus of this chapter is primarily on the family carer. The unpaid carer looking after a loved one in their own home may have the support of children, grandchildren, friends and relatives, perhaps helpers such as cleaners too, each of whom brings their own uniqueness to moving and dancing together. I mean by this the person living at home, with their loved one at any stage of the condition, who considers themselves to have an interest in the subject but has no training or experience in movement and dance. Is this possible for a family carer with no previous training in movement and dance? I argue that it is, and that this chapter can answer this question as it evolves, inspiring family carers to give the practice a go from scratch. It's inclusive, something special and may provide welcome relief to the carer to have others joining in.

The roots of this chapter lie in a lifetime's work with older people living with dementia, beginning in the day centres of Sheffield in the mid-1980s. One, the Darnall Dementia Group, which was managed at the time by Lisa Heller, was very special. Lisa recognised the value of the arts, including singing and dancing, and the very positive results for her clients, and how the spontaneity implicit in the process gave something special back to the person. People felt supported, valued and encouraged by it, all of which I was later able to study and better understand through my doctoral research (Coaten, 2009). I learned much in those early years – for example, how to use improvisatory movement and dance practices in groups, the use of props to accompany the process and the importance of maintaining relationship and connection through it. I also learned about the ways in which improvisatory movement and dance practice helped to:

- reduce social isolation by bringing people together
- reduce loneliness because people felt a strong connection with others
- reduce human suffering because they were being valued for what they could do, rather than what they could not do, with the focus primarily on accessible, non-verbal, inclusive and emotionally oriented communications. This had the effect of raising wellbeing while lowering illbeing.

What underlies the practice?

My work creates a moving and temporary state with permeable boundaries, where identity is embodied and where people are offered numerous opportunities to move. It requires willingness by the dancer to be open to change and to being touched emotionally by the creative responses, developing what I have described as a 'creative alertness' (Coaten, 2001, p.21) to their form, their content and their manner of expression. This not only informs the dancer's own felt and intuitive response to that expression, but also helps manifest how this felt response informs what happens next. This cyclical process is vital because our clients often can't speak about how they are changing and responding, so there is a primarily non-verbal requirement to be able to gauge impact and respond appropriately to it.

Just as mind influences body, and vice versa, we affect one another – continually, moment by moment. It is an iterative process. We don't simply 'make eye contact' or move with a person; we look into another's eyes, we take them in, we witness them moving moment by moment as communication flows back and forth. As this flow in communication takes place, we meet them at the permeable 'boundary' and are ourselves met by them. This is so important, because it is by way of this exploratory and improvisational process that we are learning how each is changed by the other. Emerging from our explorations as dancers, we are also re-kindling kindness, compassion, respect for a shared humanity and inspiration through shared problem-solving, at the heart of which is improvisation, playfulness and a strong sense of personhood (Kitwood & Bredin, 1992). I argue here that these qualities are not exclusive to dance workers or therapists. They are essential aspects of high-quality care and should be available to family carers, and also to paid and professional care staff working in residential and nursing homes.

The role of the family carer and the importance of music and dance

For the family carer, staying in relationship with their loved one is vital, and thus so is the need to be very resourceful and, I would also argue, improvisational in keeping their loved one occupied. It is important to discover whatever it might be that gives the person pleasure, sometimes for minutes, sometimes for hours, sometimes for only just a few seconds perhaps, before attention might need moving to something else.

The carer might be running out of ideas in supporting their loved one to stay in contact with the world and also with them. In addition, they might have shared many occasions when they danced together in the past, perhaps when courting, when married and on a regular basis, even, in dance halls and clubs. It might have been Ballroom, Latin, Northern Soul, or Rock 'n Roll that gave them much pleasure.

Under these circumstances, what might improvisatory movement and dance have to offer a family carer, or professional carer even? It is a pleasurable physical activity, it is playful, it raises wellbeing, and it is non-verbal (Coaten et al., 2013; Coaten, 2011). It engages body and mind, brings back memories (Coaten, 2001) and uses rhythm, music and a variety of different props (scarves, balloons and elastic rings). Music has been found to be particularly effective for neuropsychiatric symptoms, including anxiety (Hsu et al., 2015). In addition, in my opinion, movement and dance can bring partners together in a way they may not have enjoyed for a long time. The suggestions here require some basic theoretical and practical foundations, especially for readers who do not consider themselves to be dancers. This next section may prove helpful.

What is improvisation?

Improvisation is about being creative with the freedom to follow an impulse, while accepting the nature of the unpredictable and embracing wholeheartedly what is essentially 'not-yet-known'. It is about taking risks with old ways of doing things, about being creative and trying new things out on a whim. It's about 'doing' without necessarily having a purpose other than simply to explore, to be playful. It's about observing, while also connecting to 'self' and 'other', without being judgemental. As Matt Laurie says below (see also Chapter 20), it's being able to accept and celebrate an improvisational 'offer', in whatever way, shape or form it comes. In movement terms, it is creating a space where all movement is okay, where there is no right or wrong way of doing it, especially when it helps the relationship between 'self' and 'other', or between carer and loved one. At the heart of this process is, according to Dymoke (personal communication):

> … a dialogical form, a conversation, that opens responses and taps into the imagination – a form of spontaneous creativity – very satisfying and fluid – (awakening) body awareness, where the co-stimulus of touch and movement is a way of seeing and being seen in multi-sensory ways.

Touch and movement taken together not only facilitate relationship and connection through the joy of moving together, easing behaviours that are problematic (Coaten, 2001, 2009); they also support 'personhood' (Kitwood & Bredin, 1992). The recovery of memories, thoughts, emotions, images and feelings is also generated, because these are stored as much in the body as they are in the brain, and thus, when we move and dance, they become activated and contribute so much to our feeling valued.

The importance of improvisation

Long, long hours of loving care are very demanding and present new challenges daily, requiring new strategies, often just when one new strategy has only just been found to manage the previous one. The type, form and content of the physical activity described and presented here is that of improvisational movement and dance. It can also include any previously learnt dance style or variation of it that may lie dormant in our bodies, waiting to be rekindled by just the right music at just the right time – now! This chapter in no way seeks to deny the importance of any other kind of physical activity, such as a walk in the woods or a yoga class; nor does it seek to diminish the role of the professional dancer or dance movement psychotherapist in this field. Rather it has a particular focus, as presented in Figure 30.1, on the ongoing need on the part of the carer to be able to respond as creatively as possible to the presence of three inter-related aspects in the care relationship. These are the improvisatory nature and challenges of the dementia condition, the improvisatory nature of their own care relationship with their loved one, and the improvisatory nature of the movement and dance process itself. If a balance can be found in the practice, the place where metaphorically speaking the three aspects meet, then it is highly likely that the experience will be very enjoyable, satisfying and life-affirming, with the potential for a 'flow' experience (Csikszentmihalyi, 2014). A 'flow' experience is one that feels very enjoyable, is easy to do without stress or strain, and involves complete absorption in what is going on.

Figure 30.1: Improvisation as a key component in movement and dance, in dementia care generally and in the care relationship

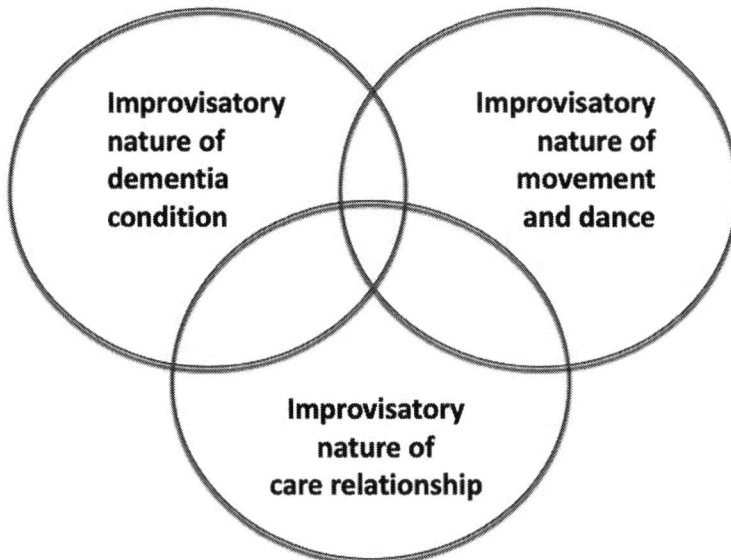

Improvisatory nature of dementia condition

Improvisatory nature of movement and dance

Improvisatory nature of care relationship

The assumption here is that improvisation and improvisatory practices are at the heart of a high-quality care relationship, and it makes good sense to apply some principles of improvisatory dance and theatre-making to support that relationship. Matt Laurie (see Chapter 20) describes a new approach to communication that he calls rapport-based communication (RBC), that is based on the improvisational 'offer', which he describes as follows:

> In rapport-based communication, the starting point for interactions are the in-the-moment interests and behaviours of the person with dementia and are called offers, a term borrowed from improvisational theatre. The concept of a behavioural offer is at the centre of improvisational theatre, a practice that also has a history of application in healthcare.

These 'offers', which Laurie describes as being presented all the time by the person with the condition, are central to his work and can be 'blocked' or 'celebrated'. In this context, 'blocked' means for them to be ignored, not seen as relevant or generally not picked up on as opportunities to connect and communicate with the person. 'Offers', in contrast, are 'celebrated' and explored together in a variety of ways and lead on to a valuing of the person. Laurie describes the nature of these offers in detail in Chapter 20. The improvisational 'offer' that he describes in relation to RBC is also at the heart of the improvisational nature and application of movement and dance in this context. Thus, it is interesting to have two chapters in this handbook that describe inter-linked approaches to communication that are fundamentally improvisatory in nature and that also support positive person work (Kitwood & Bredin, 1992) in dementia.

Learning point 1

- Read Matt Laurie's Chapter 20 in this book to better understand and gain a fuller understanding of how the author describes rapport-based communication.

- If you are a family carer yourself, think about how often in your everyday caring for your loved one you have to improvise, often very quickly, to respond to changing circumstances – for example, in finding a way to de-escalate a situation where a precious object has to be found that instant, when you are engaged in something unrelated.

Laying practical foundations for improvisational movement and dance

This section sets out practical ideas for exploring the movement and dance 'offer'. It uses improvisational approaches that can be used in the home freely and easily and that may also facilitate the family carer to be more improvisatory and playful in other aspects of their care. While different styles of dance practice can be used, the focus is more on the person and the emotional content and wellbeing that movement and dance can bring than on whether or not the person can remember dance steps. In fact, getting a 'step' right might create more anxiety, so there is no right or wrong way to do things. This is of great importance when memory is problematic in the first place.

Learning point 2

- A very wise and philosophical Jungian analyst once said the following that has helped me so much when I am stuck or trying to find a solution to a problem: 'Not to know, but through search to find a way.'

- Accepting that, in the nature of this exploration of movement and dance in the care relationship, 'not knowing' and instead searching easily together to find a way can take the pressure off to get something 'right', and lead to surprising results.

Getting started

The ideas that follow are in the service of that all-important relationship between the family carer and their loved one.

Materials

2 x bodies (or more if you like!) – any size/height/constitution etc.

1 x tube/bottle of good quality hand cream

1 x CD player/iPod/laptop & speaker

1 x favourite CD (or Spotify): for example, relaxing music – 'Songbird', Eva Cassidy; slow jazz – 'Autumn Leaves', Stan Getz; slow blues – 'Don't Let Me Be Misunderstood', Nina Simone; slow classical – 'Music for a While: Improvisations on Purcell', Christine Pluhar and L'Arpeggiatta; doo-wopp – 'The Way You Do The Things You Do', The Temptations.)

2 x chairs

2 x light, free-floating silk scarves (or similar)

2 x feathers – peacock, pheasant and/or ostrich (or similar).

Getting going – warm-up

1. Put on some relaxing music you both like.

2. Invite your partner sensitively to join you and sit in a chair opposite yours.

3. Start by massaging your own hands with the hand cream. Ask them if they would like a massage. Or, if the spoken word does not feel appropriate, try

asking the question non-verbally – if 'no', try some of the other ideas on this page. If 'yes' go on to Step 4.

4.   Gently massage their hands, working the cream in between their fingers and on the palm and back of the hands. Watch out for sensitive skin and for your own or their arms/hands becoming tired. Make sure you are comfortable before starting, and use a table between you to rest on if that might work better. Try asking how the person feels in response to the massage as you proceed. Do they have memories/sensations or images recalling past/present or even future events?

Learning point 3

- The emotional content of this work is so important, because we know that, in spite of extensive cognitive loss, the emotional, feeling aspects of ourselves are still very much alive and well. The person may forget what you say or do, but they won't forget how you made them feel.

- Physical contact through massage, as just one example, can bring many memories, thoughts and reflections. See if you can use these to further enrich the experience, giving a sense of being valued back to the person.

Dancing with hands

1.   Start by moving your hands. Next invite your partner (perhaps non-verbally) to explore how their hands might like to move too, now that they have been given a sense of connection by way of massage.

2.   Gauge non-verbally if the music makes them want to move in response, stretching fingers, rotating wrists, generally exploring movement, perhaps first with one hand, then adding the other – opening/closing movements, quick/slow.

3.   Gently 'mirror', if you can, the person's movements, meaning that you join in with this hand/finger/wrist moving experience (duet). You may like to hold their hand(s) or place your palm(s) on theirs and see where this takes you both. Try not to rush or hurry this, as it may take time for something to feel like it's happening. It may in fact take you off the chair and into moving and/or dancing together in the space you are in. There is no right/wrong to it. How does this make you feel? Reflect back to the person what you see/feel/experience and allow their responses to inform what might happen next in the dance.

4.   Change the music into something a little more up-tempo that you know your partner likes (for example, Johann Strauss's 'Blue Danube' waltz). Try using a 'floaty' silk scarf as a prop, or a feather of some kind, or a fan or balloon to pass between you, if you happen to have these.

Learning point 4

- Take pleasure in 'being with'.
- Take pleasure in the music and rhythm.
- Take pleasure in the sensations, feelings/thoughts, especially memories that may emerge during this time.

Duets

Now that you have started, try adopting a *spirit of adventure* in your movement play, meaning that you are not afraid to try out new ideas that come to you instinctively. Aim to create and maintain a sense of *trust* and *shared energy* between you, accepting *offer and gifts* you are given by your partner or a movement gift you can build on. If someone else – maybe a grandchild, a cleaner, a friend or relative – is present, try involving them in the duet too. What do they have and can 'offer' that might add to the joy and spirit of adventure of the experience for all concerned?

Figure 30.2 adds the dimensions referred to above, aiming to present them in a visual way and covering the more theoretical aspects of what lies under the surface of this approach. The outer ring in the figure below is also reflective of the atmosphere needed between all involved – one that both visually and practically contains within it the core improvisatory nature of the carer role in moving and dancing.

Figure 30.2: Underlying the approach

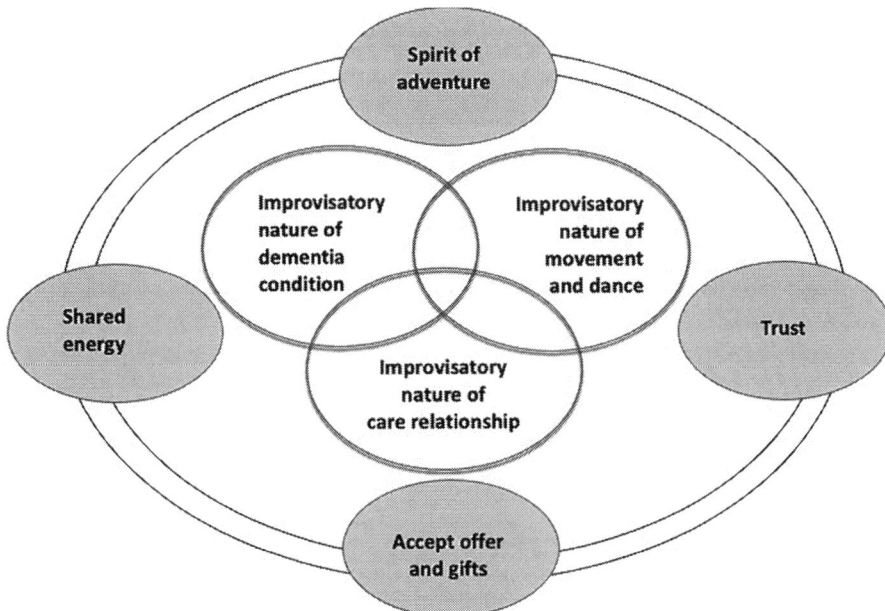

Bit of a boogie

This is simply moving and dancing with your partner. Boogie-woogie piano music (such as Hamp Garnett's 'Mississippi Boogie') that has lots of rhythm and a strong beat, or some vibrant pop (like 'I Only Want to Be with You', Dusty Springfield) will do fine. Put on the music and see what happens when you both start dancing and sharing the space together. Twisting, turning, quick, slow, forward, backward, up and down. Try soloing… one person showing the other a move they can do. Take it in turns. Use props like the scarves that you can hold between you. Take regular breaks and on you go. Above all, *enjoy.*

Going forward

This chapter has seeded new ideas about family carers taking up movement and dance in their own homes with their loved ones and helpfully widening the scope of the improvisatory nature of their role in the process – an addition that may not have been considered previously. Some might say that a dance training is necessary for carers to be able to implement these ideas successfully. I don't agree. It requires common sense, playfulness and the willingness to give it a go and see what happens. All of these are aspects that help make an effective family carer too. It is not to diminish the role and importance of the professional dancer or therapist working in this field; rather, it is to sow the seeds for more meaningful movement and dance-based approaches to assist family and perhaps even paid carers in their roles.

The focus of this chapter has been on the family carer, but there is nothing stopping professional carers in care homes and day centres from implementing these ideas. They should contribute to more spontaneity, more physical activity and more playfulness, creativity and relationship in the care of people living with dementia, nationally and internationally.

As this practice is centred in lived-body experience, it is difficult to communicate its essence in written language. If you are inspired by this chapter, I urge you to watch a film on Vimeo, *Je Me Raconte des Histoires*, by French film-maker and sociologist Gerald Assouline (2017), that continues to inspire me on this subject.[1] It contains an example of a beautiful dance between my friend and dance therapy colleague Job Cornelissen, from the Netherlands, and a resident in a care home. The dance occurs in the first five minutes of the film and demonstrates well all the aspects I have written about above.

---

1. https://vimeo.com/268436087

References

Assouline, G. (2017). *I tell stories to myself (Je me raconte des histoires)*. https://vimeo.com/268436087

Coaten, R. (2001). Exploring reminiscence through dance and movement. *Journal of Dementia Care, 9*(5), 19–22.

Coaten, R. (2009). *Building bridges of understanding: the use of embodied practices with older people with dementia and their care staff as mediated by dance movement psychotherapy*. PhD thesis. Roehampton University.

Coaten, R. (2011). Dance movement psychotherapy in dementia care. In H. Lee & T. Adams (Eds.), *Creative approaches and communication in dementia care* (pp.73–90). Macmillan.

Coaten, R., Heeley, T. & Spitzer, N. (2013). Dancemind's 'Moving Memories' evaluation and analysis: A UK-based dance and health project for people living with dementia and their care-staff. *UNESCO Observatory Multi-Disciplinary Journal in the Arts, 3*(3), 1–17.

Csikszentmihalyi, M. (2014). *Flow and the foundations of positive psychology*. Springer Publications.

Hsu, M.H., Flowerdew, R., Parker, M., Fachner, J. & Odell-Miller, H. (2015). Individual music therapy for managing neuropsychiatric symptoms for people with dementia and their carers: A cluster randomised controlled feasibility study. *BMC Geriatrics, 15*(84), 1–19.

Kitwood, T. & Bredin, K. (Eds.). (1992). *Person to person: A guide to the care of those with failing mental powers*. Gale Centre Publications.

31 Frames Of Mind: Bringing memories to life with stop-frame animation

Bo Chapman and Zoe Flynn

The creative impulse is fundamental to the experience of being human.
(APPG on Arts, Health and Wellbeing, 2017)

Seeing faces in inanimate objects, trees, domestic appliances, even toast, is a common human phenomenon called pareidolia. In stop-frame animation, we instinctively imbue inanimate objects or natural phenomena with human characteristics as we bring them to life, or 'anthropomorphise'.

Frames Of Mind is a charitable participatory arts organisation based in Newham, East London, which we established in 2019. We deliver stop-frame animation, film and digital arts programmes to support health and wellbeing, offering participants unique opportunities to learn new skills while engaging in meaningful creative processes.

We share backgrounds in television and art direction and the desire to empower communities to exploit the language of film and media as a powerful campaign tool with which to tell their stories, challenge stigma and inspire positive communication.

One of our main workstreams is dementia advocacy, along with mental health and wellbeing and digital inclusion and heritage. We have developed a resource of stimulating and meaningful activities that use stop-frame animation, digital arts and sensory engagement as an empowering communication tool to improve the health and wellbeing of participants. Whether working with participants to animate a significant object or create a digital self-portrait, the aim of our approach is to enhance experience in the moment, through humour, sensitivity and immersive play. All our projects are designed to support participants to maintain links with their skills and lived experiences.

We have pioneered stop-frame animation as a therapeutic communication and life-story tool with families living with dementia (Flynn & Chapman, 2011).

Using personal objects and photographs as catalysts for dialogue, memories can be literally animated, or brought to life.

Stop-frame animation

Stop-frame animation is produced when physically manipulated objects are moved in increments between individually captured photographs or 'frames'. When the frames are played in sequence (like a flip book), it creates the illusion of movement, as if the objects are magically moving by themselves. Anything can be animated – from peas to people. It is a very accessible art form that requires no previous experience. Anyone can do it.

When we first started making animations, it was a tech-heavy operation, with laptops, digital SLR cameras, bulky tripods, lights and endless cables. Today all you need is a smart device (phone or tablet), a stop-motion app, a remote (Bluetooth) control (optional) and a means of keeping the device stable (such as tripod, makeshift stand or adjustable phone/tablet holder).

The only thing that should physically move is the object you are animating. If the background or device moves, the whole scene will wobble – like an earthquake tremor – and the illusion of something moving on its own will be broken.

A remote Bluetooth control allows frames to be captured without touching the screen and the risk of moving the device in the process. It is a hand-held button mechanism, so it is more accessible for people who are less familiar with touch-screen technology, or who have impaired motor skills.

In an education setting, stop-frame animation is considered to be a truly 'cross-curricular' activity that embraces a range of creative and logistical subjects, from IT and maths to art, literacy and psychology. When creating an animation with people/families living with dementia, whether in a care home, community centre or domestic situation, it is no different. The levels of engagement are as multifaceted and profound. It is not only a fun, physical activity, where new skills are acquired together, but it is also an intrinsically valuable form of creative expression and an affirmation of the self.

In this chapter we explain how and why animation can be a particularly rewarding and empowering activity for carers and families living with dementia.

Immersive play

'... animation is memory that moves and evolves.'
(Tom Sherman, 2005)

Stop-frame animation provides a platform for 'play' that places the participant firmly in the moment. Its inherent alchemic and transformative nature invites suspension of disbelief. There are no rules and no linear imperative. Anything can happen.

Mary

The first time we tried animation in a care home, it was half way through a film project titled 'How You Look At it', which was commissioned by Sutton Council. We had been exploring ways of engaging residents with film-making, with marginal success, so we decided to try animation.

Our first participant was a soft-spoken Irish woman called Mary. She chose some personal objects from her room: a framed photo of her mother as a young woman, a china Shire horse and a crucifix. With a little instruction, she was able to move the objects, direct the action and capture the frames on the laptop. Our delight in seeing Mary 'doing' the animation herself and enjoying it is evident in the documentary film of the process – we are grinning from ear to ear![1]

Mary strokes the Shire horse affectionately and repeatedly, while her voice-over explains: 'I was 9 or 10 when my father bought that horse for me, at a fair… and I put it in as special place as I thought.'

She decides to move the crucifix closer to her mother's photograph.

Mary's objects were filmed on a small side table, and in the background you can see the fractured movement of another resident's knees captured incidentally. It puts the animation in the context of the care home. Ideally, objects should be placed against a plain background without interference or external movement, unless that is the dramatic effect desired (e.g. flashes of streaming traffic or moving clouds outside a window can create a dynamic backdrop).

The background for your animation can be anything or anywhere. Use what you have available. For example, a table can become a desert; a cupboard can be a dance floor; a sheet of wallpaper attached to the wall and curved onto the table can be used to create a makeshift studio backdrop.

Props related to the narrative are useful story prompts but can also provide scenic enhancement/background material – for example, an object associated with travel or adventure could be staged on a large sheet map or animated in a suitcase.

This is something that you can have fun devising together.

Jesse

Jesse, a resident at The Watermill in Walsall, chose a treasured replica of her dog Brett, which she kept in her cabinet. She told us how Brett, in a fit of canine jealousy, used to jump on her husband Norman when they played board games together on the carpet.

We re-created the scene using a chess board as the background.

Jesse began moving Brett across the squares, announcing that Norman was definitely 'on the black' and she was 'the white queen'. She watched the film over and over again, and laughed as she said: 'He looks like a different dog now altogether, doesn't he? He's a real dog! I wish Norman was here, he would love this.'

The instant playback facility of the animation held Jesse's interest, mitigating any anxiety about forgetting what she was doing or losing her place. It also allowed

---

1. See the clip on the Dementia Advocacy page of our website at https://framesofmind.uk/dementia

her to zone into the detail at her own pace and focus on certain moments that had a profound resonance.

Animation facilitates 'the slowing and stretching of time to examine or re-examine a seemingly insignificant moment, which can turn out to be a key moment in a life' (Mason, 2011).

The narrative of Brett and Norman was an evolving, playful improvisation, directed by Jesse, that enabled her to gently reconnect with memories and feelings as she brought her pet to life. The process of animating and the outcome were equally important – both integral and symbiotic. Jesse and Mary were empowered with a sense of control – deciding what to bring to life and doing it.

Learning point 1

Whether you are making the animation at home or in a care environment, collect some personal objects/photographs that are evocative of family, holidays, skills, interests, anything that catches your eye or that might spark a conversation/narrative. Surround yourself with props and choices.

- What object/s would you choose and why?
- Imagine bringing it to life – are there any potential moving parts?
- Describe what the object means to you in three words.
- What kind of characteristics would it have?
- How would it move?
- What would it say to you if it could speak?
- Where has it been? What has it seen/experienced?
- What other objects or props could it interact with?

Therapeutic communication tool

There are several stop-frame animation apps available for IOS and Android devices. Most are free or affordable and have comprehensive in-built tutorials, or you can source simple instruction videos on YouTube

We recommend capturing one photo (or frame) per movement of the object that you are animating. The smaller the distance between moves, the smoother the animated motion. The larger the moves, the faster and jerkier the animation.

To hold a position, take several frames (between four and six). You can punctuate your animation in this way and add meaning.

> The participatory arts and arts therapies can… help people to add meaning in the story of their lives and develop hopeful narratives. They can provide access to deep, nuanced feelings, communicated through metaphor and imagery. They can form part of a legacy, through the creation of artworks

to be shared with loved ones. They can give voice to those who no longer
feel able to speak and restore a sense of control to those who feel powerless.
(APPG on Arts, Health and Wellbeing, 2017)

The liberation from the literal in stop-frame animation provides an opportunity for
creative expression that can transcend language, bridge realities and communicate
sometimes sensitive and personal narratives. The process is an all-encompassing
activity that can be immensely therapeutic and improve mood and focus.

It's very easy to see people in terms of the common problems they share
e.g. old age and dementia. This animation project helped us to view people
as individuals who still have interesting stories to tell. More importantly it
makes them feel that they are still valued and worth listening to. (Family
member)

Sara

Sara had an amazing story to tell – a ready-made film script. Forced to flee her
home, Sara drove across the desert in a blue Vauxhall with her two daughters, a
tortoise, a cat and a 'bottle of fishes'. She had, she said, 'lost' her son a few years
before and was travelling through the Angolan desert to adopt a baby boy from
'the Zulus'. Initially Sara recounted several versions of her journey. She was quite
muddled and emotional. However, when we constructed the film set (a bag of sand
on the table and an imitation tortoise) she began to draw figures and animals in
the sand and her narrative became noticeably more coherent. The physical activity
and sensory engagement, reconnecting mind and body, helped Sara to focus and
tell her story in English *and* Portuguese.

Staff were not previously aware of her artistic abilities and Sara,
uncharacteristically, expressed interest in coming back the following week to do
more animation.

Edward

Edward, a former bus driver with advanced dementia, had limited vocal
communication and often became agitated. However, when we introduced him to
stop-frame animation, he showed immediate interest in the technology and 'set',
which included a map of London and a model of a vintage double-decker bus. He
helped us to move the bus and press the keys on the laptop and was calmed by the
rhythmic repetitive process of taking multiple photos. The repetition of movement
was soothing and reassuring. It helped him to disconnect and be free from the
literal – to be in the moment.

Edward was also fixated by the close-up photos of his mother and brother
when they appeared illuminated on the screen during playback. He kept saying
his brother's nickname, 'Scratch up', over and over again. Staff commented on his
smiles, changed mood and improved verbal communication: 'We don't know what
you've been doing to Edward!'

In our experience, no one has been intimidated by the technology or reticent to try something new. Men seem particularly keen to engage with the equipment. Many care providers have commented on the lack of activities aimed at men. Our approach and advice are to focus on what the technology allows you to do rather than the technology itself. What happens if you press this?

We don't know how long Edward's improved mood lasted. However, when the process of creating an animation is a positive experience, it is reassuring to know that the film can be revisited, either to be watched or continued. Similarly, if the mood/atmosphere is not conducive, the work can be resumed spontaneously at a better time.

Learning point 2

Drawing in sand or similar haptic materials can be a sensory activity in itself, especially for people with more advanced dementia.

Try collecting a selection of tactile (rice, sand, pastry dough) and aromatic (rosemary, lavender) substances and favourite edibles (e.g. sweets, grapes). Play some music to set the mood and inspire the pace of the movement. Animate the elements into faces or patterns. Change their expressions.

- What voices do they have? Record a voice-over.
- What are their names?
- What sounds do the movements make? Record some sound effects.

If the participant is absorbed in the sensory activity, don't be precious about trying to avoid capturing their hands in the animation. It can be a good effect and the process is just as important as the outcome.

Affirmation of self

Finding ways for people to express themselves and maintain a clear sense of their identity is one of the challenges of dementia care. Choosing objects that represent or link with skills and interests can be a catalyst for learned behaviour. They can provide a cognitive light switch or an external trigger, like music. Sometimes just holding the object is enough.

We worked with Alfred in the Daringly Able film project. This was commissioned by Jewish Care to ease the transition when the Ella & Ridley residential care home was moved to a new site. Staff training, their involvement in creative decision-making and planning and support from the management 'to take risks' were all key to the project's success. By chance, the objects chosen by both staff and residents for the animations were all linked to their professional skills and interests, and the film became a celebration of their expertise and stories. They included a tennis champion, an artist, a press photographer and a salmon cutter.

The Daringly Able project had a very positive effect... it broke the barrier between 'can't do' and 'can do'... it helped staff assess the balance between risk and choice. (Margaret Ofori-Koree, care home manager)

The project helped to build resilience and ease the trauma of relocation for everyone. Sharing skills and expertise deepened supportive relationships and mutual respect between staff and residents.

Alfred, salmon cutter to the queen

Initially Alfred was in a low mood and was reluctant to participate. His family had brought in his 'salmon-cutting knife' a few months before, and the care home manager allowed us to use the kitchen, so the scene was set. When Alfred walks through the kitchen door and is helped into his white coat, he spontaneously bursts into 'La donna è mobile', a canzone from Verdi's opera *Rigoletto*. When he is handed his long knife and sees the side of salmon, he straightens his back, rolls up his sleeves and is transformed. Transported back to the workplace, he is a salmon cutter to the Queen again, grinning and giving out customer service banter: 'What do you want for nothing?!'

His key worker made an animation from the cut salmon, featuring sandwiches singing the canzone, and when she showed it to Alfred, he became animated himself and started to sing again.[2] A month later, sadly, he passed away. His family has the film.

Learning point 3

Animation provokes the aesthetic decision-making and reflection associated with all creative activities. It also involves problem-solving and lateral thinking, which promote feelings of autonomy and control.

- Animate taking something apart and putting it back together – a biro, a torch, a satsuma. (Note: Playing the animation in reverse can provide a reference for the object's reconstruction.)
- Animate a jigsaw puzzle.
- Play the animations on a loop and in reverse, assembling and disassembling.
- Choose some hypnotic and calming music to set the tempo.

Conclusion

Animating objects decenters from the conventional meaning of objects... It engages humans in forming empathetic relationships with objects, by

---

2. You can watch a short film showing this at https://framesofmind.uk/daringly-able

humanising and inter-acting with them, as if experimenting with an alter ego, or a new self. Animating objects therefore has the potential to sensitise for and build empathetic capacity, not only in relation to the self-animated object, but also in relation to humans sharing a similar experience. (Budach & Sharoyan, 2020)

Animating objects or photos can be magical. It not only bridges physical and virtual realities; it also connects with the past in the present for the future. It is a fun, meaningful activity to be enjoyed together that can unearth gems of stories and anecdotes and create fresh new ones.

In a care home setting, inviting family/friends to bring in photographs or memorabilia is a very proactive way to include them. Creating the animation together can be a bonding intergenerational activity that can be re-visited on subsequent sessions – an ongoing project to help make visits meaningful and enjoyable for both parties. Technology is an enabler and cross-generational tool. Learning new skills together is a great leveller, whether at home or in residential care.

Simon, a resident, saw the potential of the activity as an incentive for his great-grandson to visit. He asked us: 'Teach me something my great-grandson doesn't know.'

Probably most importantly, the films produced, with or without a voice-over, are like gold dust.

Never underestimate what is possible, and good luck!

You can find out more about Frames Of Mind staff training courses, structured creative projects for care/community/family, consultancy and commissions at: www.framesofmind.uk

References

All-Party Parliamentary Group on Arts, Health and Wellbeing. (2017). *Creative health: The arts for health and wellbeing* (2nd ed.). Inquiry report. www.culturehealthandwellbeing.org.uk/appg-inquiry/

Budach, G. & Sharoyan, G. (2020). Exploring 'vibrant matter' in animation making. *Language and Intercultural Communication, 20*(5), 464–481. DOI:10.1080/14708477.2020.1784912

Flynn, Z. & Chapman, B. (2011). Making animated films with people with dementia. *Journal of Dementia Care, 19*(6), 23–25.

Mason, H. (2011). The re-animation approach: Animation and therapy. *The Journal of Assistive Technology, 5*(1), 40–42.

Sherman, T. (2005). Video/intermedia/animation. In C. Gehman & S. Reinke (Eds.), *The sharpest point: Animation at the end of cinema* (pp.189–197). YYZ Books.

32 Digital life-story work with people living with dementia

Kathryn Barham

There have been several studies over the past 30 years that explore the benefits of using life-story work with people living with dementia, both in the community and in care home settings. Recently, studies have looked at the benefits of expanding this work into the digital domain and creating multi-media life-story books. This means that users are able to expand their resources to include personal photographs or images from books or the internet, typed and spoken word, music and films (for example, home movies or YouTube clips). This can create a more unique, person-centred book that can tap into a person's memories in whatever way works best for them. This is particularly important for those living with dementia, as some of their senses and ways of engaging with resources can be seriously affected as the disease progresses.

Learning point 1

If you are new to the concept of life-story work, it may help you to think about the following:

- Life experiences from birth onwards. How have these experiences affected you and made you into the person you are now?
- What kind of things do you enjoy doing?
- What made you happy as a child, and what makes you happy now?
- How can revealing and sharing these things help family and carers understand what is important to you, so that they can help you to live well?

Life-story work uses a form of reminiscence therapy. A Cochrane report (Woods et al., 2018) describes reminiscence therapy as 'discussing events and experiences from the past. It aims to evoke memories, stimulate mental activity and improve well-being'. Reminiscence therapy is often assisted by props (such as videos, pictures and objects), and can take place in a group or be done with a person on their own, when it often results in some form of life-story book being created. Reminiscence therapy helps older people with depression. It may be suitable for people with dementia, because depression is common in dementia, and because people with dementia 'typically have a better memory for the past than for recent events' (Woods et al., 2018).

Recently, more research has shown that reminiscence therapy and life-story work can improve the quality of life of people living with dementia, boost their cognitive ability and communication skills, and elevate their mood in some circumstances. Life-story work can help to encourage better communication with the person with dementia, so that we can better understand their needs and wishes. This is especially important when the person with dementia is having difficulty sharing this information themselves. Sharing stories can help the person to develop closer relationships with family carers and staff. This can inform their care and ensure that it is provided in a helpful, person-centred way (Thompson, 2017).

The widely used This Is Me form[1] can often be a good starting point for a digital life story. This is a form that is used in the care profession to help careworkers and professionals better understand who the person really is, which can help them to deliver care that is tailored to the person's individual needs.

Book of You CIC is a social enterprise based in North Wales and working across the UK. Since 2014, it has used a web-based app to enable people to create their own life story via five templates: large photograph and caption; photograph and typed words (telling a story where the photograph illustrates that story); photograph and audio (using a piece of music or a person's voice to tell an anecdote or read a poem); films (new films, or uploading ones from a personal collection), and YouTube (for example, streaming a music video). By talking/engaging with the person with dementia, the experienced life-story worker, family member or carer can find out which media works best for each person, thereby building a book that can be both enjoyable and beneficial.

An evolving approach to digital life-story work is through a series of workshops or sessions in which people with dementia are assisted to play an active role in creating their own life-story book (O'Philbin et al., 2020). Book of You can organise and deliver life-story workshops in a variety of contexts – for example, in the community, or in people's own homes and care homes – to support those living with dementia, their family, friends and carers and care home staff. They have a team of committed and trained staff and volunteers to support these sessions, and the sessions are evaluated with questionnaires to find out the benefits for people living with dementia and their carers.

---

1. www.alzheimers.org.uk/get-support/publications-factsheets/this-is-me?Search=%F0%9F%94%8D&key words=this%20is%20me

Life-story work – why it is important, and why it works

Life-story work is built from our life experiences and how these have made us into the people we are today. It also helps others to understand us as individual people. When it comes to people living with dementia, looking at a life-story book can help them to stay grounded and remind them of who is important to them, thereby prompting happy memories, which helps them to communicate. Life-story work can give back some self-esteem to the person with dementia, as it is something that can be shared confidentially with others (family, friends and carers). Unlike recent memories, many of these memories from the past are clear and detailed.

Dementia can impact massively on a person's life. Family and friends can stop visiting because they feel awkward and they don't know what to say. Normal conversation can at best be stilted, is often repetitive and may even be impossible. Despite social action movements like the Alzheimer's Society's hugely successful Dementia Friends initiative, there is still a huge stigma around dementia, and sometimes friends mistakenly feel that the person won't remember or be bothered if they don't call to see them. They often say that they'd rather remember the person with dementia as they were. This can mean both the person with dementia and their family carer lose out. First of all, the person with dementia may fear the dementia itself, and what the future holds for them. They may also say that they feel lonely and forgotten. Recently, there has been growing evidence that loneliness has a clear and significant impact on people's wellbeing, with the same long-term detrimental health effects as smoking 15 cigarettes a day. Mental health issues like depression are also likely to increase (Welsh Government, 2020).

Having a digital life-story book to engage a person with dementia in conversation can be beneficial both for the person with dementia and for their friend/family member, in that it gives them snippets of good memories that can engage and stimulate them. Perhaps their mood can be improved by listening to a favourite piece of music and even singing along to it. The person with dementia could listen to a message from a family member telling them how much they love and miss them and perhaps share their own favourite memories of the person with dementia. A digital life-story book is useful in that it can tap into whatever works on a particular day.

Family members often create a 'This Is Your Life' book for their relative, combining photographs and words. Various templates are available to assist this. Such a book may be presented as a gift (Subramaniam et al., 2013). Over the years, Book of You has found that the benefits lie both in the process of digital 'book building' and in sharing the content of the book. For example, by looking at how the person with dementia reacts to particular films or pieces of music and by measuring these reactions, we can see which are the most powerful and emotive films or pieces of music for them. Benefits of using this type of life-story book can lie in the fact that it is 'Mum's Story', to be enjoyed, created and shared with the wider group of family and friends. Also, the life-story book can be used as a tool to stimulate conversation, as the relative can concentrate on memories that the person living with dementia can still recall and enjoy with their family on an equal basis. If the person with dementia is in a care home, staff can fully engage too, and have easy access to these memories and stories themselves.

Deciding what goes into a book may change over time and the digital aspect means that families can amend the content, move pages around and add more. It should also be remembered by the family that their strongest memory may not be the same as that of their relative. One daughter put a particular song by Abba into her father's book, as she always remembered that he loved it and would sing and dance around to it. But his stage of dementia meant that he had forgotten the song, and he showed no reaction to it, so it was removed. They were able to find songs that he did react to – it was a case of trial and error. We have found that a printed book, although valuable, is less flexible.

Life-story work can be one of the enjoyable and valuable activities that families can do together once dementia has been diagnosed. Starting a book before diagnosis is good, because the earlier a book is started, the more the person can choose their own content. A multi-media digital book brings extra benefits over printed versions as it can stimulate a person's different senses. Equally important is where the person is on their dementia journey, as this may also affect how much they engage with the digital book. So, for example, the sound of a granddaughter's voice recounting a spoken memory of a song that means a lot to the person with dementia can be valuable in creating enjoyment and stimulating memory. If the digital book is started at an early stage, the person with dementia is able to take a more active role in what goes into it. A rich book may also include other family members recounting their memories of the person with dementia, or of a particular event. For example, a grandfather who was living with dementia, his son and his grandson together shared a memory of a time that they all stayed up late to watch badgers in the garden. Memories such as this can easily be recorded direct to phone or tablet and immediately uploaded into the book.

Digital life-story work can often tap into long forgotten memories or re-ignite something deep down that had been assumed to be lost. Book of You has known occasions when using digital life-story work means that the person with dementia has been brought back into family conversations again. Jenny, who had not spoken for some time, was sitting in the room while her husband, Michael, recounted for a Book of You volunteer an amusing anecdote that he'd heard her tell years before, when she was a young girl. As he chatted into the tablet held by the volunteer, Jenny's face suddenly lit up, she started laughing and said, 'That's me, isn't it? I was SO naughty!' Thrillingly, the volunteer managed to catch all of this on the recording, and it went into Jenny's book. Michael was overjoyed and said that he had never expected to hear her speak again.

Learning point 2

Preparation is key to the creation of a rich, valued life-story book. Always remember to put the person with dementia at the centre. Before beginning, you should consider the following:

- How can you structure a life-story conversation?
- Who can you involve in helping you to tell the story?
- What types of media might the subject be most stimulated by?

Mum's multimedia memory book

When Mrs Peters had to move into a care home, her daughter, Frances, brought her to Ormskirk from her home town in Yorkshire so that she could visit her every day. Mrs Peters' parents had also had dementia, so she had made a memory box for them many years ago. Because of this, Frances was familiar with the concept herself and created a memory book full of words and photographs, which she would take along to the care home when visiting her mum. When she was given the option to try making a multimedia digital reminiscence book, she jumped at the chance. Mrs Peters' eyesight isn't very good, so although Frances could talk to her about what was in the written memory book, her mum couldn't see it. But she still responded very well to sound (music and spoken messages).

There were around five 'key memories' that Mrs Peters could talk about when prompted by her family, and it was clear from Mrs Peters' reaction that these provided some comfort. Using a shareable digital life reminiscence book means that staff at the home could also read about the memories and talk about them with Mrs Peters when her family weren't there, which was a huge benefit. Frances' sister still lived in Yorkshire, and she was able to record a voice message in the book. Mrs Peters responded to hearing this message by smiling and talking back to her as if she was there. The family also uploaded YouTube videos of favourite hymns, and Mrs Peters loved to sing along to these.

Mrs Peters' family was scattered around the world in different continents. The digital book was stored on the cloud and shareable by logging in with a secure, unique username and password. This meant that Mrs Peters' sister (who also had dementia) and her brother and nieces were able to look at her book from wherever they were in the world, and upload spoken messages for Mrs Peters. It was a wonderful way to keep the family in contact with each other in a meaningful way. In fact, it was the only way that they could communicate, because phone calls were not possible.

This was especially important during the Covid-19 crisis, when Frances was unable to visit her mum for several weeks. However, she was reassured that staff could play her mum the messages and Mrs Peters reacted as if her daughter were there. Frances felt that spoken words and music were most valuable in her mum's case, as she seemed to be so much happier when listening to them and she became more animated. For the time she was listening to these voices and music, Mrs Peters was calm and more grounded. She could join in with the singing and talk with the voices, and clearly found this comforting. If Frances was unable to visit at any time, she could add a new message to reassure her mum.

> **Learning point 3**
>
> Why is it valuable for care home staff to know about someone's past?
>
> - It can help staff understand why a person may react in a particular way.
> - The things in the book are the things that they can talk about safely, without upsetting the resident
> - The memories might help to calm down a distressed or a confused resident.

If the person living with dementia has no family member or carer to help create the multimedia book, and they don't have the confidence or skills to create one themselves, they can still benefit by taking part in a group and being supported by a digital 'buddy', usually a specially trained volunteer, to create the book. This has the added benefit of meaning that the person with dementia spends time with someone who has the time to listen and chat. Often, it is only when people begin to talk again about older memories that they realise that their life is full of unique experiences that are pleasurable to revisit and talk about.

Conclusion

If a person with dementia is supported to store, recall and share precious memories in a digital life-story book, they are generally happier and feel less anxious. In some cases, family relationships are strengthened. It can be useful if the person with dementia has already started their multimedia book, before they have to move into residential care, as it will provide the home with valuable information about the person they are caring for. The earlier that the life-story work is started, the better, as the person living with dementia will have more capacity to decide what is important to them that they want to record. The value of a digital book is best seen when it is used regularly and added to throughout a person's life, to show that living well continues after diagnosis and that their memories are valuable both to them and to their loved ones and carers.

References

O'Philbin, L., Woods, B. & Windle, G. (2020). Implementing digital life story work for people with dementia: Relevance of context to user experience. *The International Journal of Reminiscence and Life Review, 7*(1), 22–32.

Subramaniam, P., Woods, B. & Whitaker, C. (2013). Life review and life story books for people with mild to moderate dementia: a randomised controlled trial. *Aging & Mental Health, 18*(3), 363375.

Thompson, R. (2017). *Guidance for using the Life Story Book template.* [Online.] Dementia UK. www.dementiauk.org/wp-content/uploads/2017/03/Lifestory-.compressed.pdf

Welsh Government. (2020). *Connected communities: A strategy for tackling loneliness and social isolation and building stronger social connections.* Welsh Government.

Woods, B., O'Philbin, L., Farrell, E.M., Spector, A.E. & Orrell, M. (2018). Reminiscence therapy for dementia: An abridged Cochrane systematic review of the evidence from randomized controlled trials. *Expert Review of Neurotherapeutics, 18*(9), 715–727.

33 Music therapy in dementia care

Ming-Hung Hsu

Music is universal and has been part of everyday life throughout human history. It is played at birthday parties and ceremonies to promote excitement and joy, during candlelit dinners to enhance feelings of romance, and in times of sorrow to offer solace. As science advances, we have now learned that music may have a positive effect on our mood, motivation, stress, immunity and social bonding (Chanda & Levitin, 2013). Therefore, singing, attending music concerts or playing instruments can all be beneficial to our health and wellbeing. Singing, for example, has been found to lower levels of cortisol, known as the 'stress hormone', in people receiving treatment for cancer and their carers (Fancourt et al., 2016). Listening to music is also reported to increase relaxation in patients after open-heart surgery (Nilsson, 2009). Music therapy, a formal psychological treatment and regulated health profession, has been applied in treatments for depression (Erkkilä et al., 2011) and schizophrenia (Geretsegger et al., 2017) to enhance mood, mental state and social connection.

The use of music in dementia care has received increasing attention as hearing is thought to be the last cognitive faculty to decline over our life span. Music activates most parts of the brain and therefore enables individuals with dementia to access their remaining cognitive abilities, such as attention and memory, in order to maintain their sense of wellbeing.

Among all of the music-activated abilities, 'musical memory' seems unique to human beings, allowing us to remember music-related information, such as the title, features or content of a piece of music. One example of phenomenal musical memory was when, as she took her seat on stage, the renowned pianist Maria João Pires suddenly realised she had learnt the wrong Mozart concerto. Yet, with the conductor's encouragement, as the orchestra progressed towards the piano part, she was able to recall and play the right concerto, without missing a single note. A neuroimaging study conducted by Jacobsen and colleagues (2015) also found that musical memory appeared to be retained in people living with Alzheimer's disease.

Such findings support the application of music and formal music therapy in improving the quality of life not only of care recipients but also their caregivers. However, this raises questions about how music could be best incorporated in the daily life of those receiving care to achieve this goal. What music activities should be used, and when? What is the current evidence? How can a music therapist help? This chapter aims to answer these questions and provide caregivers with some practical methods of embedding music in daily care.

Learning point 1

Before reading further, you may like to consider the following questions:

- What have been your usual music activities (live concerts, choir singing, playing an instrument on your own or with others and listening to records or the radio)?

- What are the music genres that you and your care recipient prefer and share?

- Do you currently engage in these music activities? If yes, how often?[1]

Current evidence

In recent years, more and more research has investigated the therapeutic effects of music-based interventions in dementia care. These interventions are often divided into either music therapy – that is, delivered by qualified music therapists[2] – or music activities, which can be delivered by anyone. Music therapists can also train other people to deliver music activities or deliver them themselves. Music activities can include group singing sessions, music listening during bathing and mealtimes, or interactive live music group programmes, involving instrument playing and listening to music.

A Cochrane review (van der Steen et al., 2018) found no long-term effect for these interventions. However, it noted that providing at least five sessions of a music-based therapeutic intervention to people living with long-term dementia in care settings probably reduces depressive symptoms and improves overall behavioural symptoms. The authors also suggested that these music-based interventions may have the potential for improving emotional wellbeing and quality of life and reducing anxiety.

Current evidence suggests that active interactive singing or music-making are more beneficial than passive music listening. Additionally, music-based interventions are mostly used to ameliorate non-cognitive symptoms of dementia

---

1. See https://musicfordementia.org.uk/musicalmap/ for a map of music activities fopr dementia offered throughout the UK.

2. See www.bamt.org/training/music-therapy-courses-hcpc-approved for UK music therapy training courses.

(such as anxiety, depression and apathy). If not treated, such symptoms can quicken the progression of dementia and affect both care recipients' and caregivers' quality of life. Depression, for example, may cause reduced motivation to carry out usual activities, and may prompt withdrawal from social contact and difficulties carrying out daily tasks, such as washing and dressing. This could consequently increase caregivers' levels of burden and distress. Therefore, the management of these symptoms is a major task in dementia care. Interventions such as singing may be used during anxious or depressive episodes to help either improve or settle a person's mood. By selecting an appropriate song, singing can also re-direct a person's attention to memory recalls and generate positive emotions associated with these memories. Therefore, music-based interventions can play an important role in managing non-cognitive symptoms.

Embedding music in care

When listening to music, our attention is deployed to identifying the musical elements, including melody, tempo, timbre and so forth. In addition to using our attention, we use working memory (short-term memory that holds information temporarily). Musical semantic memory is also activated as we recognise the name and content of a specific piece. Furthermore, autobiographical memory (of one's life events and experiences, such as one's wedding and learning to play the piano) can also be triggered, as these are often associated with certain pieces of music. While playing an instrument can engage our motor planning, initiation and execution, the brain areas involved in motor function can also be activated by simply listening to music (Gordon et al., 2018). Research suggests that music can elicit communication between more parts of the brain than can any other stimuli. Therefore, listening to music can easily provide cognitive stimulation.

One caveat is that music's stimulating effect on certain cognitive abilities may only last temporarily, and for no more than 15 minutes (Rauscher et al., 1993). This may explain why people with advanced dementia can suddenly become more lucid, joyous and lively, with bodily movements, while listening to music, but appear more subdued again afterwards. Therefore, to have an effect on symptoms of dementia such as agitation and apathy, a strategic use of music is required. For example, listening to soothing music with a slow tempo may reduce levels of emotional arousal and agitation. However, it would be more effective if music listening were implemented before the onset of an episode of agitation. Some tips that have been trialled in music therapy research (Hsu et al., 2015) are outlined below for consideration.

In the right place at the right time

Caregivers are experts-by-experience. Over time they develop their own skills and strategies for managing certain symptoms, based on their understanding of the care recipients. However, there may still be occasions when caregivers may feel upset, anxious or helpless when a person's symptom catches them off guard. At these times, it may be helpful to identity potential patterns of emotions and behaviours. For example, a person with dementia might find it difficult to get up in the morning, due to apathy and lethargy. Music could be played to provide stimulation while the caregiver helps the care recipient get up. Moreover, a person might experience 'sundowning' – a state of increased confusion, accompanied with anxiety, irritability and agitation, in the late afternoons. Introducing music listening,[3] or pleasurable activities such as singing or instrument playing before an episode's onset, may help to reduce this symptom. The onset of these emergent symptoms generally indicates a place and need for this music. While this fundamental aspect guides the embedding of music within care, other aspects such as engaging care recipients' attention should also be considered.

Attention is the key

When using music to offset emergent symptoms, it is vital to choose a piece that easily engages the attention of the care recipient, after which the effect of music can be maximised to provide emotional regulation. Not all music will engage attention, which is why some songs are easier than others to hum along to. Research has shown that, when listening to recorded music, feelings of familiarity could be generated within half a second and the emotion conveyed by the music could be identified within a quarter of a second (Filipic et al., 2010). Thus, attention can be captured within a very short time-frame to identify the embedded emotion and whether the music is familiar. Certain features, particularly melodic and rhythmic patterns, may play a vital role in catching attention. Songs that are easily recalled and that engage attention often have a motif (a melodic pattern that incorporates shorter notes and a distinctive rhythm) (Müllensiefen & Halpern, 2014) and a melodic contour (the overall shape of the song) that frequently goes up and down. Many British folk songs, such as 'The Bonnie Banks o' Loch Lomond', 'Foggy, Foggy Dew' and 'The Lincoln Poacher', include these features.

It is also important to note that attention leads to the feeling of pleasure that is generated by music. This pleasurable feeling may rapidly offset the emergent symptoms. This pleasure is built on musical repetition. A repeated motif with a distinctive melodic and rhythmic pattern can make a song more satisfying and enjoyable (Service, 2016). Therefore, it would be helpful to identify from a care recipient's preferred music the songs or tunes that possess these features. Having these at hand is always helpful in managing the symptoms. Often, symptoms such as agitation can have a rapid onset, giving very little time to turn on a stereo or find a device or musical instrument to produce music. The caregiver's singing would therefore be the most efficient method to serve this purpose. If singing is not possible, The King's Singers' album *Folk Songs of the British Isles*, containing the songs discussed above, could be helpful, played from a CD or streaming platform such as Spotify or Apple Music. These songs are sung either unaccompanied or with a simple piano or string accompaniment, and use vocal harmony that may

---

3. See https://m4dradio.com/ for M4D radio, an online music station dedicated to people living with dementia.

also enhance feelings of pleasure and sustain attention. All in all, choosing the right music to catch a care recipient's attention is key to maximising the effect of music on emotion regulation. However, how the chosen song or tune is sung or played is another aspect that may require some careful considerations.

It is what you sing and how you sing it

Environmental stimuli (such as sounds, lighting and temperature) can influence the mood and physical comfort of an individual with dementia. Careful control of these should therefore be undertaken, without which, existing symptoms (including agitation, irritability or anxiety) can be exacerbated. The volume of the chosen music would be the first aspect to consider. Music that is too loud or quiet might generate discomfort and agitation or fail to engage a care recipient's attention. The timbre (the quality of the sound or voice) should also be selected mindfully. For example, an operatic voice or the sound of certain instruments (e.g. piano or tuba) might not be tolerable to some people. Music with a complex texture of complicated and changeable melodies, rhythms and harmonies might not capture the attention of a person with impaired cognitive abilities. People with dementia might find it easier to attend to music consisting of clear and simple melodic lines, rhythms and instrumental accompaniment. The folk songs sung by The King's Singers, discussed above, may be a good example.

It is also necessary to consider the music's duration. A care recipient might have a shortened attention span due to dementia and may easily become desensitised to the music and hence experience a reduced effect. Furthermore, repeatedly playing music that can generate nostalgia, sorrow and sadness may cause an enduring melancholic mood for a person with dementia who has impaired inhibitory control of emotion. Therefore, it is important to carefully observe a care recipient's responses to different pieces of music. If some negative responses or emotions appear, changing or discontinuing the music is necessary.

Learning point 2

To maximise the effect of music on emergent symptoms, choosing the right music to meet particular needs and purposes is key. It would be helpful to consider the following questions:

- During a normal day, when do certain symptoms often emerge? What might be the trigger for these? As a caregiver, how do you normally respond to the individual you care for when these emerge?

- Among your favourite music genres, are there any specific songs or pieces of music that are frequently listened to or hummed by the person you care for? Do these have a short, simple and distinctive melodic and rhythmic pattern?

- How are these pieces of music generally played or sung? How do they sound? Are they relaxing, soothing or invigorating?

- What are the care recipient's expressions when listening to or humming these pieces of music? Do they look serene, calm, uplifted or upset?

Music therapy

Music therapist is a protected title in the UK. This health profession is regulated by the Health and Care Professions Council.[4] To become a music therapist, an individual must have acquired proficient musical skills before completing the two-year Master's-level training qualification. The music therapy training in the UK is informed by psychoanalytic, psychodynamic and humanistic theories and neuroscience. Neuroscience is one of the core research areas at the Cambridge Institute of Music Therapy Research, based at Anglia Ruskin University. This has been incorporated into the university's music therapy course. The music therapy service provided in the care homes of MHA,[5] a national charity providing care, accommodation and community support services, is informed by cognitive psychology and affective neuroscience (Armony & Vuilleumier, 2013). These two disciplines allow MHA's music therapists to understand how human emotion and cognition can be facilitated using visual, haptic and auditory stimuli, including music. They can then apply the theories to assess the cognitive abilities and social, emotional, psychological or physical needs of a person with dementia. Based on their understanding of a person's needs, they then tailor the treatment in music therapy sessions and provide strategies for caregivers to use to manage symptoms and improve quality of life.

Music therapists' clinical practice follows guidelines set out by the National Institute for Health and Care Excellence (NICE). Therefore, music therapists need to keep up to date with the relevant research evidence of heath conditions, medications, care pathways and pain and symptom management. They also need to have the skills and knowledge of clinical evaluation and how to use validated outcome measures.

Learning point 3

Based on their knowledge and skills, music therapists can provide assessments and strategies to help overcome difficulties experienced by caregivers in the management of symptoms. Consider the questions below to see if you need some help from a music therapist.

- Do you find any of the care recipient's symptoms distressing and unmanageable?

---

4. www.hcpc-uk.org/about-us/who-we-regulate/the-professions/.

5. See www.facebook.com/watch/?v=320608221906844&extid=n4npxW1cbkgkFsn6 for the BBC's coverage of music therapy in dementia care.

- Do you find it hard to identify suitable music activities?
- Have you tried some music or activities, but they have not worked?

Conclusion

This chapter has discussed some suggestions as to how music may be used in alleviating the non-cognitive symptoms of dementia. Music's potential may be maximised if used in small amounts whenever a need or a symptom arises, rather than as a prolonged period of music listening. The selection of music should be based on the features of music that can capture attention. In addition, singing or playing music with an appropriate timbre and volume, as well as observing a care recipient's response, can help the caregiver determine the music's effectiveness. In dementia care, the role of music therapists is not limited to delivering therapy sessions. Their problem-solving skills can help implement music activities and improve quality of life for people with dementia and their caregivers.

References

Armony, J. & Vuilleumier, P. (Eds.) (2013). *The Cambridge handbook of human affective neuroscience.* Cambridge University Press.

Chanda, M.L. & Levitin, D.J. (2013). The neurochemistry of music. *Trends in Cognitive Sciences, 17*(4), 179–193.

Erkkilä, J., Punkanen, M., Fachner, J., Ala-Ruona, E., Pöntiö, I., Tervaniemi, M., Vanhala, M. & Gold, C. (2011). Individual music therapy for depression: randomised controlled trial. *British Journal of Psychiatry, 199*(2), 132–139.

Fancourt, D., Williamon, A., Carvalho, L.A., Steptoe, A., Dow, R. & Lewis, I. (2016). Singing modulates mood, stress, cortisol, cytokine and neuropeptide activity in cancer patients and carers. *ecancermedicalscience, 10*, 631. doi: 10.3332/ecancer.2016.631

Filipic, S., Tillmann, B. & Bigand, E. (2010). Judging familiarity and emotion from very brief musical excerpts. *Psychonomic Bulletin & Review, 17*(3), 335–341.

Geretsegger, M., Mössler, K., Bieleninik, Ł., Chen XJ, Heldal, T.O. & Gold, C. (2017.) Music therapy for people with schizophrenia and schizophrenia-like disorders. *Cochrane Database of Systematic Reviews, 5*(5), CD004025. doi: 10.1002/14651858.CD004025.pub4.

Gordon, C.L., Cobb, P.R. & Balasubramaniam, R. (2018). Recruitment of the motor system during music listening: An ALE meta-analysis of fMRI data. *PloS One, 13*(11).

Hsu, M.H., Flowerdew, R., Parker, M., Fachner, J. & Odell-Miller, H. (2015). Individual music therapy for managing neuropsychiatric symptoms for people with dementia and their carers: A cluster randomised controlled feasibility study. *BMC Geriatrics, 15*(1), 84.

Jacobsen, J.H., Stelzer, J., Fritz, T.H., Chételat, G., La Joie, R., & Turner, R. (2015). Why musical memory can be preserved in advanced Alzheimer's disease. *Brain, 138*(8), 2438–2450.

Müllensiefen, D. & Halpern, A.R. (2014). The role of features and context in recognition of novel melodies. *Music Perception: An Interdisciplinary Journal, 31*(5), 418–435.

Nilsson, U. (2009). Soothing music can increase oxytocin levels during bed rest after open-heart surgery: A randomised control trial. *Journal of Clinical Nursing, 18*(15), 2153–2161.

Rauscher, F.H., Shaw, G.L. & Ky, C.N. (1993). Music and spatial task performance. *Nature, 365*(6447), 611.

Service, T. (2016, April 29). Stuck on repeat. Why we love repetition in music. *The Guardian.* www.theguardian.com/music/2016/apr/29/why-we-love-repetition-in-music-tom-service

van der Steen, J.T., Smaling, H.J., van der Wouden, J.C., Bruinsma, M.S., Scholten, R.J. & Vink, A.C. (2018). Music-based therapeutic interventions for people with dementia. *Cochrane Database of Systematic Reviews, 7*(7):CD003477. doi: 10.1002/14651858.CD003477.pub4

34 Poetry: Telling it like it is

John Killick

I began writing poetry with people with dementia more than 25 years ago. The stimulus to initiating an approach came from the observation that, at a certain stage of the development of the condition, the breaking down of language resulted in the release of poetic possibilities that appeared to have been latent in the person's earlier life. This I attributed to the challenge dementia offers to the reasoning faculty and the need for the person to find a new expressive outlet for their feelings.

When, in the past couple of years, my wife began to show characteristics of dementia, I wondered if my theory would be borne out in her own speech patterns. It has been, as I hope the following examples will illustrate:

> I like music that is a nice warm walk.
> That question has crumbled me out.
> My message is: our clocks are timeless.
> Rain is chuck-a-puddle.
> That meal was full-up to its memory.

I submit that these small units of language have a vividness and ambiguity that in other contexts we would acknowledge as poetry.

The question I was faced with at the outset was how to harness such creativity into the shaping of whole poems.

Becoming a true listener

It soon became clear to me that what was required was an intensity of listening so that one could begin to piece together ideas and expressions that at first might appear disparate. Interruptions in the form of questions were unhelpful to this process. Writing down or recording a person's words over a period of time and then reflecting on them was the most productive way to proceed. But first of all, you had to gain the person's confidence. Relationship-building in most instances came first, and then the words would begin to flow. The individual's preferences or preoccupations dictated the subject matter. It was undesirable to mention poetry when you were setting this up one to one; it was only necessary to establish that one's role was that of a listener, and to seek permission to record the words because they would be of value.

Cultivating silence

In many ways, the most difficult task I faced was keeping silent; we are so used to observing the conventions of conversation. But anything that might distract the speaker proved unhelpful. All that was required was occasional encouragement, which could be offered by way of a sound or a gesture. By far the most difficult aspect of this was becoming comfortable with the silences that punctuated the monologues; these could be quite protracted, and the instinct to leap in and fill a gap was difficult to resist. Nevertheless, I had to learn quickly that keeping quiet was essential to giving the person the time and space for marshalling their thoughts and feelings.

Learning point 1

You might like to try to answer the following questions:

- Think of a conversation you have had with someone where you were aware of having been listened to intently. What did it feel like? How would you have felt if you had been interrupted?
- Think of a time when you were completely absorbed by what someone else was saying. What did it feel like? Did you want to interrupt?
- Have a conversation with another person. Practise silence. How did it feel? Ask them how it felt for them.

An example and its qualities

Here is a poem by Peter Van Spyck, a man attending a day centre, which comes from my book *The Elephant in the Room* (Killick, 2009):

It can be done

This is heaven
because for a lot of people it helps them.
You do it on a one-to-one
and that's right.
I feel I'm very lucky
because I've got something like poetry.

I've lots of memories, good and bad.
Most of my friends, they never say a thing ---
I think they're frightened:

I've got a friend in London
and he's only phoned once in three years.
We've just come back from Madeira.
My wife noticed it and told me.
I said 'I've got Alzheimer's.'
I could see the same signs.
He was there with his wife.
She had it. On the last three days
we stayed together,
we found a rapport.

Some people can't handle it.
They think, how can they carry on?
But I don't think I want these things round my neck.
I want to live!

I'm not wanting to get rid of myself,
I've never even thought of it.
I really mean it.
If you take your courage in both hands
it can be done!

Now this poem has a logical structure. It has a theme, and it isn't dependent on sensual language or unusual imagery. But it shows Peter's attitude towards his diagnosis, and the reactions of others. We learn of the nature of his resolve to stay in charge of his life, and we can encourage him on this basis. So there can be a practical as well as aesthetic outcome of this work.

Learning point 2

You might like to try answering the following:

- Choose a subject and ask someone to write down your words as you speak. What did it feel like?
- Now ask the other person to speak on a subject of their choice while you write down their words. How did that feel?

Two kinds of outcome

I consider there are two main and contrasting characteristics of the poems produced by people with dementia. The first is that of entertainment and reminiscence, and these poems can be valued for their outward-looking storytelling nature. In the following, 'Watching Grandmother Dress' by Mary Williams, the feelings are implicit in the telling:

Once I slept with my grandmother and watched her dress.
First one petticoat, then another, then another,
then another, then another. And I said, how many
do you wear, grandmother?
And she said, only
one more.

She'd start with her flannelette one – always wool
next to the skin – then her linen ones, and then
her skirt. And over the top she'd wear her apron.
She was a tiny little woman.
And in her hat she'd wear
a long hatpin
to hold it on.

This poem comes from the book *Bee's Knees and Pickled Onions*, which I edited (Killick, 2014), and the poem was transcribed by one of the four poets I mentored at the Courtyard Centre for the Arts in Hereford, for the In the Pink project.[1]

Now here is a poem that reflects a more inward and therapeutic approach:

All you got

All come out fresh
Today
Just for one day
You give all you've got and
You can't give no more

Mustn't grumble
You know.
Things here got it ---
Got to do this, do that
But that's what's got to
Happen
You've got to sacrifice.

This poem comes from the book *The Things Between Us*, an anthology from the Living Words project in London, of which Susanna Howard is the founder, artistic director, and also editor of this collection (Howard, 2014). The name of the composer is not given.

The first poem appears spontaneous and genial. The second is more awkwardly phrased and sombre. These are the two extremes, and they are both equally valid. The vast majority of the poems produced and published in the first project are of

---

1. https://www.dementiapositive.co.uk/poetry-in-herefordshire.html

the fluency of the Mary Williams' poem. The vast majority of the poems produced and published in the second partake of this striving nature. It is almost certain that the differences between the two sets of work are the results of the approaches of the projects and the poets working in them. In that sense, it could be said that there is a bias that is controlled by the facilitators and does not come from the people with dementia themselves. They reflect the bias, but that does not mean that the emotions that they express and that the poets shape are not genuine.

Other factors that may influence the nature of the work produced are the expectations of the institutions in which the projects take place, and the degree of difficulty in expression experienced by the clients in the scheme. For example, attempts to engage with people who are less likely to come forward may result in different emphases to what emerges from work with people who have only recently received a diagnosis.

Also, although both poems printed above come from one-to-one sessions, the In the Pink project does a great deal of group work, and this may set a collaborative tone, which is then followed throughout the scheme. The first book tells us more about the pasts of individuals, and the second tells us more about dementia and how people are coping with it. Both are confirmatory in effect in their own way, but it is impossible to assess the degree to which the people with dementia are satisfied by the experience, except where they have given utterance to their appreciation, as in this passage from another poem in *The Things Between Us* (Howard, 2014). Again, the composer is not named:

After you've gone, it's quiet
But my brain is still going.
I speak my mind, my feeling
It comes naturally ---
Everybody can have it,
Anybody can have it ---
You are a human person, that is all.

What is this work for?

These are just some of the complexities we encounter in weighing up the instrumental value of poetry produced in such projects. A further layer is supplied by an answer to the question, what is this work for? Few people need convincing that, of all mental and physical conditions, dementia is the one that carries the most stigma. Some of this comes from the persistent negativity of the media in presentation of the subject, which produces a debilitating effect on people with the condition and on their carers, and affects the reception of people with dementia in social settings. There is still talk of people having 'gone away' and having lost the very qualities that make them human. The findings of projects such as these and the dissemination of the work can serve to counteract this unthinking stance. On this basis, however, questions may need to be asked as to how far the Living Words approach may run the risk of reinforcing stereotypes, rather than dispelling them.

Who is the author?

Moving from consideration of the process and its efficacy, there are issues to be raised over the product – the poems themselves and their viability. One of these concerns ownership. Very few of the poems in the 10 or so books ostensibly by people with dementia published in the UK have been written down by the people with dementia themselves. Most are the work of poets, who are transcribing and editing the speech of those with whom they are working. There are people with the condition who can and do write for themselves, but most of the residencies that have resulted in publications have been based in care homes, day centres and hospital wards – places where such individuals are few and far between.

It is necessary to write down the words of those who can no longer do it for themselves, and this provides opportunities for mishearing and misinterpreting, which can only be corrected by the speaker him or herself, and when they are presented with the finished text, they may not even remember what words they have used. Also, the poets have the freedom to select from the samples of language offered them and arrange these extracts on the page. In poetry, as we all know, paring down and shaping are essential elements of the meaning, and these come from the facilitator and not from the progenitor. Whose poems are they, then? The best one can say is that they are the fruits of a collaboration.

An example of editing

The nature of this collaboration is an unusual one. An example from my own practice may serve to illustrate this. The following is the full text of a one-to-one collaboration I did at a time when I was not allowed to attach names to the poets, so he is anonymous. I did not suggest subjects to him; nor did I ask any questions; I just waited quietly, encouraging him and showing by my concentrated attention how much I valued his words.

> You're on 50 now, and in all the years I've only had one or two chats with you.

> Such unselfish lives, just putting themselves last in all walks. No bitterness or anguish, all loving kindness. Now the evening is coming to its close for me.

> Have you been up to the crematorium lately?

> You don't see your family much now. Like a carrier bag on your back, one way or another.

> Has Jock been to Liverpool?

But you can't barge it or dish it, all of it was everwell. You've always had a house to go back to.

The left eye was always a bit touchy. One day I woke up and said 'This eye isn't alright'. There's a small recess in the eye, and they took it out, and I've never seen the same again.

Have you any craving to stay in one of the Shropshire places? I am a Salopian. In the War I saw nothing that wasn't a waste of time and life. The door opened to dust, and I thought it might be me tomorrow.

I'm 86 I think, but I might be exaggerating --- it's only because I don't know.

I've had a drink, a little liverer. But I'm almost teetotal.

It's a good idea, this writing it down; it's got a bit of merit. It's tantamount to saying that you're speaking from your memory all the while.

Learning point 3

You might like to try answering the following:

- Take the first piece you dictated in Learning point 2 and ask the other person to edit it. Discuss with them the result.
- Take the second dictated piece and attempt to edit it yourself. Discuss the result.
- Who is the author of either dictated piece?

And this is the poem that I made from the above collaboration, which is published in the *You Are Words* collection (Killick, 1997):

Writing it down

It's a good idea,
this writing it down;
it's got a bit of merit.
It's tantamount to saying
you're speaking from your memory all the while.

In the War I went around
and I saw nothing that wasn't
a waste of time and life.

The door opened to dust
and I thought it might be me tomorrow.

Such unselfish lives,
just putting themselves last
in all walks. No bitterness
or anguish, all loving kindness.
Now the evening is coming to its close for me.

You don't see your family
much now: like a carrier bag
on your back, one way or another.
But you can't barge it or dish it ---
all of it was everwell.

Now it is obvious that I made some important decisions in the editing job I did, and that another writer might have put the emphases elsewhere. For example, I chose the comments on writing first; someone else might have put them last or missed them out altogether. For me, it was a significant statement, and I wanted it stressed. I never ask participants what they think of the process, so when a spontaneous evaluation is forthcoming, it is especially valuable. In the rest of the poem, I chose the passages that hung best together and seemed to me most universal and emotional.

Expecting the unexpected

Of course, those who approach individuals with stimulus materials, such as pictures, music or objects, may well get more thematically coherent responses, but they must realise that they are affecting the resultant poem in a more dominant manner. And, whether there is a planned or a spontaneous approach, there is always the possibility of a person completely confounding expectations by composing a poem aloud that needs no editing other than arrangement on the page. This happened to me once when a participant in a group that was responding to a picture suddenly uttered one of the most profound poems about dementia that has ever been vouchsafed to me, and I could see no obvious connection with the stimulus provided. These experiences may be rare, but they are memorable when they occur.

Here is the entire poem. It was composed by Joan Davies and has not been published before:

Deep currents

It's your feelings, isn't it?
It's not catching
it would be like a river
with its whirlpools
and you're pulled in

the thing pulls you down
down down down
so that you could drown
you can't save yourself
not unless you've something around you
something attached to something
we've got to keep going
or else.

This is a poem that is both thought provoking and metaphorical.

Acknowledging ownership

We are still faced with the question of who is the author of a work composed in this way. In the first years of my working in this area, I published all the poems under my own name, because the company I worked for would not allow their residents to be identified. I changed this practice as soon as I could, and for the last decade I have not permitted any poem to be afforded publicity without the person's name attached. I see that the US poet Karen Hayes has sometimes adopted the practice of acknowledging joint authorship of poems. These practices chime with the more enlightened times in which we live regarding combating stigma and the labelling of people with the condition as 'sufferers' or 'patients', rather than people. It is all the more surprising, then, to see one of the later books of poems, Susanna Howard's collection *The Things Between Us* (2014), which I have previously quoted from, reverting to anonymity. Maybe there were special problems surrounding the participants in the Living Words project; if so, these are not explained in the book.

Judging quality

Finally, there is the huge issue of how poems and projects are to be judged. Do they conform to the accepted standards by which poems from writers from outside the dementia world are appreciated? Or do we have to develop a special aesthetic based on a series of allowances for mental and emotional deficiencies? When I submitted the first manuscript of dementia poems to the then poetry editor at Faber, 17 years ago, he pronounced the poems 'not mad enough'. His criterion was certainly based on expectations that would not have come into play if the poems had emanated from a more orthodox source. The poems, of course, are the work of amateurs, filtered through the sensibilities and techniques of professionals. In the best of them, the poets have resisted tampering and achieved a clarity of exposition of the material presented to them. As such, the poems are a contribution to what Peter Elbow advocates as 'vernacular eloquence' in his book of that title (2012). They are restoring to writing qualities that have been overlooked in the rush to literacy: an authenticity of language and feeling that is to be treasured alongside the more formal achievements of literary tradition.

References

Elbow, P. (2012). *Vernacular eloquence.* Oxford University Press.

Howard, S. (Ed.). (2014). *The things between us.* Shoving Leopard.

Killick, J. (Ed.). (1997). *You are words.* Hawker Publications.

Killick, J. (Ed.). (2009). *The elephant in the room.* Cambridgeshire Libraries.

Killick, J. (Ed.). (2014). *Bee's knees and pickled onions.* The Courtyard Centre for the Arts.

35 The magic of paint

Susan Liggett and Megan Wyatt

The purpose of this chapter is to demonstrate how painting can enhance the wellbeing of people living with dementia. Arts in health is a developing area that is now recognised as a means to improve people's health and wellbeing while supporting current major health and social care demands. With dementia being the largest social and health care challenge in the United Kingdom, it is imperative to develop new, creative ways of improving the lives of those living with or affected by the condition.

Painting can provide new forms of purposeful experience and engagement for people living with dementia, which can improve their wellbeing. This is important and should be recognised as an alternative pathway in supporting people living with the condition to create meaningful experiences.

Learning point 1 – Expression of memories and feelings

We all have memories that are fuelled with emotions, and these can at times be hard to communicate verbally. Before you read the next section, you may want to consider the following points to help you to relate to the experiences that are described. Consider the following questions in relation to your own experiences, or those of other people you know who are living with dementia:

- When you think of a memory, does it make you feel a certain way?
- Do you have a favourite colour, and if so, can you say why this is?
- Do different colours remind you of different things?
- Do you ever look at a piece of art and find it reminds you of something?

As humans, we constantly reflect on our memories and feelings within our daily lives. However, for people living with dementia the ability to draw upon and verbally communicate these experiences can become restricted, and sometimes it is not possible to communicate with others (Alzheimer's Association, 2018). This can cause numerous difficulties for those living with or caring for someone living with the condition.

Painting can provide a new avenue of communication for people living with dementia, which can create feelings of reassurance and relief. Colour, form and gesture can all be used as a means of expression in painting and can be accessed even when verbal ability may be compromised.

This process of expression is unique to the creator and, regardless of whether the painted form appears representational or abstract, painting encourages emotive and spontaneous expression.

People living with dementia often maintain a rich inner life; their emotional capabilities may be preserved even when they are no longer able to communicate verbally. Painting allows an expression of these emotions without a reliance on words.

The role of colour in painting is important in expressing memories and feelings for people living with dementia. Colour is flexible in the painting process and can be used as a means of intuitive, emotional or representational expression. For example, a green may be used to depict the leaves on a visible tree, or the artist may have a particular preference for bright orange but cannot say why. People living with dementia often have the ability to relate colours to specific memories or feelings but may not be able to articulate the reasonings behind this. Painting provides an alternative means of expression and the choice and application of colour allows people living with dementia to make non-verbal decisions. This in turn can enhance their self-esteem (Killick & Craig, 2012).

The importance of colour can be seen in the following words, spoken by Mary, a lady living with dementia who attended an arts workshop that we ran:

> Because the thing is – as I'm doing the pink cloud, I find myself cheering up, it's not been a good day for me, I had a dreadful night, a lot of pain, up with pain, I don't think they are pink, but I'm not fed up anymore, I've cheered up as I went on.

The recall of memory can make people living with dementia feel a specific way (Alzheimer's Society, 2020). The emotive process of painting can therefore support people living with dementia to reconnect with memories and feelings, which in turn can provide immersive and meaningful experiences that do not rely on words.

James, who attended the same art workshop for people living with dementia, painted a small man-like figure in the corner of the piece of paper (Figure 35.1). Although James found it difficult to verbally communicate, his wife linked what he had painted with a poem that he had recited earlier that morning:

He recited a poem this morning that he remembered. He said a friend of his did this verse, blue legs with black teeth and blue legs. He's done his with blue legs now.

The use of motor skills in painting can encourage the recollection of memories in alternative ways. Therefore, painting should be thought of as a mechanism for people living with dementia to access and experience memories and feelings.

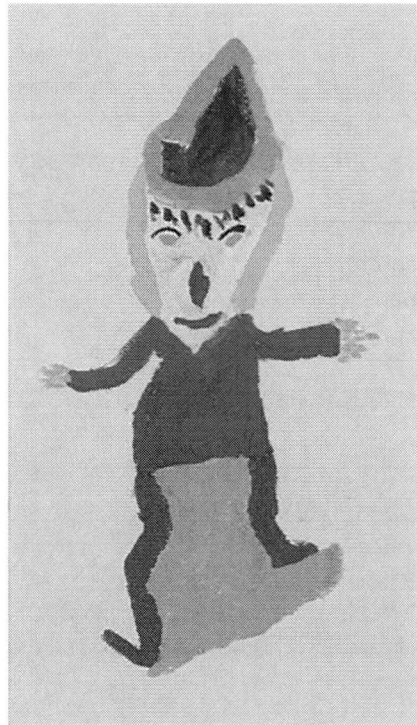

Figure 35.1: 'Blue Legs', by James

Learning point 2 – Reflection

Within the creative process (for example, while painting), naturally you will be constantly reflecting on the development of your work. This might be a conscious thought process, or it might be an experience that defies verbal articulation. Consider the following questions in relation to your own experiences, or those of other people whom you know who may live with dementia:

- How do you decide when you have finished a painting?
- Do you ever feel that your painting work feels 'just right'?
- Do you ever know what needs to be added to your painting but are unable to say why?

At times the process of reflection in painting can be easily verbally articulated. For example, the artist may be trying to paint something representational and will be able to say why a certain colour needs to be added. However, there is a second type of reflection in the painting process that provides a much more intuitive form of knowing. This involves feelings of correctness, even if the reasoning behind it cannot be communicated. Wilson (2010) suggests that, when painting, the artist engages in a constant feedback loop whereby every mark is both different to and influenced by the previous one. These reflections are based on an intrinsic relationship between the colour, marks and composition within the work, with each influencing the others.

Throughout the art workshop, Mary regularly stopped and looked at her painting and made comments such as 'that needs to be straighter' or 'I need to add another pink flower there' (Figure 35.2). She would then carry on painting, and this process would be repeated. It was evident that this reflective process was beneficial for Mary, and at the end of the art workshop, she looked at her painting and said, 'I think it's magic.'

Figure 35.2: 'Pink Clouds', by Mary

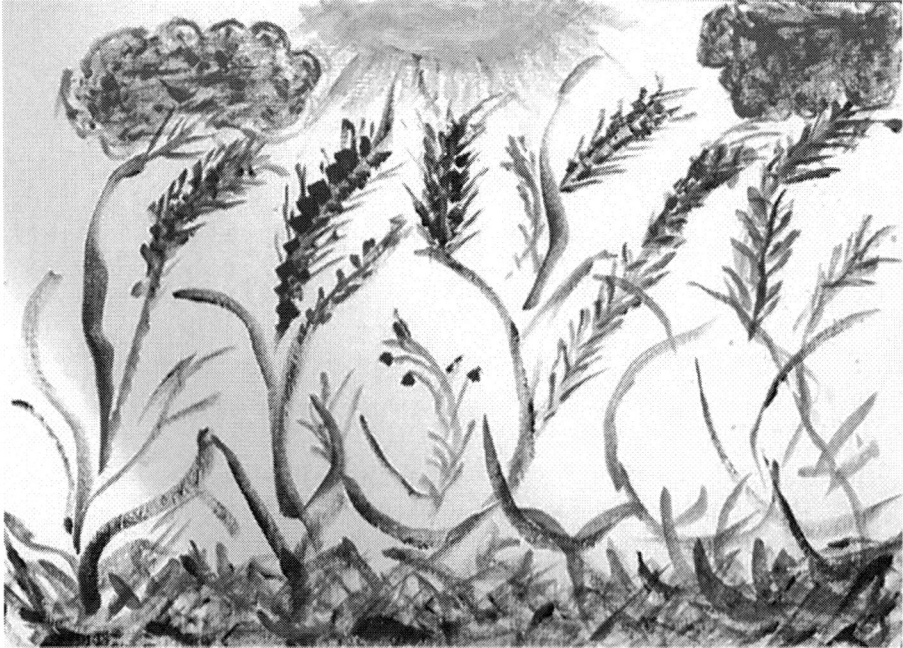

People living with dementia have the potential to access this mode of reflection within the painting process, even if they are unable to communicate this verbally. Furthermore, people living with dementia can have feelings of certainty about when their painting is finished. Elkins (1999, p.14) describes this moment for the creator as a 'magical point' where there is an intuitive understanding that the painting is complete. The importance of this experience of knowing and reflection for people living with dementia should not be underestimated. Reflection within the painting process can facilitate non-verbal modes of thought that support people living with dementia to make decisions and contemplate thoughts. This is something they may not always be able to do easily otherwise.

What's more, the constant cycles of reflection that occur within painting facilitate feelings of freedom and spontaneity. This promotes a developmental process where there are no rules or pressures to adhere to. Feelings of wrongness can be easily overcome through the ever-evolving activity of applying paint in different ways. This non-verbal mode of thought allows people living with dementia to make numerous decisions without the feeling of incorrectness. Painting should therefore be used to promote feelings of autonomy for people living with dementia and used as an alternative pathway to supporting them to maintain some levels of control even after their verbal abilities have declined.

Another participant in the art workshop was Daisy, who had advanced dementia. Although Daisy had limited verbal ability, it was clear that, while painting, she reflected on her artwork throughout. She would stop and look at her painting and then add tiny marks to specific areas. This provided Daisy with the opportunity to make decisions without the need to verbally articulate anything.

Learning point 3 – Immersion

It is likely that we have all had an immersive experience where there is a complete focus on the task at hand and a lack of awareness of external realities. Think about the following questions in relation to immersive experiences within the creative process and consider your own experiences, or those of other people you know who may live with dementia:

- When in the past have you experienced a feeling of immersion?
- How do you feel when you are engaged in an immersive experience?
- Do you find that these immersive experiences provide relief from any negative feelings?

Painting can facilitate immersive experiences for people living with dementia, which in turn can increase feelings of self-esteem and confidence.

The creator's own thoughts and feelings, in combination with the physical engagement of paint, can provide an experience whereby there is a full focus on the present moment.

Mary described how she was painting her old garden. Throughout the workshop, Mary's full focus was on the painting, and when asked if she found the process relaxing, she replied:

> I do, I not only find it relaxing, I find it, the picture that's in my head
> is cheering me up, I mean it's not exactly coming out because I'm not a
> talented painter you see, but I think that actual painting like this is relaxing,
> you see the very stroke gives it expression.

The nature of dementia can mean that it is often difficult to cognitively process the future or past, which can force people to live in the present moment. Immersive experiences within painting can embrace this focus for people living with dementia and subsequently embrace a person's abilities rather than focusing on their challenges and losses (Killick & Craig, 2012).

Painting can also be used as a mechanism to provide relief for negative emotions, such as anxiety and grief, for people living with dementia. Engaging in an immersive experience can provide a distraction from negative feelings and promote relaxation and calm. Painting can therefore be used as a tool to ease the frustrations or anxieties of a person living with the condition. Furthermore, the focus on a person's abilities will support the re-integration of those living with dementia within society through creating a sense of purpose.

For example, when James entered the room, he was visibly upset and began to cry. Although he could not communicate fully, it was clear that he felt frustrated about how he had become dependent on his wife and felt a loss of independence. However, when James was supported to paint, he became immersed in the process, and he stopped crying. The process of painting provided an immersive experience that helped ease the negative emotions that James was facing.

Conclusion

For people living with the condition, painting can provide a communication and stimulation of emotions and memories, an embracement of feelings of uncertainty, experiences of reflection and an immersive experience. This can provide new, individualised forms of engagement that access a fundamental part of the emotional being of a person living with dementia.

Painting should be acknowledged as a means to support people living with dementia to access new experiences and develop their knowledge and understandings. This focus on a person's abilities rather than their difficulties can support them to feel a sense of purpose and integration in society.

References

Alzheimer's Association. (2018). *Memory loss and confusion.* [Online]. Alzheimer's Association. www.alz.org/help-support/caregiving/stages-behaviors/memory-loss-confusion

Alzheimer's Society. (2020). *How do people experience memory loss?* [Online]. Alzheimer's Society. www.alzheimers.org.uk/about-dementia/symptoms-and-diagnosis/symptoms/memory-loss-in-dementia

Elkins, J. (1999). *What painting is.* Routledge.

Killick, J. & Craig, C. (2012). *Creativity and communication in persons with dementia: A practical guide.* Jessica Kingsley Publishers.

Wilson, A. (2010). *Practising uncertainty in search of something strangely attractive.* PhD thesis. Unitec New Zealand. https://www.researchbank.ac.nz/handle/10652/1441

36 Teleplay: Approaches to digital clowning for dementia care

Richard Talbot and Claire Dormann

In this chapter we offer some creative ideas for dementia care that draw on clowning practices designed to improve the wellbeing of people living with dementia. We introduce playful methods for interaction via online platforms. Widespread access to digital platforms is relatively new, but the number of older people who are able to use digital media, iPads and screens is increasing. Apps and digital games are being developed for people living with dementia (Dormann, 2016), and digital literacy is expanding in applied performing arts. Online interaction has become particularly important where older people are isolated due to cognitive decline, diminishing social networks, or under the constraints of healthcare 'shielding', such as during the coronavirus pandemic. The approaches presented here should benefit anyone interested in creating a space for playfulness and laughter in interactions with people living with dementia. The practices outlined here are suited to people living with dementia with a less advanced condition, usually those living at home or in private sheltered housing, but may also apply in residential care home settings.

The relevance of clowning to dementia

The benefits of laughter include strengthening the immune system, offering relief from pain, and improving mental health. People continue to use humour and laughter into older age. Humour can be used to lift moods and to facilitate interaction with peers, family and friends. In fact, humour and playfulness have many functions in social interactions.

Clowns make us laugh; they are playful and can bring joy to our lives. Studies have shown that exposure to stand-up comedy and clowning can increase positive attitudes and improve socialisation among people living with dementia, and can encourage an acceptance of ageing. An interest in absurd situations and satirical comedy may increase in response to the predicaments faced in ageing.

Clowns are known for their physical difference. They seem poorly adapted to their environment, frequently tripping, falling and bumping into things. A clown's use of language may also be scrambled. Peculiar phrasing, unusual words, rude words and gibberish are all comic 'material' to the clown.

This behaviour may reflect the experience of anyone whose perception of time and reality is becoming distorted through physiological difficulties, memory loss and speech control. So the clown can be understood as a stereotypical manifestation of declining faculties. In practice, by embodying difference, the clown actually creates a *distance* from behaviours associated with dementia. Through objective and innocent antics, the clown enacts behaviours that are difficult to accept in a more serious mode. The clown can create a zone for rethinking the experience of the illness, and this can provide a release.

Learning point 1

In contrast to a character comedian, the clown-performer can acknowledge their 'failures': they can 'flop' for comic effect. As we laugh at the clown's 'flops', the clown makes us laugh at ourselves, at our ideas and assumptions. And so we learn to laugh with, not at, strangers and strange behaviours:

- Clowns don't *tell* jokes; they *are* the joke. What is the crucial difference?
- The next time you 'get something wrong', try smiling – how does it make you feel?

Elder clowns and ageing

You may have reservations about the suitability of clowning for older people and for people who are struggling with cognitive decline. Clowns are generally assumed to be zany, noisy and contrary, and you may be concerned about an automatic negative reaction. You may associate clown doctoring with children, and there may be some resistance to introducing clowning into elder care, perhaps for fear of seeming to infantilise people living with dementia. These are understandable reasons, and they account for the emergence of 'elder clowning'. This is a form of clowning specifically designed for the needs of older people. Elder clowns generally work in pairs or small groups and visit residents in care homes and present gentler and quieter modes of play. They deploy a combination of rehearsed material and skills that can be drawn on spontaneously. They may bring a repertoire of gentle songs, simple games, non-verbal play and nostalgic dialogue. They explore universal themes such as personal grooming, everyday household chores, the workplace, pets, children and marriage (Balfour et al., 2017).

Just like 'clown doctors' in paediatric care, elder clowns have been found to have a positive impact on people living with dementia. Elder clowns can reduce levels of anxiety, and the experience of loneliness or institutionalisation (Killick, 2013). Interactions with elder clowns can reduce aggressive or mocking humour as well as low mood (Baumgartner & Renner, 2019).

Teleplay: Setting-up online comical interactions

Entering a private space, someone's home, or going online requires some ground rules and preparation.

Learning point 2

Think about visiting a person living with dementia:

- How many people are there with you?
- How do you prepare?
- How do you enter their personal space?
- Do you introduce yourself, even if you know the people living with dementia well?
- How do you encourage a response?

Now imagine that meeting online. How does this change these 'ground rules'?

Online interactions with people living with dementia are also more effective if they allow for direct engagement and clarity. We prefer to work with two participants – the caregiver and person living with dementia – and two clown performers. Before beginning an interaction, performers and participants can reduce the chance of noise distractions. Try to create a calm space. Switch off digital announcements on your computer, such as email sounds. If possible, use a room with carpet and curtains – something to soak up reverb and echo. This will make your voice softer. Test your microphone and video beforehand. Switch off any software programmes that you don't need as some of these update automatically and this can drain your bandwidth, reducing the quality of the video image and sound.

Try to avoid clutter in the image in the application window. Think about how your face is positioned on the screen in the window. You do not need to fill the frame, but your expressions need to be easily visible. A medium-to-close-up 'headshot', with one or two faces at most in each 'window' of the gallery view, helps create a clear image of each person involved in the interaction. Think how you are positioned in relation to the viewpoint of the webcam, rather than what you can see on your own screen.

Think about this encounter in terms of engaging with someone's personal space. When a clown looks directly into the webcam lens, it can seem more innocent or more 'stupid', and this is potentially funny. If they look right down the webcam lens, it helps the clown to appear to 'clock' the response of the viewer. It shows they are listening. It helps everyone to 'tune in' to each other's words and feelings. However, the closer to the screen that the clown appears to be, the bigger they look and therefore the more intimidating, so the clown needs to consider this too. When the clown steps back, it is experienced as an invitation for the participant to engage and participate.

Then think about how the clown introduces themselves. The performers should use short, familiar phrases and should wait for responses, taking account of the digital delay and any echoes. A discussion about what you are wearing is a good starting point for conversation. Clowns may be strangely dressed, but they take care with their appearance, and elder clowns especially tend to be more formal. Check whether participants are comfortable with the use of a red nose. A red nose especially can seem 'unreal', and this can be disturbing for people who are uncertain about what is real and what is not.

You can use a mediator to control how long the clowns engage with the participant. A mediator can translate the wishes of the person living with dementia. They can be a social care representative or any caregiver, such as a partner or grandchild. A mediator can encourage the person living with dementia to participate, based on how well they know them. The clown can have a strong presence and energy and sometimes they need to be 'managed', but this can be part of the fun. The mediator can intervene gently to deflate overexcitement or unhelpful triggers from either side. An experienced clown performer should be able to 'play with' these constraints and should have new material ready to deploy – a new topic, a new object. The clowns can contradict and banter with the mediator. This will create a hierarchy between the people living with dementia, the mediator and the clown.

When there are two clowns working together, they should take it in turns to be the one to approach the webcam. This helps to shift the focus between each of them and affects the perception of their status as a duo. The one who tends to lead the interaction with the viewer will appear to be the boss, and the one who follows will have low status. The boss can be closer to the camera. Their assistant can stand or sit further away. But this status can be played with. The assistant can come close to the camera to confide with the viewers, perhaps whispering to the people living with dementia. Negotiating the screens and playing within this hierarchy generates some of the fun with technology that we will discuss later.

Giving and getting permission – laughter

In a dementia café setting where the clown is interacting with a group, the sense of the performance and its purpose can easily be lost. Distractions and sudden noises can lower individual engagement with the performer. By contrast, in an interaction online with participants in their own home, it may be easier to create *complicity*. Complicity is a feeling of trust and mutual understanding that allows people to play together. In focused interactions, the clown can elicit permission to play and keep the trust going by listening very closely. Focused activities in pairs

– that is, two clowns on one side of a digital screen and two participants on the other – can be more effective than large group settings in creating a zone for play. This is precisely because the clown uses *individual* responses to gain permission to carry on playing.

A clown can bring a positive mood into a room and, like anyone else, people living with dementia respond well to a positive affective environment (Kontos et al., 2017). In standard clown performance, the clown uses laughter as a 'barometer' that indicates permission to stay with their audience (Gaulier, 2006). But laughter can be an unreliable signal; it can indicate bafflement, nervousness or conformity. A clown's 'stupidity' may be frustrating, or they may only make us laugh 'inside'. With people living with dementia, the laughter response may be very quiet, delayed or absent. So the clown must be especially sensitive and allow for all kinds of response. During a standard clown performance, you will see people looking around to check whether others are laughing too. Clowns work with this need for reassurance; they try to get people to laugh at each other in order to build up communal hilarity, because laughter can be contagious. In online elder clown performance, the mediator/carer can help create a positive mood too. They can laugh at the clown, encouraging the participant to laugh too, and creating contagious laughter.

Learning point 3

So elder clowns don't need to act funny. They don't need to force hilarity:

- Like good actors, clowns *re-act*.
- Trust is earned by paying attention to the reciprocal exchange at the individual level.

Try this practical exercise:

- Begin a simple action. Listen carefully for a response. Be patient.
- When you notice any signal, 'look' directly down the lens, moving slightly closer to the webcam. Have the feeling of seeking *permission*, with a smile.
- After a short pause – no more than a beat – repeat the same action precisely. Stay positive even if you don't hear a response. Repeat and build.

Creating content for your online interactions

We have seen that elder clowns adapt clown material to the specific circumstances of their audience. People living with dementia have a wealth of knowledge and experience and can offer ideas, observations and suggestions for the clown. Carers can help too: knowing facts about the life story of participants means that they can offer ideas, stories and songs for the clown to pick up.

Many performers, professional or not, worry about improvising because they want to 'get it right'. But when the *clown* gets it 'wrong', they can acknowledge their failure. Having a practical 'problem' encourages people to join in. Rather than over-planning material, the clown can work with *spontaneous* comedy from unexpected or *accidental* comedy (Baumgartner & Renner, 2019) Think of an everyday 'problem', such as putting on a big, heavy coat, or folding a large bed sheet, or drinking tea without slurping. Try an abstract 'problem' like a body that moves to musical prompts. The people living with dementia can make suggestions to help with the coat and bed sheet. They can clap or play music to get the clown's body moving.

It can be useful to set a time limit for the interactions, especially where people living with dementia have a limited ability to sustain focus. Where attention may drift, there is little time to develop complex characters or storylines. Short skits generate simple actions and easy-to-understand gestures. These 'jokes' can be used as a simple repertoire that the clown can repeat to reinforce a playful habit.

Learning point 4

If you do not feel confident with making up material on the spot, a game structure can help:

- Games with limited or flexible rules are perfect for players who can't remember the rules very well.

Try this practical exercise:

- Hat Snap is a game of Snap for two people, who take it in turns to pick a hat out of a suitcase without looking. This game can be played by people in the same room (sharing a screen), or between rooms. The objective of Hat Snap is to call out a coincidence simply by looking at the hat on your partner's head.
- Shout 'Snap!' for *every* hat.
- Savour the names of hat styles, colours and textures. Play with vocalisation by repeating words, copying each other's tone and rhythm and finding unexpected associations.

You can find a video recording of the Hat Snap game at https://youtu.be/xjesegCm588

Playing with the limitations of technology using make-believe

Online calls can be frustrating and there might be problems with bandwidth. How do we deal with digital glitches and interruptions that occur during a call?

The objective of the next scenario, 'The Driving Lesson', is not to present a realistic illusion of driving together, but to conjure up the world of driving using rudimentary resources. This is the essence of play. If the connection is broken, this too can be understood as a 'make-believe' accident connected to the situation: a crash, a broken-down vehicle. Play will then help create a transition; while the connection is being re-established, the mediator/caregiver and people living with dementia can talk about a real experience of driving, until the clowns return. Finally, online displays typically locate participants in a 'window', and these can be played with too: arrange them side by side to create a single 'windscreen'.

Learning point 5

Clowns can work with unpredictability as content:

- Unexpected audio interruptions, or visual distortions can be incorporated into play.
- This requires a serious investment in 'make-believe' by everyone playing.

Try this practical exercise:

- Set-up: The carer and people living with dementia sit in front of the computer, having 'dialled up' the clowns online.
- Make-believe: They are looking at one clown in one window playing the role of a 'chauffeur' miming a steering wheel. In the other window is a passenger.
- Improvise: the chauffeur and passenger bounce up and down, check the 'mirror', look left and right, make the sound of a horn, an exhaust or brakes.
- The people living with dementia can call out 'turn right', 'slow down' or 'look out!'

You can find a video recording of 'The Driving Lesson' at https://vimeo.com/285901856

Enhancing with additional recorded elements

Live online interaction with clowns creates an experience of a 'clown world'. Recorded media can be used to enhance this world. Your online improvisation can be recorded. You can create a further personalised element by curating external music and video playlists in an online 'cloud'.

This supplementary material can be incorporated in your interactions or played *asynchronously* to revisit clowning and the topics that came up.

Learning point 6

Be playful with supplementary media:

- Recordings can help the people living with dementia gain confidence with online play.

Try this practical exercise:

- Record your online interactions and allow participants to 'encounter' clowns in their own time. Make a recording and upload it to YouTube, Vimeo or similar (use the privacy tools, of course).
- Record yourself improvising: with Hat Snap, try wearing a pile of hats, moving with a funny hat on, using a bell instead of shouting 'Snap!' Get one clown to cross from one 'window' into the other and back again, stealing their opponent's hats on the way.
- Keep a handy playlist of external video clips or the music used by the clowns.

Conclusion

We have introduced teleplay with elder clowns and proposed some learning points with practical ideas for interactive clowning performance. This approach to playful interaction online can be directed by caregivers and family members as both mediators and participants, alongside people living with dementia. These clowning principles can be applied by anybody and promote the advantages of co-creativity, reciprocity and spontaneity in playful online interactions to support the wellbeing of people living with dementia and their caregivers.

References

Balfour, M.,Dunn, J. & Cooke, M. (2017). Complicité, le jeu and the clown: Playful engagement and dementia. In S. McCormick (Ed.), *Applied theatre: Creative ageing* (pp.105–125). Methuen Drama.

Baumgartner, G. & Renner, K. (2019). Humor in the elderly with dementia: Development and initial validation of a behavioural observation system. *Current Psychology.* https://doi.org/10.1007/s12144-019-00455-y

Dormann, C. (2016). Toward ludic gerontechnology: A review of games for dementia care. In *DiGRA/FDG '16 – Proceedings of the First International Joint Conference of DiGRA and FDG,* 13(1). Digital Games Research Association/ Society for the Advancement of the Science of Digital Games. www.digra.org/digital-library/publications/toward-ludic-gerontechnology-a-review-of-games-for-dementia-care/

Gaulier, P. (2006). *Le gégeneur (The tormentor).* Editions Filmiko.

Killick, J. (2013). *Dementia positive.* Luath Press.

Kontos, P., Miller, K.L., Mitchell, G.J. & Stirling-Twist, J. (2017). Presence redefined: The reciprocal nature of engagement between elder-clowns and persons with dementia. *Dementia, 16*(1), 46–66.

37 Dementia-friendly museums: How cultural activity benefits people with dementia, carers and communities

Rosie Barker and Louise Deakin

From fossils to contemporary art and Egyptian mummies to 1960s dresses, museums and the millions of objects they hold tell stories about the people who made, bought, used, wore and worked with them. At Birmingham Museums Trust (BMT), we care for more than 800,000 objects and use the richness of these stories to help entertain and educate people of all ages.

More and more museums worldwide are running activities to support wellbeing. Within the museum sector (which here also refers to art galleries, historic houses and heritage sites), there has long been an understanding that being able to touch objects, get up close with paintings or step inside historic buildings can leave people feeling happier and more connected, and that taking part in creative activities can increase wellbeing. In 2019, the World Health Organization (WHO) published a review of more than 3,000 studies looking at the impact of arts (including performing and visual arts, culture, literature and digital arts) on wellbeing, and concluded that there is 'a major role for the arts in the prevention of ill health, promotion of health, and management and treatment of illness across the lifespan' (Fancourt & Finn, 2019, p.ii).

With funding for the arts decreasing, there is increased pressure on museums to demonstrate their value and social worth. Supporting the health and social care sectors and individuals with wellbeing needs is one way museums have raised the profile of their relevance and use. This growing challenge to museums to contribute to wellbeing has been supported by *Creative Health*, the report of a UK All-Party Parliamentary Group (APPG) (2017), which emphasises the need for the arts and health sectors to work together and sets the idea into public policy. With social prescribing on the rise, the arts and heritage are now being taken seriously as places that can provide cultural prescriptions for health.

What is a museum dementia programme?

For many people, the idea of visiting a museum with people with dementia might seem unhelpful or pointless, and there is often little awareness of what exactly museums can and do offer for these groups.

Learning point 1

Before you continue reading, think about your own experiences of museums:

- Do you have positive or negative memories and associations of museums?

- What are your assumptions about the kinds of activities that take place in museums?

Museums today go far beyond static displays of art and objects and visits by quiet school children. In recent years at BMT, we have held drag storytelling for children, Fright Nights, Christmas carolling, silent discos and a contemporary art exhibition about the decriminalisation of homosexuality, and we've exhibited a giant dinosaur – often at the same time. As part of this broad offer, programming for people with dementia is part of the everyday for many museums.

In museums, 'dementia programming' refers to any activity targeted at those with dementia, whether alone or with those who care for them (friends, family or care workers). The programmes use artefacts, artworks and exhibitions as a stimulus for conversation and creativity, and may include objects that can be handled, music, movement, taste, smell and more. The programming provides an informal, social learning activity in unusual but welcoming surroundings, led by museum staff experienced in using objects to engage.

Programmes can take place on site (in-reach), with people with dementia coming to the museum, often with carers or support staff. This has the benefit of maintaining the feeling of being part of a community, but is labour intensive for care staff, and new settings can be challenging for people with dementia. Outreach, where the museum takes its objects and activities to clinical settings, such as hospital wards or care homes, requires more capacity from museums. Outreach can be easier for the person with dementia, as they are in a familiar setting, but restricts their engagement opportunities with the wider world.

Wherever it is carried out, there are two main strands to museum dementia work: reminiscence programmes and 'in-the-moment' activities. Reminiscence programmes are designed to help people recall past memories. For most people with dementia, memories from long ago last longer than more recent memories, so activities can reinforce and value past life experiences by using objects as memory triggers. Often a set of themed objects will be used (for example, objects based on work, leisure or domestic life in the past), to remind participants of their lived experiences.

'In-the-moment' programmes offer new, unfamiliar activities and objects to people with dementia and their carers. This helps reduce any potential negative emotions around difficulties in recall. Camic and colleagues (2019) highlight how reminiscence can also be difficult for those with painful memories of the past, or people from different cultural or ethnic backgrounds who do not have the same experiences. These 'in-the-moment' programmes allow for equality between the person with dementia and their carers, as the experience is new to both.

The Museum of Modern Art in New York (MoMA) was one of the first cultural institutions to run dementia programmes with 'Meet Me at MoMA', which launched in 2006. MoMA takes an 'in-the-moment' approach, offering new experiences, although the phrase actually originated three years after their programme began, coming from a carer's comment that, although there may be no lasting change from a museum dementia programme, 'you do it for the moment' (MacPherson et al., 2009, p.748). Kinsey and colleagues expanded on this:

> the focus is not on 'remembering' but on the person's views and feelings
> in that moment, with the aim that this way of questioning and discussing
> allows people with and without dementia to participate on an equal basis.
> (Kinsey et al., 2019, p.2)

Poignantly, Camic quotes a participant with dementia who responded to this approach, saying: 'Thank you for not thinking us old people are only interested in remembering our pasts' (Camic et al., 2019).

Another approach offered by a select few museums is dementia awareness training, such as the award-winning House of Memories (HoM) programme at Liverpool Museums. HoM offers training to carers and health/social care staff in using objects with people with dementia, with the aim to upskill health and care staff to develop their own object-based programmes.

Programming at Birmingham Museums

BMT manages nine historic venues in Birmingham, and has initiated dementia programming in two venues to date. The first dementia programme took place at Soho House Museum, a Georgian house. The programme's content was based on the museum's collection, with themes for each session chosen to represent rooms that were part of a typical tour – food, entertainment, decoration, gardening, fashion, education and the story of Birmingham's growth. Monthly sessions included a tour and creative activity and were based not around reminiscence but on the idea that finding out about new areas of history would be of interest to those with dementia and carers equally – an 'in-the-moment' approach.

Participants at the very first session confirmed our non-reminiscence approach was right. They included three people of African Caribbean heritage with dementia – the white British facilitator would not have been able to relate culturally to their histories. As the group grew in numbers, it became increasingly obvious that the non-reminiscence approach was more inclusive and what participants had in common was their enjoyment in learning about the historic house and taking part in activities relating to it.

The second wave of dementia programming took place at Birmingham Museum and Art Gallery, a large, purpose-built museum with a varied collection. This completely different setting provided a new opportunity: to invite staff and volunteers, who already possessed high levels of engagement skills, to be involved and educate them about dementia. The emphasis again was on new experiences, and responses demonstrated how much participants valued learning something new.

Learning point 2

Thinking about the care settings you may work in:

- How could you use objects, touch, sound and imagination to create new 'in-the-moment' experiences for people with dementia?

- What local cultural resources are near to you? New surroundings can offer both people with dementia and carers fresh perspectives. By forming relationships with cultural organisations, you are opening up to new possibilities.

Practicalities – what makes a good session

Much of the research on dementia programming has captured what makes a session work well. Key factors to consider include group size, length of session and number and type of objects (for guidance, see Age & Opportunity's publication on exploring greater inclusion of people with dementia in museums and galleries (2012)).

One aspect highlighted in all research is the need for skilled facilitation. Facilitators must not only know about the objects and the impacts dementia can have on cognition, communication and behaviour, but also understand how to bring out the best in people with dementia through open-ended questions and be able to support each individual's learning approach and needs (e.g. Camic et al., 2019; Ander et al., 2013; MacPherson et al., 2009).

Allowing participants to engage all of their senses is also important (e.g. Sharma & Lee, 2020). For our programmes at BMT, we used a mix of resources: pictures, replica food, musical instruments, examples of Georgian fabrics and furniture, audio tracks, costume, a mouse trap – all enhanced the experience. Scents and tastes were also incorporated, to engage all the senses.

Being actively engaged is important, so we included creative activities suitable for all abilities. We created spice pouches, practised calligraphy, played with wooden toys, printed wallpaper and arranged flowers. The facilitator did not act as an expert in the activity, but encouraged participants to share their own knowledge, skills and experience with one another. As one participant said: 'We learn together, no pressure to be right.' Carers commented on the positive and lasting impact of the activities: 'The ladies talk about it when they get back and show their work to other people in the care home.'

The social aspect of a programme is vital to its success (e.g. Camic et al., 2016; Windle et al., 2018). During our sessions, barriers were broken down and bonds were created between participants. It was notable during object handling and activities that participants with dementia would have long conversations, enjoying one another's company, not realising they'd spoken at previous sessions.

Having an accessible space (and refreshments!) added to the relaxed atmosphere, and the word 'dementia' was rarely used – something recommended in the MoMA guidelines (Age & Opportunity, 2012, p.13). We had not come together to talk about dementia; this was about people engaging with the museum collection and learning in a nurturing space that had been designed specifically to meet their needs. One carer commented: 'These creative sessions are good – we can do them together and take time to just be.'

Learning point 3

If you were planning to take an individual or a group with dementia to a museum:

- What practical challenges do you think you would encounter? Think about group needs in terms of seating, toilets, signage, refreshments, transport and more.
- How could you work with the museum to communicate and resolve these access needs? What benefits are there to the museum from your support?

The impact of dementia programming in museums

There are several reasons behind the positive impact of dementia programmes. These programmes involve touching objects, which supports those who have impaired hearing or vision to engage with the world. Sessions can prompt memories, with objects, experiences or conversations acting as triggers to recall. A multi-sensory approach leads to deeper processing and increased learning, and touch is linked to emotional systems in the brain (Camic et al., 2019). There is also evidence that being trusted to touch precious objects from the past gives people a sense of being valued and special (Ander et al., 2013).

Well-executed museum programming for people with dementia can:

support communication, encourage creative capabilities, stimulate new learning particularly 'in the moment', improve cognitive function, increase confidence and self-esteem, social participation… and generate a sense of autonomy. (Sharma & Lee, 2020)

Interestingly, Johnson and colleagues found that object handling and art viewing had a greater impact on wellbeing than the social aspect of a programme alone: providing opportunities to connect over objects appears to be more effective than simply providing opportunities to connect (Johnson et al., 2017).

A final benefit moves beyond the individual participant: research shows that museum programmes also affect public perceptions of dementia. Windle and colleagues (2018) report four studies that showed an impact on those facilitating a museum programme, from artists to school children taking part, while Camic and colleagues (2016, p.1038) also found that a programme 'dispelled some commonly held beliefs about dementia' in facilitators. We saw this ourselves, in comments from volunteers, such as: 'I discovered how easy it can be to interact with other people who are "different".'

Evaluation

Most museums will regularly evaluate their programmes to ensure they are meeting their own aims and the needs of their audiences. Current research points to the validity and usefulness of Visual Analogue Scales for people with dementia (e.g. Johnson et al., 2017; Camic et al., 2019), and they are quick and simple to administer so they can be used at several points during a session if required (Johnson et al., 2017). Many museums may use University College London's purpose-designed wellbeing measures toolkit for museums (Thompson & Chatterjee, 2013), which was trialled in part with people with dementia.[1]

Carers are also an important judge of the impact of museum sessions on people with dementia. Museum staff may only meet participants for an hour or so and won't recognise changes in engagement and behaviour. Carers, with their greater knowledge of participants, are best placed to help museums understand their impact. Carer feedback regarding increased interest and positive changes in mood after the session supports museums to develop programme content further.

Conclusion

In 2018, Age UK's report, *Creative and Cultural Activities and Wellbeing in Later Life*, found that creative and cultural participation was the greatest contributor to wellbeing in older age (Age UK, 2018). While not every older person will develop dementia, the idea that creative and cultural activities have a greater impact on wellbeing than marriage, material resources or friends, is a testament to the power of these activities. The WHO report (Fancourt & Finn, 2019), based on a review of

---

1. www.ucl.ac.uk/culture/projects/ucl-museum-wellbeing-measures

thousands of pieces of research, adds further weight to this. For anyone planning to work with people with dementia, we hope this chapter highlights the real benefits of using culture and creativity, and that the considerable evidence of museum dementia programmes' positive impact on participants' wellbeing can and should be used to make the case for the health and social care sector to work more closely with the cultural sector.

Through high quality programming, everyone can benefit: the person with dementia, through improved confidence, greater social connection and improved communication; the carer, by seeing the person with dementia in a new light and understanding their experiences, and wider society, through normalising the participation of people with dementia in daily life and challenging perceptions of the disease.

Our first dementia-friendly programming, the Dementia Café at Soho House, prompted this response from one family carer: 'When you get a dementia diagnosis, the health service would do well to direct families to the Dementia Café experience.'

References

Age & Opportunity. (2012). *Exploring greater inclusion of people with dementia in museums and galleries in Ireland.* Dublin: Age & Opportunity.

Age UK. (2018). *Creative and cultural activities and wellbeing in later life.* Age UK. www.ageuk.org.uk/bp-assets/globalassets/oxfordshire/original-blocks/about-us/age-uk-report--creative-and-cultural-activities-and-wellbeing-in-later-life-april-2018.pdf

All-Party Parliamentary Group on Arts, Health and Wellbeing. (2017). *Creative health: The arts for health and wellbeing* (2nd ed.). Inquiry report. www.culturehealthandwellbeing.org.uk/appg-inquiry/

Ander, E., Thomson, L., Noble, G., Lanceley, A., Menon, U. & Chatterjee, H. (2013). Heritage, health and wellbeing: Assessing the impact of a heritage focused intervention on health and wellbeing. *International Journal of Heritage Studies, 19*(3), 229–242.

Camic, P.M., Baker, E.L. & Tischler, V. (2016). Theorizing how art gallery interventions impact people with dementia and their caregivers. *Gerontologist, 56*(6), 1033–1041.

Camic, P.M, Hulbert, S. & Kimmel, J. (2019). Museum object handling: A heath promoting community-based activity for dementia care. *Journal of Health Psychology, 24*(6), 787–798.

Fancourt, D. & Finn, S. (2019). *What is the evidence on the role of the arts in improving health and well-being? A scoping review.* WHO Regional Office for Europe.

Johnson, J., Culverwell, A., Hulbert, S., Robertson, M. & Camic, P.M. (2017). Museum activities in dementia care: Using visual analog scales to measure subjective wellbeing. *Dementia: The International Journal for Social Research and Practice, 6*(5), 591–610. doi: 10.1177/1471301215611763

Kinsey, D., Lang, I., Orr, N., Anderson, R. & Parker, D. (2019). The impact of including carers in museum programmes for people with dementia: A realist review. *Arts & Health, 13*(2), 1–19.

MacPherson, S., Bird, M., Anderson, K., Davis, T. & Blair, A. (2009). An art gallery access programme for people with dementia: 'You do it for the moment'. *Ageing and Mental Health, 13*(5), 744–752.

Sharma, M. & Lee, A. (2020). Dementia-friendly heritage settings: A research review. *International Journal of Building Pathology and Adaptation, 38*(2), 279–310.

Thomson, L.J. & Chatterjee, H.J. (2013). *UCL museum wellbeing measures toolkit.* University College London.

Windle, G., Gregory, S., Howson-Griffiths, T., Newman, A., O'Brien, D. & Goulding, A. (2018). Exploring the theoretical foundations of visual art programmes for people living with dementia. *Dementia, 17*(6), 702–727.

38 'Our friends can't believe all the things we're doing': The role of culture in supporting people to live well with dementia

Nicky Taylor and Gabrielle Hamilton

Leeds Museums and Galleries, Leeds Playhouse and Leeds Libraries established the Peer Support Cultural Partnership with Leeds City Council's Peer Support Service in 2010 to offer regular, bespoke cultural experiences to people living with dementia and their partners. Drawing on 10 years' learning and reflection, here we outline the challenges and successes encountered in this unique partnership, through three key elements: museum, theatre and library resources and expertise of *partners*; contributions by and impact on *participants*; and *processes* of refining practical models of delivery, including creating safe spaces, evaluation, funding and organisational transformation.

Partners

Our story starts modestly in 2010 – five men, each recently diagnosed with a form of dementia, gather in a meeting room in Leeds Art Gallery. They are drawn together by referrals from the Leeds Peer Support Service for people living with dementia – a new adult social care service in Leeds, one of 40 Department of Health pilot projects exploring the potential of peer support among people with dementia, established as part of the National Dementia Strategy for England (Department of Health, 2009). Over the following six weeks, guided by artists and creative facilitators, they will talk, laugh and reflect on their lives and the events and people who are important to them, and each will create art in the form of a suitcase full of visual and tactile memories and stories.

The idea of dementia-related peer support is still an emerging one at this time, as interventions for people with dementia have traditionally been offered by medical professionals. Peer support presents a different model, in which acknowledgment and openness around lived experience of a health condition is valued, and the sharing of experiences, challenges and coping strategies is encouraged. Crucially, the Leeds Peer Support Service focuses on maintaining and developing connections among participants, building a supportive network that operates in stimulating, social environments. An evaluation of the national peer support pilot networks established through the dementia strategy showed that involvement in peer support enabled people with dementia and their supporters to gain confidence, maintain independence, find meaning and purpose in life with dementia and feel more socially connected and included, and also raised awareness and uptake of other services (Clarke et al., 2013).

With an established tradition of partnership working, colleagues from Leeds Museums and Galleries, Leeds Playhouse and Leeds Libraries were swift to research and learn more about the potential of using existing resources to engage people with dementia. There is demonstrable evidence of the effectiveness of using arts and culture to engage people with dementia in community-based, failure-free activities (Fritsch et al., 2009; Young et al., 2016). Our initial gallery programme was influenced by an internationally renowned model of museum engagement at the Museum of Modern Art (MoMA) in New York. Within such programmes, activities such as object handling, art viewing and art making can offer opportunities for creative expression (Rosenberg, 2009) and improved social experiences between group members and care partners (Camic et al., 2014).

In Leeds, the Cultural Partnership extends beyond museum and gallery settings to use the resources of libraries and theatres. While object handling and viewing of collections plays a key role in the offer, the approach is broadened by the expertise of library and theatre staff and enhanced by a range of programmes not usually found in museums. Participants can experience researching hyperlocal library records and historic archives, as well as live performance and performing arts mechanisms, such as costume, props, song and improvisation. Projects have included time spent in Leeds' ornate Central Library exploring rare book collections in research rooms that are usually off limits to the public. Participants have also followed the production of numerous theatre shows at Leeds Playhouse, influencing the development of dementia-friendly performances. As a producing theatre, the Playhouse is able to welcome people with dementia into rehearsal rooms as a show is created and share with them the process of play-making, from initial ideas and designs through to set-building and costume-making processes. In Cultural Partnership programmes, attendees are just as likely to be participating alongside an actor, librarian or curator. Each partner organisation brings specific expertise and possibilities, making the project as a whole greater than the sum of its parts.

Partnering with the Peer Support Service means that many of the usual barriers to participation in the arts are removed or lessened. Attendance and participation at arts institutions are traditionally highest among middle-class communities (Jancovich, 2011), yet this programme attracts a more diverse socio-economic demographic. People are brought together by the common experience of dementia and through engaging with a social care service. Participation in the programme is not means-tested and is free – all partner organisations offer the sessions without charge as part of their strong commitment to community outreach and engagement. Small donations towards tea, coffee and biscuits are accepted from participants. It is notable in sessions that participants have a broad range of life experience and that the programme brings people into contact with others outside their usual demographic. This too is part of the strength of the programme as people learn to understand and get along with others while acknowledging different backgrounds and experiences.

Learning point 1

- What are the resources and skills within your organisation? Who might you partner with to fill any gaps in knowledge?

- Could you invite people with dementia and their supporters to help you plan or assess your offer?

- What can you do to ensure that your information is accessible? Will it reach trusted people who can guide people with dementia to your activity?

- How can you ensure you are welcoming to people of different backgrounds and communities who may experience additional barriers in opting in to your activity?

Participants

Our first five intrepid explorers paved the way for many more over the following 10 years. Originally a service that was established for people in the early stages of dementia, the consistent support offered to participants by the two full-time members of the Peer Support team – Debbie Marshall and Debbie Catley – meant that some participants were able to maintain attendance at activities for up to eight years as their dementia progressed. Others experienced a more rapid progression of symptoms and so entered different support systems, and ultimately residential care settings or hospital.

Our initial programme was specifically for people with a diagnosis of dementia, although we soon recognised that the format had much to offer people in care partnerships, and we now welcome people either alone or with a partner, depending on their preference and support needs. People participating in cultural programmes as couples or care partners can feel released from the dynamic of carer and cared for; they are offered the equal status of artists, within which their roles are less rigid. It is not uncommon for a person with dementia to take the lead in a creative activity while their partner without dementia might sit back. In these activities people with dementia are freed up to offer a different version of themselves, rewriting the story that their diagnosis has inscribed on them.

While it is difficult to quantitatively measure the sense of joy, pleasure and fun that the sessions bring, it is a palpable element of the experience, felt by participants and staff alike. Laughter and wonder are plentiful, as we explore bizarre museum collections or marvel at gloriously elaborate costumes. June and Len tell us: 'Our friends can't believe all the things we're doing!' As they recount their experience at the theatre, museum or library to friends, they recognise that a new world has opened up. They identify that they are doing things they never would have done before. They have a connection to the major cultural institutions in their city, are on first-name terms with the people who work there and gain an insight into behind-the-scenes processes, which they feel is a privilege. In embracing these opportunities, participants demonstrate that life with dementia can be fulfilling and enjoyable and challenge the prevailing narratives of dementia as solely devastating and tragic.

For people who have not previously come into contact with arts and cultural institutions, the programme can open up a new world of cultural possibilities at a point when investment in personal wellbeing is crucial. During a period of adjustment to a life-changing diagnosis, a sense of something new beginning can energise people with dementia and their supporters, offering relief and distraction from the worry of their changing world.

Learning point 2

- How will you manage the different needs and expectations of people with dementia and their partners?

- How can you help participants feel welcome, safe and comfortable? Could you invite people with dementia to help carry out an access audit?

- Can you identify the different skills and talents that participants bring? How will you draw on these to enhance experiences within your sessions?

Processes

Our aim is to connect people with dementia with the rich cultural offer of their city's museums, theatres and libraries. These collections and programmes belong to everyone, and it is our responsibility to adapt if some people need to access them in different ways, so they don't miss out. We focus on themed projects in order to have a thread running through sessions, and aim to engage people in the long-term, rather than in a one-off activity. This affords participants the time to find and meaningfully explore their personal spark of interest.

Staff feel privileged to be involved in a project that brings enormous fun and joy, yet there is significant emotional investment in designing, facilitating and holding each session. Designing themed activities across multiple sites and disciplines takes dedicated time and can be a challenge. Detailed planning is needed, and care is taken to provide varied experiences without inadvertently causing participants stress or pressure. Inevitably, attendance figures vary due to health issues, although staff-to-participant ratio is always high. We accommodate between 15 to 25 people, supported by five members of staff, balancing demand for places with ensuring participants have a meaningful experience.

Projects are carefully curated to allow for a mixture of new learning, reminiscence and connection to current cultural events, and are focused on local stories, while embracing broader national and international angles. Each session runs for two hours, allowing time for arrivals and greetings. There is a main focused activity linked to the overarching theme, and a crucial half hour of social time with refreshments before the session closes. During this time, peer support is abundant as participants share their challenges and successes and friendships are solidified. Sessions take place at different cultural venues, creating an exploration of the city, sometimes with transport assistance or agreed meeting points at less familiar venues. This means that people gain confidence in using public transport or entering new spaces, and this also ensures that access for people with dementia is not restricted to one familiar venue; rather, its importance is recognised and acted on across a number of sites.

We constantly consider the ethics of our approach. There are few truly safe spaces for people with dementia and we have worked determinedly to create more. As leaders of this programme, we take our responsibility as gatekeepers seriously in deciding when it is appropriate to open the gates. We receive many requests to observe our sessions, but the presence of a newcomer – especially an observer who arrives with a specific agenda – can disrupt the precious dynamic of the group. For some participants, our weekly sessions provide their only opportunity to think differently about themselves, step away from the restrictions of dementia and feel free. We choose to share learning from our programmes through regular presentations and exhibitions of participants' creative work hosted at partner sites, in particular Leeds Playhouse and Leeds Museums Discovery Centre.

The range of experiences of participants can be vast. Someone who has received an early diagnosis in the previous month may be participating alongside someone who received a diagnosis eight years ago. This might result in those with more advanced symptoms feeling exposed, or those with less advanced symptoms being confronted and frightened by an insight into their potential future. Staff are mindful of the emotional impact of this, offering focused support to individuals when needed. The intention is always to celebrate what people *can* do, rather than highlighting what has been lost. We offer a short description of each week's activity in advance, which gives people the opportunity to opt out if they feel it isn't for them. However, we feel conflicted about this, as it can result in people taking less risk in the activities they choose, despite all sessions being designed to be failure free. Staff pay close attention so as to build a sense of community, to give choice around involvement in certain activities, and to seat people with others in similar situations or where a friendship is developing.

Activities focus on in-the-moment experiences, and each session stands alone. We have worked hard to move away from the trap of introducing sessions based on what we did 'last time', as many people cannot recall this. We avoid words like 'remember' so we do not highlight people's difficulties, instead focusing on what people 'think' and 'feel'. It is clear that the language around factual memory is deeply embedded in our culture, and it takes effort to retrain ourselves in the language we use. But this is necessary to ensure we are offering a failure-free setting and an equal starting point for people with dementia and their partners without dementia. An important aspect of the delivery of sessions is that everyone joins in as equals, including staff, volunteers, visitors, family supporters, paid carers and people with dementia.

Funding for the project has come from each partner organisation's existing budget. We have operated on a shoestring and drawn on existing resources, with a consistent staff team able to apply dementia-specific adaptations to our delivery. There has been only one change of staffing in our team of six professionals during 10 years of partnership working. This consistency has undoubtedly led to mutual understanding, trust and a shared ethos among staff while also contributing to meaningful, reliable and playful relationship-building with participants. In our experience, too little attention is given in research and evaluation to the consistency and relationship-building that is involved in the delivery of cultural activities with people with dementia. The whole experience of arts engagement is relational and depends on a stable, reliable base, which provides the conditions for people to feel free to explore their creativity. A feeling of security and familiarity enables people to express themselves with less fear. We advocate strongly for a relational approach and model it within our staff and participant interactions.

Each 12-week project is evaluated informally week by week, with feedback from participants and observations from staff given equal weight. We have learned about approaches we can use again and those we need to adapt further or abandon entirely. We notice the general mood of the group while identifying individuals who may need specific attention, whether that's to contribute in a different way, to be assisted to shine or to stay safely in the background.

Learning point 3

- How will you develop an activity that is failure free and inclusive of people with dementia?
- How many people can you meaningfully engage in your activity?
- Can you create a safe space by closing a section of the venue to the public, to maintain privacy and lessen distractions?
- How might you adapt and continue to support participants as dementia-related changes occur?

Conclusion

Our organisations have benefitted from the time spent developing this programme and the contributions of people living with dementia. We have cultivated pockets of expertise and highlighted lived experience, which has broadened the understanding of dementia-friendly cultural provision beyond the sessions themselves. Each organisation in the Cultural Partnership has experienced elements of transformation – bolder programming, greater staff understanding, the confidence to present new public events to raise awareness of dementia, and the continued, respectful and meaningful involvement of people living with dementia.

References

Camic, P.M., Tischler, V. & Pearman, C.H. (2014). Viewing and making art together: A multi-session art-gallery based intervention for people with dementia and their carers. *Aging & Mental Health, 18*(2), 161–168. doi: 10.1080/13607863.2013.818101

Clarke, C., Keyes, S., Wilkinson, H., Alexjuk, J., Wilcockson, J., Robinson, L., Reynolds, J., McClelland, S., Hodgson, P., Corner, L. & Cattan, M. (2013). *Healthbridge: The national evaluation of peer support networks and dementia advisers in implementation of the National Dementia Strategy for England.* Project report. Department of Health.

Department of Health. (2009). *Living well with dementia: A national dementia strategy.* Department of Health.

Fritsch, T., Kwak, J., Grant, S., Lang, J., Montgomery, R. & Basting, A. (2009). Impact of TimeSlips, a creative expression intervention program, on nursing home residents with dementia and their caregivers. *The Gerontologist, 49*(1), 117–127.

Jancovich, L. (2011). Great art for everyone? Engagement and participation policy in the arts. *Cultural Trends, 20*(3–4), 271–279.

Rosenberg, F. (2009). The MOMA Alzheimer's project: Programming and resources for making art accessible to people with Alzheimer's disease and their caregivers. *Arts & Health, 1*(1), 93–97.

Young, R., Camic, P. & Tischler, V. (2016) The impact of community-based arts and health interventions on cognition in people with dementia: A systematic literature review. *Aging & Mental Health, 20*(4), 337–351.

Conclusion

The principal purpose of this practical handbook is for it to be useful, easy to use and a go-to source of state-of-the-art knowledge, advice and inspiration in the field. Going forward, we hope it will help in enabling people to live well with their dementia. It is our fervent wish that these purposes will be fulfilled in the quality of thought, knowledge, experience and especially the practical ideas presented here.

The handbook throughout draws attention to some very rich seams of knowledge and practical advice, and offers up some emerging threads that point to future directions for practice and research. Working in this field is, as John Killick says in Chapter 34, so often about 'an intensity of listening', where we need to become 'a true listener' for those arising, often momentary 'threads' or fragments of memory, songs, ideas, thoughts and feelings. Over time, we learn how it is possible to listen in such a way that what at first may appear to be 'non-sense' is not at all. It's just that we haven't tuned ourselves in sufficiently to the true nature and purpose of that communication, so at first we may not understand, especially if we are full of our own personal noise or chatter that we haven't yet learnt to hush. Creatively and imaginatively, we can become more adept at listening for and paying attention to these fragments and threads, which we can learn to weave together. In so doing, we can help create a 'mosaic' from them, where the fragments may become, metaphorically speaking, 're-framed', in often very satisfying and life-affirming ways.

Matt Laurie, in Chapter 20, has described this process well in relation to his rapport-based communication (RBC), where he argues that empathy and the building of rapport are at the heart of communicating in 'person-centred care'. His use of improvisatory techniques, together with the three Cs of accepting 'offers', is essentially about going with whatever fragments or 'threads' are offered in the moment by the person and so building rapport and facilitating communication. John Killick, again in Chapter 34, describes some wonderfully evocative phrases that his wife has used and 'submit(s) that these small units of language have a vividness and ambiguity which in other contexts we would acknowledge as poetry' (p.281). He might also describe Laurie's RBC, in his words, as another way of 'becoming a true listener'.

The handbook began with an introduction that drew attention to another personal – and also family – experience of living with dementia by Isla Parker, and to her relationship with her grandmother, Vera. It describes how she was inspired by John Killick's approach, and how she used his techniques with Vera. Parker also links creative writing and the importance of the home as a hub for this creative activity. We would argue that the home is also the centre of what could be described as intimate relating. It is within the home that so many of the chapters are located and it is within the home that so many people living with dementia are being cared for in the UK and around the world, rather than in hospital or residential or nursing care settings. It is also the focus of Gary Lockhart's (Chapter 5) moving experiences in caring for his parents in Australia, and the heartfelt difficulties and triumphs of Peter Hemsley's role (Chapter 6) as a single carer looking after his wife.

The 'home' is, in addition, the context within which the intimate relating takes place that is so crucial in best practices in the field. The philosopher Martin Buber (Buber, 1937/2004) drew attention to the roots of this intimate relating, which he described in terms of an 'I/Thou' relationship, and its importance in communicating the necessity to truly see the person for who they are and not simply for what they represent. This simple, yet paradoxically highly complex dictum, when put into practice, is at the heart of John Kitwood's last and pioneering work, *Dementia Re-considered* (Kitwood, 1997). It is still repeated in references throughout these pages, years later.

A brief example of what is meant by useful and a go-to-source of up-to-date advice occurred soon after we received Lisa Austin's Chapter 17 on insomnia. Richard Coaten, one of this book's editors, works on an inpatient unit for older people with mental health problems. Two nurse colleagues were struggling to find a suitable assessment tool for a person with insomnia. He referred them to the two tools quoted in Austin's chapter, which they were able to access and found helpful in the person's care. This is just one small example of how the information contained here can be useful.

It has been a deliberate strategy on the part of the editors to ask authors to come up with key Learning Points as they go along. This is in order to help the reader stay focused on the key messages that the authors are seeking to communicate. It also means that, at a later date, each chapter can be revisited for the key learning points, as a quick reference. We consider that these two elements taken together make this practical handbook of particular value.

However, the usefulness and value of any handbook has to be seen in the context of the times from which it emerges, and the months of the Covid-19 pandemic, of self-isolation and lockdown have placed an enormous burden on the mental health of every one of us living through it. None more so than those living with dementia in care homes, in the community and in hospital inpatient wards. The isolation and loneliness, the loss of life, the carer stress, both professional and unpaid, has been unprecedented and, indeed, intolerable in this generation. If this handbook and the rich variety of contributions contained within it can go some way towards creating a better world for people living with dementia following the pandemic, then it will have been worth every ounce of effort in producing it.

We want to acknowledge what Caroline Cantley achieved in her handbook, published more than 20 years ago (Cantley, 2001). A lot has happened since then, of course, but her book has not gathered dust on a shelf: the work of these authors is deeply rooted in past best practice, sound and up-to-date scholarship and the all-important necessary practical experience within their respective fields.

The care of people living with dementia is such a complex, challenging and critically important task in society right now, it is vital that, in addition to it having deep roots in dementia care practice, there is a wide range of perspectives present in this book, and that they cover, as far as possible, the full range and depth of the field. Immediately of note is a thread that appears to link all the chapters together – namely, a strong focus on how a richer sense of humanity, of hope and human expression is being constellated, and on what in the literature is described as an 'ecology of human flourishing' (McCormack & Titchen, 2014) – a concept that goes back to the work of Aristotle. As McCormack and Titchen say:

> Human flourishing happens when persons interconnect with their physical, social, spiritual, creative and natural being through meaningful and intentional practices. (p.20)

All these chapters kindle messages of inspiration and hope in their different ways. They range from the lived experience of people with dementia and their carers in Part 1, through to inspiring creative approaches found in Part 4. All these, including the work to support people living with dementia in Part 3, go way beyond attempting to ameliorate symptoms and instead refer to the conditions that need to be created in order for human beings to flourish.

For instance, in the context of gardening, in Chapter 24, Sarah Swift and Margaret Brown are sharing ways not only to create 'empowering and enjoyable' garden spaces, but also, by way of their practice, a strong affirmation of the dementia activism movement, expressed in the phrase, 'nothing about us without us' (Bryden, 2015). This is a key theme expressed through the co-creation, co-design and co-construction that are also present, and by way of these, how gardening can become part of a further thread encouraging activism in the everyday business of finding enjoyment in life in spite of the condition. In the words of Swift and Brown:

> … the garden becomes a space for the expression of identity and selfhood, the embodied articulation of agency, and the development of lasting social connections. (p.201)

Here in the garden is a time and a space for an 'ecology of human flourishing' to grow, where all involved may share in a richer conception of our interdependences, and where we may find profound value in each other and in nature and our place within it. We can also experience this daily, when finding ourselves in garden spaces however small, all of which are echoed in Wendy Brewin's Chapter 25 on the same subject. She also notes that these benefits are predicated on barriers to access being overcome, and on the basis of the provision of varying degrees of intensity in their application, both of which are helpful pointers.

There is so much to draw attention to in these pages that this conclusion could run away with itself in attempting to name them all. However, a brief critical reflection on the gaps must look also at its potential weaknesses. For example, an editorial decision was taken not to describe the many different types that make up what is known collectively as the dementia syndrome. This was made because, at time of editing (2022), there is so much information available on the internet and some very good definitions. For example, a first port of call would be the Alzheimer's Society UK's website and their helpful fact-sheets.[1] To have attempted to replicate this would have taken up precious space, reducing the number of different perspectives that we were able instead to include here. We also chose to concentrate on the very practical and experiential ways in which best practice in dementia care can be captured and communicated.

Another gap that emerged during the course of the handbook's creation is the need to understand more about how the unpaid family carer can be best supported to cope with the grief and loss associated with the death of their loved one. In fact, it goes further than this. How can they be helped to find their own place in the world again, having had to transition from long-time partner or spouse to full-time carer, often for many years, and then to being on their own once more? As with all aspects of dementia care, there are no simple answers to this question. However, Karen Harrison Dening's call in Chapter 13 for us all to be more pro-active is relevant here: we need to be proactive not only in recognising signs and symptoms early on, but towards the end, as people reach the palliative care stages. Sascha Bolt and colleagues similarly point out in Chapter 14 how an integrated palliative care approach made a huge difference for 'Fiona' in her last years. There is also a need for researchers to focus on understanding life beyond dementia, in particular for family carers. For example, to what extent can a grieving family be assisted to re-adjust to a new life without the partner of a lifetime?

While as editors we do not possess a crystal ball to view the future, it is not difficult to see that technology is going to play an increasing role in care practices going forward, and nowhere perhaps more so than in the home. John Woolham in Chapter 22 argues convincingly that technology should support a wider range of activity than simply keeping people safe. He argues that it should be able to facilitate social contact, hobbies and preferred lifestyles and in the process be much more interactive and customisable to meet changing individual needs. He also argues that telecare should be much better at exploiting new technologies, and these should be designed around the person, rather than fitting the person to the technology, which is perhaps too often the case at the moment.

---

1. www.alzheimers.org.uk/get-support/publications-factsheets

The message is clear from Woolham's chapter in particular that, while the care of people living with dementia has come a long way in the past two decades, there is still much that needs to be improved. There are still many challenges to overcome and opportunities for learning. One key opportunity here is the extent to which co-design, co-creation and co-production can play an integral part in improving dementia care going forward. This sentiment is also echoed in Richard Talbot and Claire Dormann's Chapter 36 on digital clowning and telecare, and how clowning can be used very effectively online to engage and improve wellbeing, and in Kathryn Barham's Chapter 32 on digital life-story work. Research and developments in the field today have clearly mandated that now, and in future, people with lived experience have to be at the heart of any research and development that takes place.

As a whole, the huge amount of knowledge, skills and experience condensed in these fascinating chapters points to a need for a much more nuanced understanding of what it means to live with and care for someone living with dementia. While bio-medical science and research continue their attempts to better understand the science and mechanisms underlying the condition, so that we are better able ultimately to find a cure for dementia syndrome, there is much that can and must still be done to help people live to their full potential with dementia, while we wait for that cure to be found.

This much more nuanced understanding also means engaging more proactively and on many different levels with all aspects of life that affect people living with dementia. We are particularly delighted to have a chapter on the subject of spirituality – arguably much neglected in people with dementia – by North American pastor Kathy Fogg Berry (Chapter 8). Here she offers her perspective on how this essential element in so many people's lives can be acknowledged, nurtured and maintained in person-centred dementia care. She notes the importance of local faith communities proactively coming forward to welcome and continue to include people with dementia in their churches. She also helpfully takes the reader through practical suggestions for working from a spiritual perspective in the early, middle and late stages of the condition and offers what could be the first spiritual assessment tool in the field.

It is clear too that in the UK today there is much very good advocacy and support work going on to ensure people with dementia have their say and their citizen's rights are not overlooked. One such initiative is the Dementia Engagement and Empowerment Project (DEEP),[2] that seeks to empower people living with dementia to influence attitudes, services and policies that affect their lives. The Dementia Friends Champion initiative, John's Campaign and YODA (Young Onset Dementia & Alzheimer's) are others that, via social media, also facilitate a great deal of communication and advocacy work, helping to reduce stigma and more. Chapter 9 by Anthea Innes, John O'Doherty and Helen Rochford-Brennan builds on this in relation to early onset dementia, providing moving personal accounts

---

2. www.dementiavoices.org.uk/

that address the challenges and change needed to enable future generations with the condition to live more supported lives.

This is also relevant to employment issues, as reported by Louise Ritchie, Debbie Tolson and Mike Danson in Chapter 21. While research indicates that the majority of people with dementia do not continue in employment post-diagnosis, this chapter argues that, if provided with appropriate support, people do want to continue to do meaningful paid work. It is important post-diagnosis to the maintenance of a sense of belonging and worth and the continuation of social interaction and physical activity, in addition to income, which has to be welcomed. This is yet another thread pointing to how the future of dementia care can be best influenced and changed for the better, through the use of well-focused and co-produced research on how people can be maintained in employment post-diagnosis.

Part 4 has a rich focus on creative approaches, ranging from Cath Arakelian and Jonathan Barker's Chapter 28 on mindfulness through to Ming-Hung Hsu's exposition of his work as a music therapist in Chapter 33. Bo Chapman and Zoe Flynn's quite remarkable stop-frame animation work, described in Chapter 31, which they have developed and refined over years now, similarly reflects the great diversity in the field. However, the penultimate words must be taken from Nicky Taylor and Gabrielle Hamilton's description of the ground-breaking partnership-working in Leeds, where a range of cultural institutions have worked so inspiringly with the peer-support service for people with dementia, making a huge difference to individual lives and also to awareness of dementia in the cultural sector (Chapter 38). At the heart of the work has been consistency, respect, stability in terms of consistent professional staff involvement, sound evaluation, great partnership working across the city and a strong ethical focus. As they say, there is present in the project 'a sense of something new beginning (that) can energise people with dementia and their supporters, offering relief and distraction from the worry of their changing world' (p.316).

Finally, this snapshot of best practices in the field will, we hope, energise and support new beginnings in the strong relational and forward-thinking movement expressed so clearly in the empowering phrase 'Nothing about us, without us!' These are new beginnings that can educate and inspire all involved in this remarkably challenging and rewarding field. We commend this book to all those working in the field who are seeking new, practical ideas that can help them take their work forward towards a better world for all living with dementia and those who care for and work with them.

Isla Parker, Richard Coaten, Mark Hopfenbeck

References

Bryden, C. (2015). *Nothing about us, without us! 20 years of dementia advocacy.* Jessica Kingsley Publishers.

Buber, M. (1937/2004). *I and thou.* Continuum.

Cantley, C. (Ed.). (2001). *A handbook of dementia care.* McGraw-Hill Education.

Kitwood, T. (1997). *Dementia re-considered: The person comes first.* Open University Press.

McCormack, B. & Titchen, A. (2014). No beginning, no end: An ecology of human flourishing, *International Practice Development Journal, 4*(2), 1–21.

Afterword

Julian C. Hughes

My good friend Professor Steven Sabat, in the Foreword to this volume, invoked the work of Martin Buber (1878–1965). In his book *I and Thou*, Buber says: 'All real living is meeting' (Buber, 1923/2004, p.17). I am inclined to say this could be the message of this book. This might seem to underplay everything that has been written in these pages. I hope to persuade you that it does not.

I am tempted to start with the question 'What really helps?' Again, there is something mischievous about the question, since the book is a 'practical handbook', so by now we should know what helps. But what *really* helps? One answer that suggests itself is to say that there is, of course, no one thing that helps. As this book has amply demonstrated, there are numerous things that all seem of more or less importance. I must apologise to the authors of the book if, in the space available, I do not highlight their particular chapter. Yet – to select somewhat randomly – it is obvious that we need good nutrition, the invaluable advice of speech and language therapists, help with sleep, assistive technology (robots even), good design, and so forth. We need the judicious use of medications of various sorts, where the operative word is 'judicious', suggesting the need for good judgement and sense. We need good quality palliative care and advance care planning to help to put this into effect. We need, in short, the full panoply of the multidisciplinary team readily to hand. But what *really* helps?

To answer this question, it seems right and proper to turn, as this book has done, to the experience of people who are affected by dementia: those who live with a diagnosis and those close friends or family who live with them. What do we then find? Well, we find unique individuals, who wish to engage, to participate, to be heard, to enjoy companionship, to visit the coffee shop; we find those who honour and support others who live with dementia, and we see the importance of friendship. Perhaps 'all real living is meeting'!

Art and culture

But in these pages, we have found a whole lot more. It turns out, albeit unsurprisingly, that there is a vast array of creative and cultural activities that can help people living with dementia: music, gardening, mindfulness, yoga, dancing, digital art, museums, painting, poetry, playing, clowning and so on. So, what is this all about? It's certainly not about doing all of these things. You just wouldn't have the time! And we also have to recognise that, in considering art and dementia, we are dealing with 'deeply psychosocial, idiosyncratic, and experiential issues' (Beard, 2012). Different art and cultural activities will appeal (or not) to different people. Just as they might for any of us.

Nevertheless, what we cherish in considering such creative and cultural activities are our different ways of being. As has been mentioned in these pages several times, quality of life is key. But this leads me to two cautionary notes.

First, quality of life is not one thing that can be measured. For sure, there are aspects of it that can be measured, but it is, rather, an amalgam of all that makes life worthwhile. That amalgam is deeply idiosyncratic. Our particular ways of being cannot be circumscribed by the domains of quality-of-life measures. The second caution is that it is dangerous to judge someone else's quality of life from the outside. We know this can prove to be wrong. Many people would judge that having a disability (including dementia) would mean that the person's quality of life was poor. But, as we know, people with disabilities deny this and achieve great things when they have appropriate support. So this caution is also a caution against any action or attitude that might tend to undermine the standing of people living with dementia as full human persons. There is a German word, *Menschenwürde*, which roughly means 'human worth', but which conveys the notion of 'unconditional inherent human dignity' (Woodruff, 2016, p.227). Such a conception of dignity could be a guiding light in our meetings with any and everyone, but should have particular traction in meeting people living with dementia. However, the point to which I wish to return is, in a way, the point made by another friend, Keith Oliver, in Chapter 1, when he emphasises the unique person. Creative and cultural activities speak to our unique, idiosyncratic selves, to which I shall now turn.

Persons

Buber, whose work greatly influenced Tom Kitwood and should therefore underpin true person-centred care, wrote near the start of *I and Thou*:

> Every *It* is bounded by others; *It* exists only through being bounded by others. But when *Thou* is spoken, there is no thing. *Thou* has no bounds.

> When *Thou* is spoken, the speaker has no *thing*; he has indeed nothing. But he takes his stand in relation. (Buber, 1923/2004, p.12).

So we start with the unique person, but the thrust of Buber's idea is that the unique person, once understood properly as *Thou*, or more properly as *I-Thou*, is no mere thing but is part of relationships.

This contrasts quite starkly with the characterisation of the person that emerges in the work of empiricist philosophers such as John Locke (1632–1704) and David Hume (1711–1776), where the key thing is memory – or, as the more contemporary philosopher Derek Parfit (1942–2017) put it, psychological continuity and connectedness (see Hughes (2011) for further discussion). But such a view is too narrow (as if what makes us persons is simply memory), because we are not isolated atoms or islands. Rather, we are situated in the context of our relationships with others and with the world. Indeed, we are uniquely situated in more ways than we can name: culturally, politically, spiritually, socially, ethically, psychologically, and so on and so forth. We are also embodied (our bodies are important in themselves and because of how they represent us) and we are agents, so that even in the advanced stages of dementia our movements may have what Pia Kontos (2004) has called 'gestural significance'.

This situated, embodied agent view provides a broad picture of what it is to be a person with dementia (Hughes, 2001). So, as we have seen in these pages, there is little about us that can be ignored when it comes to supporting or maintaining our personhood – and, contrariwise, there is much that can be undermined egregiously or by stealth and subtlety. Hence, Kitwood and Brooker (2019) spoke of 'malignant social psychology' and Sabat (2001) of 'malignant positioning'. And much of what has been presented in this book amounts to bulwarks against the possibility of undermining the person's standing as a self or unique person.

To suggest another philosophical underpinning, Martin Heidegger (1889–1976), who characterised our being as humans as *being-with*, spoke of solicitude to describe the way in which human beings have, or should have, a significance for each other (Heidegger, 1927/1962, p.158). Once again, 'All real living is meeting.'

Social citizenship and authenticity

Our unique personhood, therefore, reveals itself in the multifarious ways in which we can interact with others. Moreover, personhood is shored up by a great variety of social and cultural endeavours, as we have seen in the preceding chapters. We've seen the importance of social networks, social inclusion, of validation (which builds relationships and communication) and of safety with others. We've seen the ways in which we can practise so as to uphold the rights and values of people with dementia. And we have even seen the importance of connecting with the natural world.

Much of this feeds into a newer understanding of what it is to be a person with dementia, which is to look at matters through the lens of social citizenship:

> … a relationship, practice or status, in which a person with dementia
> is entitled to experience freedom from discrimination, and to have
> opportunities to grow and participate in life to the fullest extent possible.
> It involves justice, recognition of social positions and the upholding of
> personhood, rights and a fluid degree of responsibility for shaping events at
> a personal and societal level. (Bartlett & O'Connor 2010, p.37)

Enabling people with dementia to continue to work, therefore, is right on message. Yet the challenge is to encourage social citizenship all the way through the course of dementia, and to try to understand how this might be possible. Seeing the person as embedded in his or her personal, familial and cultural context will be a start.

Yet, there is also a type of seeing and hearing the person – really seeing and hearing – that underpins everything else. You could say it's a type of meeting. To pick up on the wisdom of another friend who has written in this book, John Killick (Chapter 34) suggests we need 'an authenticity of language and feeling'. Such authenticity should perhaps pervade all interactions with people who live with or care for those who live with a diagnosis of dementia. We might, then, wish to amend Buber's claim and write it as the motto for all that we do: 'All real living is authentic meeting.'

References

Bartlett, R. & O'Connor, D. (2010). *Broadening the dementia debate: Towards social citizenship*. Policy Press.

Beard, R.L. (2012). Art therapies and dementia care: A systematic review. *Dementia, 11*, 633–656.

Buber, M. (1923/2004). *I and thou* (R.G. Smith, trans.). Continuum.

Heidegger, M. (1927/1962). *Being and time* (J. Macquarrie & E. Robinson, trans.). Blackwell. (First published as *Sein und zeit* in 1927.)

Hughes, J.C. (2001). Views of the person with dementia. *Journal of Medical Ethics, 27*, 86–91.

Hughes, J.C. (2011). *Thinking through dementia*. Oxford University Press.

Kitwood, T. & Brooker, D. (Ed.). (2019). *Dementia reconsidered revisited: The person still comes first*. Open University Press.

Kontos, P.C. (2004). Ethnographic reflections on selfhood, embodiment and Alzheimer's disease. *Ageing and Society, 24*, 829–849.

Sabat, S.R. (2001). *The experience of Alzheimer's disease: Life through a tangled veil*. Blackwell.

Woodruff, R. (2016). Aging and the maintenance of dignity. In G. Scarre (Ed.), *The Palgrave handbook of the philosophy of aging* (pp.225–245). Palgrave Macmillan.

Contributors

Cath Arakelian currently works as a dementia counsellor in Oxford. In 2008, she trained with the Alzheimer's Society and designed and delivered psycho-educational dementia programmes for carers and people living with dementia. Cath is a trainee therapist member of BACP and UKCP.

Dr Lisa Austin is a research management professional who has worked in university, NHS and Department of Health settings. She is currently based in the Humanities Faculty at the University of Bath, where she is the Department for Health Research Manager. She is also an NHS research manager to local primary and community care. Lisa has a professional doctorate in health and is interested in sleep and dementia. She is passionate about extending research to everyone and is the equality, diversity and inclusion lead for the Research Design Service South West, helping researchers to develop grant applications with patient and public involvement. Lisa lives in between Bristol and Bath and is a firm fan of country walks and all things vintage.

Kathryn Barham is co-founder and CEO at Book of You CIC. After a career in the civil service, she built her own successful sales team with a major national company and worked at the award-winning DangerPoint Safety Centre. Kathy is also a published author and presents a 'new music' radio show.

Jonathan Barker is a qualified mindfulness teacher and has taught at the University of Reading and in secondary schools and a homeless persons' hostel. In 2016, he and Cath Arakelian developed a mindfulness programme for staff and people living with dementia in care homes. Jonathan also works as a TV documentary director.

Rosie Barker is Participation Manager for Birmingham Museums Trust, with more than 20 years' experience in museums. She has a particular interest in working with communities to make museums accessible, representative and inclusive, and in using museums to support and improve wellbeing.

Sascha Bolt, MSc, PhD is a senior researcher and knowledge broker at the Academic Collaborative Center Older Adults Tranzo, Tilburg University, in the Netherlands. She has Master's degrees in neuropsychology and clinical and health psychology. Her doctoral research focused on improving palliative care for people with dementia and their families.

Wendy Brewin has created a successful model for using nature interventions in dementia care through the Sensory Trust's Creative Spaces project, working with researchers to evaluate and refine techniques. Her passion for highlighting the benefits of nature connections has increased during nearly 30 years of working to enable people of all ages and abilities to access nature.

Dara Brown is a specialist speech and language therapist in mental health of older adults and dementia, South London and Maudsley NHS Foundation Trust. She supports people with communication and swallowing disorders on acute mental health wards and dementia assessment services for older people across south London. Dara began her career working for the Alzheimer's Society and the Dementia Friends initiative, before moving into speech and language therapy.

Dr Margaret Brown is a researcher, educator and practitioner in the field of dementia and mental health care for older people. She authored the first report in Scotland about housing and dementia and has a lifetime achievement award for outstanding commitment in the field of dementia care.

Dr Rachel Butterfield is a clinical psychologist who has worked in mental health services for older people in north London for 20 years. She has undertaken training in a range of psychological approaches and has a strong interest in Open Dialogue and dialogical practice.

Bo Chapman received an MA in art history from Edinburgh University and attended École Internationale de Théâtre Jacques Lecoq Paris. Bo has an eclectic background in art, music and performance. Before co-founding Frames Of Mind, she worked as an art director and stylist for stills, music videos, commercials and short films, and was a singer-songwriter and performer.

Dr Richard Coaten is a dancer and registered dance movement psychotherapist (RDMP) with the Association for Dance Movement Psychotherapy, where he was a director on the Governing Council 2013–2016. He has spent the past 16 years working clinically as a DMP in an NHS older people's psychiatric ward in West Yorkshire and in day centres. He completed a doctoral thesis on dance movement psychotherapy and dementia at Roehampton University and delivers workshops and conference presentations in Canada, the US and Europe, supporting the training of the next generation of DMPs. He is on the editorial board of the peer-reviewed international journal *Dementia*. He also sits on the Board of the Creative Dementia Arts Network.

Mike Danson, DLitt, FAcSS, FIED, FRSA, FeRSA is Professor of Enterprise Policy at Heriot-Watt University. Mike is an economist, researching and publishing on ageing, demographic changes, Just Transition, Basic Income, Kawasaki disease, microbreweries and rural and islands economies. Formerly Treasurer of the Academy of Social Sciences, he is on the council of charities and professional and learned societies and an advisor to national and international governments.

Louise Deakin is a learning, engagement, and outreach officer working in the cultural sector. Inclusivity, food, British telly, and her cat Winston are her passions. She believes museums are for everyone: to increase expression, discussion and co-production and to celebrate our differences and shared heritage.

Vicki de Klerk-Rubin is the Executive Director of the Validation Training Institute and a certified Validation master. She authored *Validation Techniques for Dementia Care* and *Validation for First Responders*. Together with her mother Naomi Feil, the founder of the Validation method, she co-authored the revisions of *Validation: The Feil Method* and *The Validation Breakthrough*. She holds a BFA from Boston University, an MBA from Fordham University, and is a Dutch-trained registered nurse.

Claire Dormann is Senior Research Fellow at University College London, researching the junction of artificial intelligence and human-computer interaction. A large part of her research relates to serious games, and playful interaction. She also has a strong interest in humour and has published quite widely on the subject.

The Reverend Kathy Fogg Berry has been a chaplain for 22 years. She received a BS in mass communications, an MS in patient counseling, and a postgraduate certificate in aging studies from Virginia Commonwealth University. Her Master's in religious education is from Southern Seminary in Louisville, Kentucky. She frequently speaks on spirituality and dementia and her book, *When Words Fail*, was published in 2017.

Zoe Flynn completed her BA Hons in photography, film and video at Westminster University. After graduating, Zoe worked in television and the advertising industry, on a variety of programmes, documentaries and cinema trailers. Before co-founding Frames Of Mind, she ran her own production company, Eyesaw Productions, specialising in social documentaries, multi-media projects and training in filmmaking.

Robert Freudenthal is a general-adult and old-age psychiatrist, based in London NHS mental health services. He has pursued further training in peer-supported Open Dialogue and in group work via the Institute of Group Analysis, which informs his clinical work.

My name is **Gail Gregory** and I'm 57 years old. I was diagnosed with early onset Alzheimer's at the age of 54 on 14 February 2019. I don't look at my diagnosis negatively. This is a new chapter in my life. My dementia chapter. Over the past three years I have entered a whole new world. New ways to keep me occupied and keep my brain active. Dementia does not have to be the end. This is my new beginning.

Gabrielle Hamilton spent some years working in the third sector in Leeds in supported housing services before transferring to the heritage sector, heading up the Community Engagement Team for Leeds Museums and Galleries. Since retiring, she has become a trustee at SKIPPKO, where she is committed to exploring different ways in which involvement in the creative arts enhances people's health and wellbeing.

Dr Dylan Harris, FRCP, MSc, FAcadMEd is a consultant in palliative medicine in South Wales and a lecturer at Cardiff University. He was closely involved in originally establishing a partnership between dementia services and Hospice of the Valleys in Blaenau Gwent (Wales) in 2014, to facilitate collaborative support for people with a dementia diagnosis and their families.

Dr Karen Harrison Dening is a nurse with 45 years' experience in dementia care. Karen completed her PhD at University College London on advance care planning in dementia. Head of Research and Publications at Dementia UK, she has influenced national dementia (e.g. NICE) guidelines. Research interests include dementia care, palliative and end-of-life care and advance care planning.

My name is **Peter Hemsley** and I was made redundant at 63. My wife had early symptoms of dementia. I was in denial of this, but very slowly the realisation dawned that we were both on the crest of rapid decline. Help by human kindness from unexpected sources made me eternally grateful.

Nina Herrington is a qualified dietitian and is registered with the Health and Care Professions Council. Nina has specific interests in nutrition and mental health, nutrition in older adults and palliative care nutrition. Nina has worked with people who have dementia in a variety of NHS and charity organisations across London.

Mark Hopfenbeck is a social anthropologist specialising in health and social policy, an assistant professor at the Norwegian University of Science and Technology (NTNU), visiting fellow at London South Bank University (LSBU) and individual partner at the Collaborating Centre for Values-based Practice in Health and Social Care, St Catherine's College, Oxford University. At NTNU, he teaches mindfulness and is a member of the Wellbeing and Social Sustainability research group. For the past 20 years, he has been teaching and supporting the implementation of the Open Dialogue approach in mental health care. Mark is co-editor of *The Practical Handbook of Hearing Voices* and *The Practical Handbook of Eating Difficulties*. He is currently co-investigator on a large-scale programme of research into crisis and continuing mental health care within the NHS (the ODDESSI study).

Dr Ming-Hung Hsu is a music therapist and a senior research fellow at the Cambridge Institute for Music Therapy Research, Anglia Ruskin University. Ming's research interests are mainly in dementia care, looking at how the role of music therapists can help personalise dementia care and support caregivers.

Professor Julian Hughes was an NHS consultant in old-age psychiatry, working mostly in Newcastle and North Tyneside. He was honorary professor of philosophy of ageing at Newcastle and professor of old age psychiatry at Bristol. Among other things, he served on the Nuffield Council on Bioethics, including as Deputy Chair.

Anthea Innes is Professor, Health, Aging and Society, Gilbrea Chair in Aging and Mental Health and Director of the Gilbrea Centre for Studies on Aging at McMaster University, Ontario, Canada. Anthea is a social scientist who has specialised in the area of dementia for the past 25 years.

Dr Amy Jebreel practises old age and adult psychiatry in London. She trained in peer-supported Open Dialogue in 2014 and has since been working with the approach. She is a British-Iranian queer Jew who in her spare time enjoys cooking, eating, silent meditation retreats and adrenalin sports.

Dr Rachael Kelley is a senior research fellow in the Centre for Dementia Research at Leeds Beckett University. Before becoming a researcher, she worked as a mental health nurse, supporting people living with dementia. Her research focuses on improving the care and support offered to people living with dementia and their families, primarily in general hospital settings.

John Killick has been writer, teacher and researcher. For six years he was Research Fellow in Communication Through the Arts at the University of Stirling. He has written eight books on communication, creativity and dementia. Forthcoming is an anthology, *The Poetry of Dementia*, from Sheffield Hallam University.

Sally Knocker, PgDip Dramatherapy and BA Law & Society, works part-time with Meaningful Care Matters, an international culture change organisation, and with Plan with Care, a wellbeing and care consultancy. She is the author of a range of publications in the field of older people's care and on the needs of older LGBTQ+ people. She facilitated the Opening Doors Rainbow Café for its first two years from 2017–2019.

Matt Laurie has since 2001 worked as a community artist, special needs trainer and consultant, supporting many people with complex needs arising from dementia, autism, learning disabilities and mental health issues. He specialises in working in collaboration with services to embed person-centred practice and has developed the approaches of Rapport-Based Communication and Rapport-Based Music. *www.mattlaurie.com*

Dr Susan Liggett is Reader in Fine Art and Associate Dean for Research in the Faculty of Art, Science and Technology at Wrexham Glyndŵr University. She has a

PhD from the University of Wales, a postgraduate diploma in painting (MA) from the Royal Academy Schools, London and a BA (Hons) Fine Art from Nottingham Trent University. Her work as a practising artist includes paintings, fine art films and arts in health collaborative research projects, resulting in her artwork being exhibited in different and varied contexts, including galleries, public spaces, conferences and festivals. As a curator, she has organised exhibitions, chaired conferences and published work on the interface of art/science. She is a member of the Royal Cambrian Academy and SUITE Studio Group, Salford.

Gary Lockhart is an outreach youth program manager for a Sydney-based youth service that specialises in assisting homeless and disaffected youth. He has worked with young people for more than 20 years. Since 2015, he has been a carer for his parents, who are both in their 90s. His mother has vascular dementia and requires constant supervision. He has a Bachelor of Social Science and is currently completing his Master's of Social Work. He currently lives in Sydney with his parents and balances these responsibilities. Gary talks with candour and insight about his experiences and the challenges he faced when relocating his parents interstate.

Professor Mary Marshall has worked with and for people with dementia for 40 years. She was the director of the Dementia Services Development Centre at the University of Stirling for 16 years and then worked as a design consultant for a further 10. She has written widely on dementia design.

Judith Meijers, MSc, PhD is a nurse, epidemiologist and associate professor at the University of Maastricht and Zuyderland. Her research line focuses on nursing interventions to improve care at the end of life in long-term care and nursing education – for example, end-of-life communication (ACP) and interprofessional and transmural collaboration. She has received national and international grant applications. The research uses co-creative context-related designs (mixed methods).

Josephine Norrbo is a Swedish yoga teacher and landscape architect trained in hatha yoga and Trauma Center Trauma-Sensitive Yoga. She is one of the co-founders of the NGO Yoga for All that aims to offer yoga to people who do not have easy access to it, such as elderly people with dementia. She is currently undertaking a PhD in landscape architecture, focusing on aesthetics and social sustainability.

John O'Doherty is dedicated to improving the care of people living with dementia. He has served on many national and regional advocacy forums, including the Alzheimer's Society, 3 Nations, the Greater Manchester Combined Health Group and the Dementia Associate Panel at the Salford Institute for Dementia.

Keith Oliver is married with three grown-up children and three grandchildren and lives in Canterbury. He worked for 33 years as a teacher, headteacher and school advisor. On New Year's Eve 2010, aged 55, Keith's life changed dramatically when a diagnosis of Alzheimer's disease was confirmed. He now uses his energy, drive and remaining skills towards public awareness around dementia, which was recognised by the award of an Honorary Doctorate by Canterbury Christ Church University. He's written or co-written three books, spoken at many conferences, and addressed the UN in Geneva on dementia. Keith receives support from his wife and friends, including Jess, Lucy and Lydia, who helped enormously with his chapter.

Isla Parker is a pen name. Isla is a freelance editor and writer who promotes the understanding of health issues and wellbeing. She undertook a degree in English and found it interesting to study how literature explores illness. This led to Isla writing a novel about anorexia for teenagers called *Size Zero?*, which is loosely based on her own experience. Isla has co-edited *The Practical Handbook of Hearing Voices* for PCCS Books and *The Practical Handbook of Eating Difficulties*. In her free time, Isla enjoys playing the piano. She also takes part in an online writing group that has introduced her to writers from different countries.

Marieke Perry is a general practitioner in the Netherlands. As a senior researcher, she is employed at the Radboudumc, studying complex processes in integrated primary care for people with dementia and their informal caregivers. This includes projects on interprofessional collaboration and the interaction between social health and cognitive decline. Marieke has contributed to several Dutch dementia guidelines, written columns for persons with dementia and carers about her experiences with dementia care in daily practice, and is involved as an expert on the website of the Dutch Alzheimer Association.

Louise Ritchie, PhD, BA(Psy), PGCert is a reader in the Alzheimer Scotland Centre for Policy and Practice at the University of West of Scotland, leading on dementia employment and careers research. She is an executive member of the Scottish Dementia Research Consortium, with a particular focus on research involvement. Other interests include creative evaluation through the eyes of people with dementia.

Helen Rochford-Brennan is a global dementia ambassador. Helen was diagnosed with dementia in 2012 and is a collaborator with Global Brain Health Institute and many other organisations. She is also Vice Chair of the Irish Dementia Working Group, and a member and former chairperson of the European Working Group of People with Dementia, and its nominee to the Board of Alzheimer Europe.

Professor Steven R. Sabat is Professor Emeritus of Psychology at Georgetown University. He is the author of *The Experience of Alzheimer's Disease: Life through a tangled veil* (2001) and *Alzheimer's Disease and Dementia: What everyone needs to know* (2018), and co-editor of *Dementia: Mind, meaning, and the person* (2006).

Dr Sarah Swift did her doctoral research exploring the experience of participation in a community gardening project for people with dementia. Her research interests include the role of gardening and the outdoors in the lived experience of dementia, the sociocultural impacts of community gardening, and facilitating the meaningful involvement of older people in research.

Dr Marianne Talbot, since September 2021 happily retired, was the Director of Studies in Philosophy at the University of Oxford's Department for Continuing Education. Marianne was a carer for 14 years for her beloved parents, both of whom had dementia. She chronicles the love and laughter, and tears and traumas of caring in her book, *Keeping Mum: Caring for someone with dementia.*

Richard Talbot is a performer, senior lecturer and Programme Leader in Comedy Writing and Performance at the University of Salford. He has trained in clowning with Pierre Byland and Philippe Gaulier. His research interests include physical comedy and participatory performance, with a focus on collaborations with older people.

Nicky Taylor is Theatre and Dementia Research Associate at Leeds Playhouse, where she has led ground-breaking creative practice with older people and people living with dementia since 2005. Her study of creative co-production processes in theatre with people with dementia forms the basis of her doctoral research at Leeds Beckett University's Centre for Dementia Research. Nicky created the world's first dementia-friendly theatre performance, and initiated and directed *Every Third Minute*, a pioneering theatre festival curated by people living with dementia. She is an Atlantic Fellow for Equity in Brain Health at Global Brain Health Institute, Trinity College Dublin.

Deborah Thompson is a qualified dietitian and registered with the Health and Care Professions Council. Deborah has a special interest in mental health and has worked as a specialist mental health dietitian for 11 years at South London & Maudsley (SLaM) NHS Trust. Deborah provided a dietetic service for adults and older adults with dementia. Her client group included a Lambeth-based specialist care unit for older adults with dementia.

Debbie Tolson is the Alzheimer Scotland Professor of Dementia and Director of the Alzheimer Scotland for Policy and Practice at the University of the West of Scotland. She is the executive lead for the living with dementia research theme within the Scottish Dementia Research Consortium.

David Truswell BSc, MSc (Econ), MBA is an author, consultant and trainer with a background in mental health and dementia care in NHS, local authority and community organisations. Executive Director of the Dementia Alliance for Culture and Ethnicity and Chair of Dementia in Dub, David serves at board level in a number of third sector organisations working to reduce racial inequity in health and care services and the criminal justice system.

Jenny van der Steen, MSc, PhD, FGSA is an epidemiologist and associate professor in the Netherlands who studies how to improve care at the end of life, and in particular in dementia. She has received national and international awards. Her research uses rigorous quantitative, qualitative and mixed methods, employing international comparative and parallel methodological work.

Eleonore Stenqvist Wesén is a yoga teacher and stress therapist based in Ljungskile, Sweden. There she runs a yoga studio, offering courses, classes and private lessons in Hatha Yoga, yin yoga and breathwork. During this past year she has been offering yoga at a day centre for people with dementia through the project Yoga for All.

Lucy Whitman cared for her mother with dementia and has worked with people with dementia and carers for 15 years. She was Dementia Engagement Officer at Opening Doors from 2019 to 2022. She has published two anthologies: *Telling Tales About Dementia: Experiences of caring*, and *People with Dementia Speak Out*.

Toby Williamson is an experienced independent consultant working in adult mental health, dementia and mental capacity. He has managed frontline mental health services and worked in research, education and training, service and policy development for charities, central government and statutory services, as well as having experience as a family carer.

John Woolham is a visiting senior fellow at the Health and Social Care Workforce Research Unit at King's College London, where he was employed between 2015 and 2021. Before this, he held posts at Coventry University and worked as a researcher in local government adult social care.

Dr Megan Wyatt is a practising artist and researcher. Her PhD research (University of Wales) investigated how people living with dementia engage with painting while working alongside an artist researcher (herself). She also has an MA in art practice and a first-class honours degree in fine art. She is currently working as a research associate at The Geller Institute of Ageing and Memory, University of West London.

Name index

Subject index